An Atlas of
DERMATOLOGY

THE ENCYCLOPEDIA OF VISUAL MEDICINE SERIES

An Atlas of
DERMATOLOGY

Lionel Fry, BSc, MD, FRCP

St. Mary's Hospital,
London, UK

Foreword by

John J. Voorhees, MD

Duncan O. and Ella M. Poth Distinguished Professor
University of Michigan, Ann Arbor, Michigan, USA

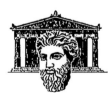

The Parthenon Publishing Group
International Publishers in Medicine, Science & Technology

NEW YORK   LONDON

Library of Congress Cataloging-in-Publication Data
Fry, Lionel
 An atlas of dermatology / Lionel Fry.
  p. cm. -- (The Encyclopedia of visual medicine series)
 Includes bibliographical references and index.
 ISBN 1-85070-461-9
 I. Title. II. Series.
  [DNLM: 1. Dermatology--Atlases. 2. Skin Diseases--
diagnosis-- atlases. 3. Skin Diseases--therapy--atlases.
WR 17 F946ad 1996]
RL81. F958 1996
616.5'0022'2--dc20
DNLM / DLC
for Library of Congress   96-15108
                                              CIP
British Library Cataloguing in Publication Data
Fry, Lionel, 1933–
 An atlas of dermatology. – (The encyclopedia of
 visual medicine series)
 1. Dermatology – Atlases
 I. Title
 616.5

ISBN 1-85070-461-9

Published in the USA by
The Parthenon Publishing Group Inc.
One Blue Hill Plaza
PO Box 1564, Pearl River
New York 10965, USA

Published in the UK and Europe by
The Parthenon Publishing Group Limited
Casterton Hall, Carnforth
Lancs. LA6 2LA, UK

Copyright ©1997 Parthenon Publishing Group

Printed and bound in Spain by T.G. Hostench, S.A.

Contents

Foreword

This book is an atlas of dermatology, as indicated by its title but, in fact, is also much more than an atlas. The book includes most of the common as well as the rarer disorders that may be encountered in patients with skin disease. Particularly noteworthy is the large number of high-quality color photographs, which have been carefully chosen because they best depict the typical appearances of each condition.

Over the years, several atlases of skin disease have been published, but these pictorial guides were either too all-inclusive or too brief to be of great value to the user. This atlas, in contrast, is just the right size and hits its target audience squarely. The targeted reader is not the trained dermatologist such as myself or Dr. Fry, the author of the book. Rather, this volume has been prepared to meet the needs of internists, general practitioners, emergency-room physicians and medical students. There is a requirement in university dermatology departments in the United States to organize short courses in dermatology for medical students, for whom this atlas will undoubtedly prove to be most helpful. The book should also be invaluable to physicians during the first year of training wherein they undertake subspecialty training in dermatology.

However, the ideal coverage and high standard of color photography in this book constitute only a fraction of its true value. The first chapter provides an explanation of how to perform a history and physical examination on skin. Because a poorly performed history and physical inspection can only produce a similarly poor result, the inclusion of such a chapter is particularly appropriate. In addition to the clinical photographs, each disorder is carefully discussed in terms of cause and natural history. These descriptions provide precisely the amount of detail which, together with the illustrations, will permit the reader to arrive at an appropriate diagnosis.

In his preface, Dr. Fry mentions the importance of the chapter on treatment, an opinion with which I most wholeheartedly concur. This chapter, although brief, contains all the information necessary to initiate proper therapy. As the purpose of a correct diagnosis is to allow the initiation of an equally correct treatment, this is a keynote chapter, the likes of which are usually not included in books of this type. In addition, an atlas such as this is no better than its index and, in this book, the index is remarkable in that it is arranged according to lesion type and body location as well as by the more traditional disease entities.

Finally, it is clear that a book can be no better than the expertise of its author. In this case, Dr. Fry has made major original worldwide contributions to dermatology at both the clinical and basic-science levels. As the head of the dermatology unit at a major London hospital and as a consultant dermatologist, Dr. Fry has diagnosed and treated thousands of patients suffering from a multitude of skin diseases. His clinical skills are widely recognized as peerless in the United Kingdom and are among the very best in the world. It is with these credentials that this book has been written. Indeed, Dr. Fry has produced an atlas that is the very best of its kind.

John J. Voorhees, M.D.

Duncan O. and Ella M. Poth Distinguished Professor
University of Michigan
Ann Arbor, 1996

Preface

This volume is a follow-on from *Dermatology: An Illustrated Guide*, which was first published in 1973, with subsequent editions appearing in 1978 and 1984. The book now has a new publisher, but continues with the same format that was responsible for the success of its previous editions. The text has been fully updated with particular emphasis on treatment; the old has been discarded and the new added.

There are 439 color illustrations in this atlas, most of which are related to the more common disorders as this book is intended for medical students, primary-care physicians, casualty officers and dermatologists teaching students in the outpatients clinic, where pictures of conditions may be particularly helpful. Color illustrations should now be the norm, especially in dermatology textbooks, and I am grateful to the publishers for allowing the use of so many. However, this book also contains a text that is essential reading for both students and practicing physicians.

The inclusion of such a large number of color pictures provides an opportunity to 'see' a large number of patients and does not imply neglect of the basic approach to making the clinical diagnosis, namely, the taking of a good patient history. I have found that when students are asked to give a case presentation of a patient with a dermatological disorder, they omit such a history and immediately describe the condition with numerous Latin and Greek terms which may have little relevance in establishing the diagnosis. However, once a full and adequate history has been obtained, the diagnosis can usually be confirmed by what is seen. In this book, therefore, the text is designed to give the reader an understanding of the natural history of the various conditions and how they present.

Dermatology is not a difficult subject, but too little time is devoted to the subject in the majority of undergraduate medical schools. With this in mind, it is hoped that students will find the tips presented in the first chapter helpful in establishing a diagnosis. Furthermore, the last chapter, which covers simple facts pertaining to the preparations most commonly used in dermatology as well as how to use them, should do away with some of the mystique attached to dermatological treatments.

I am grateful to the following people for the loan of their slides and allowing their use in this book: Philip Rodin, Arnold Levene, R.R. Davies, C.W. Marsden, C.D. Calnan and the Institute of Dermatology, K.W. Walton, Counsellor-Specialist Guidance in Public Relations and Marketing, Gerald Haffenden, P.P. Seah and J.N. Leonard, The Leprosy Study Centre and the Wellcome Museum of Medical Science.

Lionel Fry
St. Mary's Hospital
London, 1996

1
History and examination

Even in this age of medical technology, the definitive diagnosis of dermatological disorders is still made, in the majority of cases, on clinical grounds alone. In disorders of other systems, the clinical diagnosis can be confirmed by measurement and the answer expressed in mathematical terms; the limits of normality are also known. In dermatology, one has to rely on a visual impression; even if the lesion is biopsied and histopathology used as an aid, one still relies on visual impressions and not definitive mathematical limits.

HISTORY

Before beginning the examination of the skin, an adequate history should be taken. Particular attention should be paid to the duration and extent of the lesions, whether they are persistent or intermittent, and if there is irritation. It is important to enquire into the past medical history, particularly for skin disease, and into the family history (one often gains a clue to the diagnosis of scabies if other members of the household are known to have similar symptoms). The occupation of the patient is important, and enquiry should be made concerning specific exposure to irritants or allergens, including bubble-baths.

As in disorders of other systems, it is necessary to enquire about any recent stressful situations. Although it is all too common for skin disorders to be attributed to 'nerves', in some diseases, stressful conditions are a contributory factor in susceptible individuals.

No history of a skin disorder is complete without determining what treatment the patient has already had for the condition, and what systemic medication is being taken for any other complaint. The former is important because the potent topical steroids (the supposed panacea for all skin disease) can alter the appearance of a bacterial or fungal infection so that it may well be misdiagnosed. Furthermore, patients develop sensitivity to topical antibiotics and antiseptics

(which are added to the steroid preparations) or even to the bases of the topical preparations and this perpetuates or exacerbates the original condition.

Eruptions caused by systemic medication are not uncommon and the rashes can be bizarre in appearance, leading to difficulty in diagnosis. Direct questioning concerning drug taking is necessary as patients do not consider aspirin, laxatives, slimming pills, cough mixtures, etc. as drugs and therefore will not admit to taking any drugs. Patients also mistakenly believe that if they have taken a drug for a considerable length of time, it cannot be responsible for a skin rash which has only been present for a short time and, thus, they will not volunteer the required information.

EXAMINATION

As the diagnosis in dermatology is made visually, it is important to make sure the lighting is adequate.

Type of lesion

Macule
This is a flat circumscribed discoloration of the skin (Figure 1.1). If larger than several centimeters, it may be referred to as a patch. A macule may be red (alteration in blood supply) or brown due to a pigment (melanin or hemosiderin). Examples of this type of macule are freckles, flat moles or 'staining' following purpura.

Papule
This is a discrete lesion raised above the skin surface (Figure 1.2) and arbitrarily classified as being less than 1 cm in diameter. The majority of warts are papules.

Nodule
This is a raised discrete lesion measuring more than 1 cm in diameter (Figure 1.3). It also may refer to a lesion deeper and firmer than a papule.

Blister

This is a discrete collection of free fluid in the skin. If it is small, e.g. 2–3 mm, it is usually referred to as a vesicle (Figure 1.4) and, if larger, it is termed a bulla (Figure 1.5). Although there are specific diseases, such as pemphigus and dermatitis herpetiformis, which are sometimes termed the bullous dermatoses, it should be remembered that blisters are commonly seen in acute eczemas (particularly pompholyx eczema), in common viral diseases – herpes simplex and herpes zoster (Figure 1.4) – and in fungus infections of the feet and erythema multiforme (Figure 1.5).

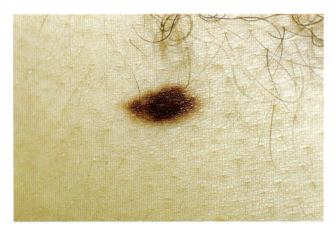

Figure 1.1 *Macule. Melanocytic nevus*

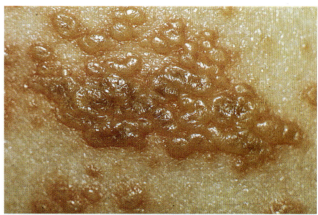

Figure 1.4 *Vesicles. Small blisters in herpes zoster*

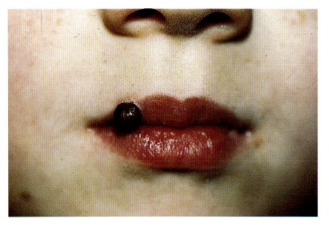

Figure 1.2 *Papule. Pyogenic granuloma (acquired hemangioma)*

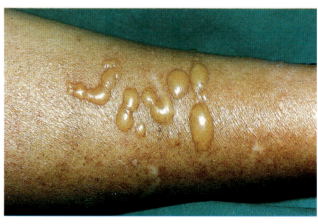

Figure 1.5 *Bullae. Large blisters in erythema multiforme*

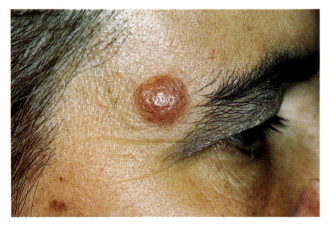

Figure 1.3 *Nodule. Lymphocytic infiltration of the skin*

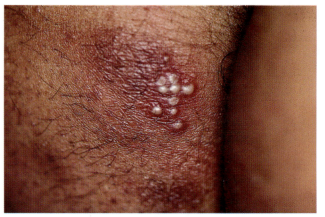

Figure 1.6 *Pustules in herpes simplex*

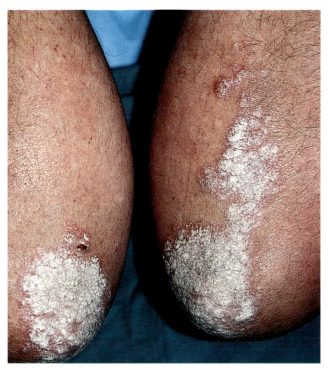

Figure 1.7 *White scales as seen in psoriasis*

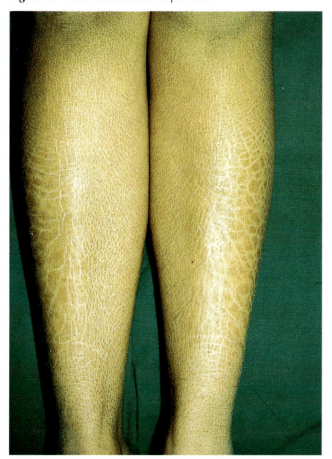

Figure 1.8 *Brown scaling as seen in some forms of ichthyosis*

Pustule
This is a skin elevation containing pus (Figure 1.6).

Scaling and crusted lesions
Scaling represents abnormality of the uppermost layer of the skin, the stratum corneum (horny layer or keratin). There may be abnormality in the formation of the keratin or it may not be shed normally. Certain types of scaling are characteristic, e.g. the white scales of psoriasis (Figure 1.7), the yellowish scaling of seborrheic eczema and the brown scaling of some forms of ichthyosis (Figure 1.8).

Crusts
These are the dried remains of serum, which may occur in an acute inflammatory condition, such as acute eczema or impetigo, and have a yellow color (Figure 1.9).

Distribution of lesions

Considerable help in arriving at the correct diagnosis can be gained from the distribution of the lesion; certain common diseases show a predilection for certain sites, e.g. psoriasis – elbows, knees, sacrum and behind the ears; atopic eczema – flexures of the limbs; acne – face and upper trunk; pityriasis rosea – the trunk, with the long axis of the oval lesions along the lines of cleavage; scabies – wrists, between the fingers, genitalia in men and breasts in women; erythema nodosum – extensor surface of the legs (and occasionally arms).

Configuration

Certain patterns may be suggestive of a diagnosis, although none is absolutely diagnostic.

Linear
Lesions of this type, particularly in lines of trauma (Koebner phenomenon), occur in viral warts, psoriasis and lichen planus (Figure 1.10). Some nevi are also linear.

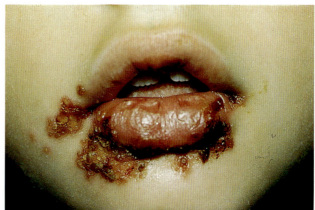

Figure 1.9 *Crusts in impetigo*

Annular

Fungal infections are the best known annular lesions (e.g. ringworm; Figure 1.11), but a common mistake is to diagnose all annular lesions as fungal infections. Partially treated or clearing psoriasis often has an annular pattern (Figure 1.12). Urticaria, pityriasis rosea and a condition of unknown etiology called annular erythema can all be represented by annular lesions.

Grouped lesions

Grouped blisters are characteristic of herpes simplex, herpes zoster and dermatitis herpetiformis (Figure 1.13), and grouped papules are commonly found in molluscum contagiosum.

Symmetry and asymmetry

Disorders due to external factors such as certain viruses (Figure 1.14), bacteria and fungi (Figure 1.15) tend to give rise to asymmetrical eruptions. Diseases due to internal factors, so-called endogenous disorders, e.g. lichen planus, vitiligo (Figure 1.16) and the 'internal' eczemas (Figure 1.17), usually give rise to symmetrical eruptions.

Additional points

It is often well worthwhile examining the buccal mucosa and nails, either for confirmatory evidence or a clue to the disease. For example, in lichen planus there is often involvement of the buccal mucosa as evidenced by white streaks or patches (*see* Chapter 9), and small pits (like pin-pricks) are often found in the nails in psoriasis (*see* Chapter 8).

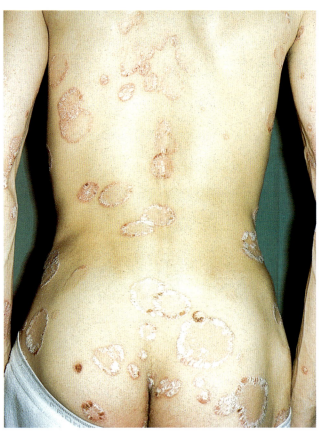

Figure 1.12 Annular lesions in resolving psoriasis

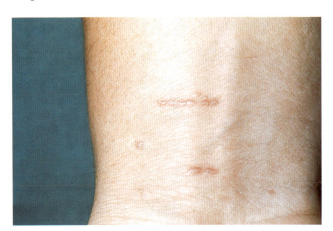

Figure 1.10 Linear lesion. Koebner phenomenon in lichen planus

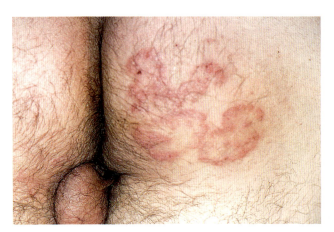

Figure 1.11 Annular lesions as seen in fungus infections

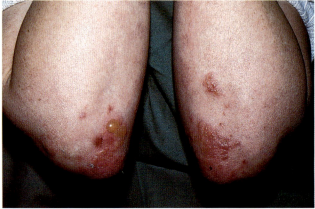

Figure 1.13 Grouped blisters on the elbows in dermatitis herpetiformis

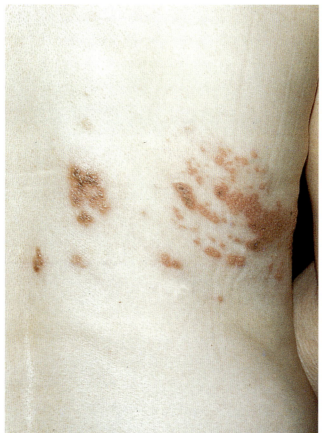

Figure 1.14 *Asymmetrical eruption in herpes zoster*

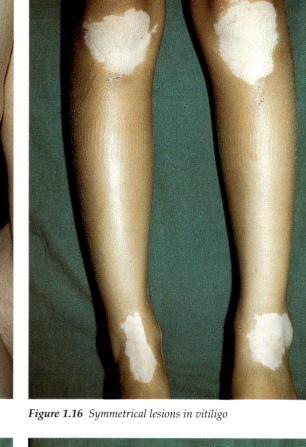

Figure 1.16 *Symmetrical lesions in vitiligo*

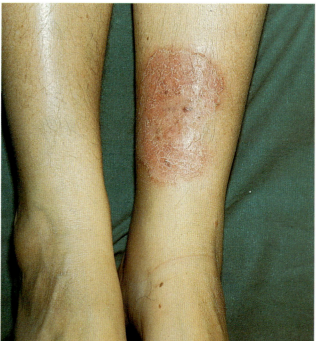

Figure 1.15 *Asymmetrical eruption in a fungal infection*

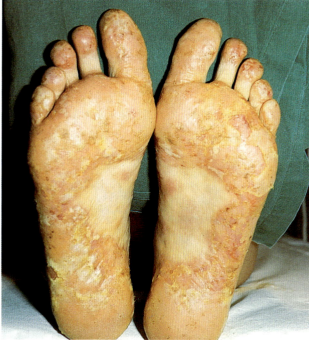

Figure 1.17 *Symmetrical eruption in endogenous foot eczema*

2

Eczema: Clinical features and classification

The terms 'eczema' and 'dermatitis' tend to be used synonymously, although eczema is more common in the UK and Europe, and dermatitis in the USA. Eczema is derived from the Greek word *ekzein* meaning to boil over or break out and, in this book, eczema will be used in preference to dermatitis.

DEFINITION

Eczema denotes a special sequence of inflammatory changes in the skin which, though similar, can vary from patient to patient. Likewise the clinical features can vary depending on the severity and/or chronicity of the disease and the site involved. The principal signs are redness, swelling (papules or edema; Figure 2.1), blisters (large or small; Figure 2.2), scaling, which may be loose and thin (Figure 2.1) or thick (hyperkeratosis; Figure 2.3), depending on how the normal process of keratinization is affected, and exudation of serum, which may be severe leading to weeping, or moderate and mixed with scales of skin to form crusts (Figure 2.4). Fissures or splits (Figure 2.5) may occur particularly on the palms or soles. Thickening of the skin, referred to as lichenification (Figures 2.6 and 2.7), is particularly likely to occur as a result of continued scratching in atopic eczema.

Changes in pigmentation may occur, and this may be seen as hyperpigmentation (Figures 2.6 and 2.7) or hypopigmentation (Figure 2.8). This physical sign is most apparent in black patients and is sometimes the most obvious sign of the eczema. Purpura or bleeding into the skin is not common but may occur after continual scratching, particularly on the leg

The appearance of any particular case of eczema may include one, two or several of the above features; thus, one case of eczema may vary from another. In addition, the eczema in a given patient may vary from one site of the body to another, e.g. an acute weeping eczema on the hands may spread to the forearms and trunk to appear there as an erythematous papular eruption.

CLASSIFICATION

The classification of eczema is difficult and not very satisfactory. This is because, in the past, some of the terms used to describe eczema have been based on the appearances of the eruption while others have been based on so-called etiological factors, or specific sites of the eruption. Thus, there has been considerable overlap in the terminology, with one type of eczema having three or four names depending upon which criteria are used.

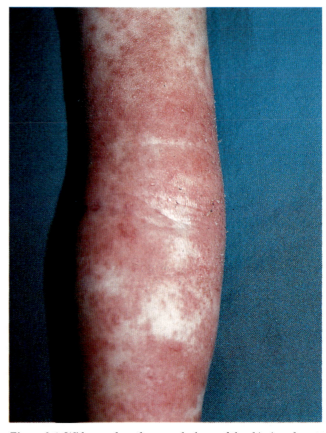

Figure 2.1 *Widespread erythema and edema of the skin in subacute eczema*

At present, the eczemas are divided into two main groups: eczema due to specific *exogenous* factors; and eczema with no specific exogenous factors, sometimes termed *endogenous* (Table 2.1). This subdivision is important because, if there are exogenous factors, they must be identified because, if they can be avoided, this in itself may result in a cure.

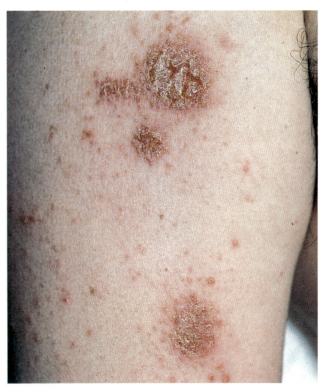

Figure 2.4 *Yellow crusts in subacute discoid eczema*

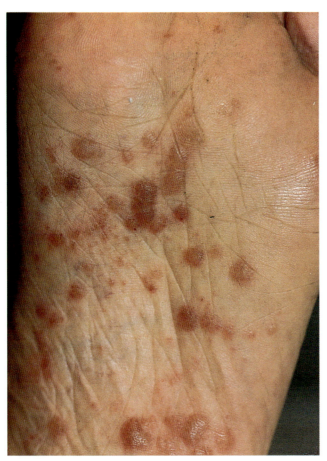

Figure 2.2 *Blisters on the sole in acute pompholyx eczema*

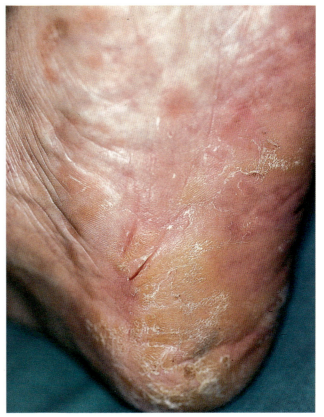

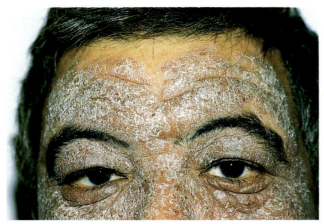

Figure 2.3 *Hyperkeratotic scaling in chronic eczema*

Figure 2.5 *Fissuring on the sole in chronic eczema*

Table 2.1 Classification of eczema

Exogenous	Endogenous
Primary irritant	Atopic
Allergic	Seborrheic
	Nummular or discoid
	Leg (hypostatic or varicose)
	Pompholyx of hand and foot
	Asteatotic

Unfortunately, exogenous eczema does not have a specific morphological pattern but shows the same features that may be exhibited by an endogenous eczema. However, the distribution of the eczema (Figure 2.9), occupation of the patient, and direct questioning concerning self-medication with topical preparations and cosmetics, etc. may well give a clue as to whether or not the eczema is due to exogenous factors. In some instances, such as eczema caused by metal earrings, lipstick or an article of clothing, the distribution and localization of the eczema suggests the diagnosis. Eczema due to a constituent of an ointment, either the drug itself (Figure 2.10) or the base, may be

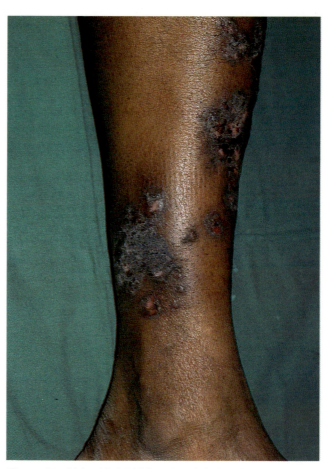

Figure 2.7 *Lichenified (thickened scaly) skin due to continual scratching in adult atopic eczema*

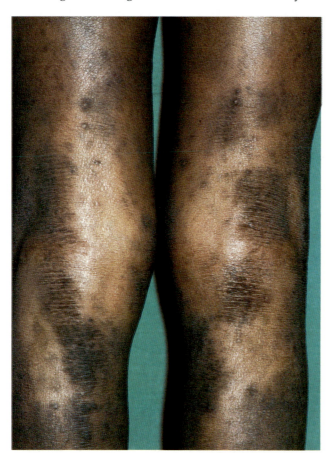

Figure 2.6 *Lichenification and hyperpigmentation in chronic atopic eczema*

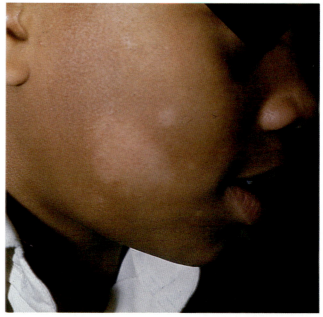

Figure 2.8 *Hypopigmented areas on the face secondary to eczema*

extremely difficult to diagnose unless one is aware of the possibility, as there are no specific sites and it is often superimposed on an endogenous eczema to which the patient has been applying the ointment.

Exogenous eczema is usually subdivided into the following categories:

(1) *Allergic* eczema, in which an antigen is recognized by specific T lymphocytes, resulting in their activation, release of cytokines and subsequent inflammation; and

(2) *Irritant* eczema, in which the chemical substance causes direct damage to the stratum corneum (the skin barrier). Once the skin barrier is breached, the same chemical will penetrate to the remaining epidermis and dermis, resulting in an inflammatory response; no antigen-specific T cells are involved.

The classification of endogenous eczema is more difficult because it is based not on any scientific principle but on gross morphological appearances and sites of the body affected. Confusion often arises because more than one term is used to describe one particular type of eczema, e.g. atopic, infantile, flexural; the blistering eczema that occurs on the palms and soles is referred to as dyshidrotic eczema, pompholyx, or hand and foot eczema. Until we understand more about endogenous eczema the classification will have to remain arbitrarily based on the following clinical criteria:

(1) *Atopic eczema* This is the most common type of eczema seen in childhood, and is often associated with a family history of asthma or hay fever;

(2) *Seborrheic eczema* This derives its name from the fact that the sites involved are those with the greatest sebum production per area of skin surface, e.g. scalp, face, back and chest;

(3) *Nummular or discoid eczema* This derives its name from the clinical appearances, i.e. small circumscribed areas of eczema;

(4) *Leg eczema* This occurs on the lower leg and is associated with impaired venous drainage of the limb;

(5) *Pompholyx eczema of the hands and feet* This tends to be symmetrical, occurring on the palms and soles, sides of the digits and over the backs of the distal two phalanges; and

(6) *Asteatotic eczema* This term implies degreasing of the skin, and refers to loss of lipid from the stratum corneum, seen usually on the legs of the elderly.

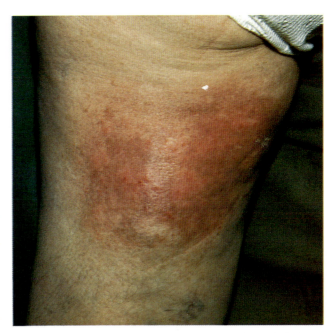

Figure 2.9 *Well-demarcated eczema on the back of the thigh due to contact eczema from an antiseptic applied to a toilet seat*

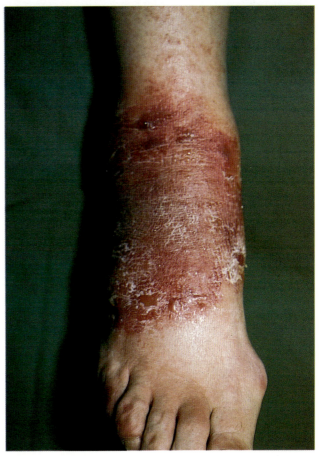

Figure 2.10 *Localized eczema on the dorsum of the foot due to an antiseptic ointment*

It should be emphasized that this classification may not be complete enough to cover all the endogenous patterns of eczema encountered, but it does serve as a useful guide for further discussion. It should also be stressed that eczema often does not appear in the clearly defined patterns described in any classification. Any type of eczema (endogenous or exogenous) may lead to spread of the eruption, so-called autosensitization (Figure 2.11), with more general involvement of the skin which, if complete, is referred to as *erythoderma* or *exfoliative dermatitis* (Figure 2.12).

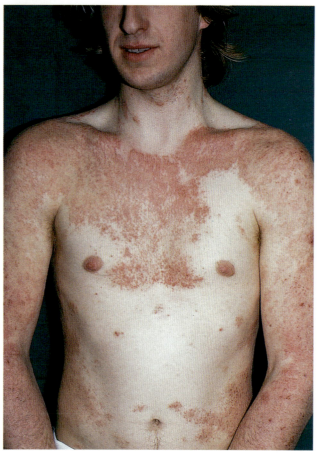

***Figure* 2.11** *Widespread eczema on the arms and trunk due to autosensitization from pompholyx eczema on the hands*

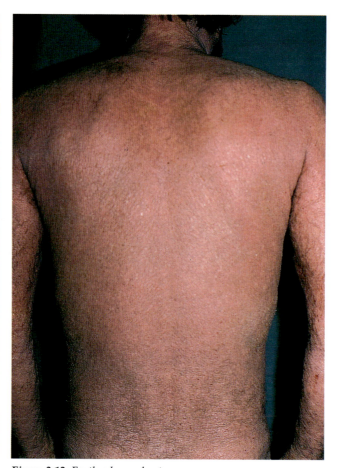

***Figure* 2.12** *Erythroderma due to eczema*

3

Exogenous eczema

Eczemas in this group are caused by the skin coming into contact with chemicals, natural or synthetic. There are certain clues which may be present and should be looked for when establishing a diagnosis of exogenous eczema. In the early stages, a sharp delineation between affected and normal skin may be apparent (Figure 3.1).

Some sites are more commonly affected than others, and three factors determine these sites. Certain parts of the body are more likely to be in contact with chemicals, e.g. hands, face, neck and genitalia (by transfer of the chemicals from the hands).

The thickness of the skin varies. If the hands are exposed to chemicals, the eruption is more likely to appear first on the backs of the hands, then on the palms, as the skin is thinner on the backs of the hands and chemicals will be more easily absorbed (Figure 3.2).

Absorption of chemicals into the skin is enhanced by moisture and, thus, parts of the body which secrete larger amounts of sweat, or where the evaporation of sweat is impaired by opposing skin surfaces and lack of air (e.g. groins, axillae and flexures of the limbs), are more likely to be affected.

This point is well illustrated by contact eczema due to stockings in which the eruption first appears on the feet and popliteal fossae due to greater absorption of the allergen into the skin at these sites.

Contact eczema has also to be considered when the distribution of the eruption is localized to one particular area and is asymmetrical.

SPREAD

The eruption in contact eczema ranges from a faint erythema to an acute blistering. It should always be borne in mind that eczema may subsequently appear at sites of the body that have not been in direct contact with the chemical. This spread of the eczema may be due to 'autosensitization' from the primary eczematous skin or to absorption of the exogenous chemicals which affect the skin at distant sites. Although this secondary spread of eczema may affect any part of the skin, some allergens have a tendency to spread to certain sites. For example, eczema due to nickel sensitivity frequently spreads to the skin around the eyes and antecubital fossae (Figure 3.3). This may be the pattern presenting to

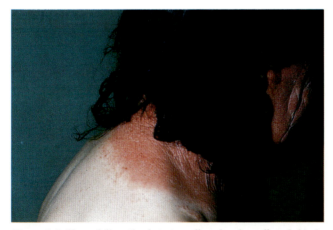

Figure 3.1 *Sharp delineation between affected and unaffected skin in contact eczema due to hair dye*

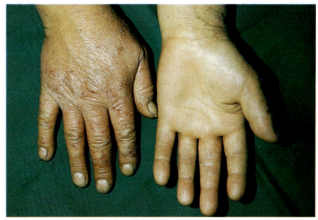

Figure 3.2 *Contact eczema on the back of hands but not the palms due to thinner skin at the former site*

11

the physician and the patient may not mention the 'suspender rash' she may have had for years. At present, the factors which cause eczema to spread to secondary sites are not fully understood, but some eczemas spread after a matter of days and others only after months or even years with continuing eczema at the primary site.

CAUSE

The cause of contact eczema may be a primary irritant (non-allergic) or allergenic (sensitizing) agent.

PRIMARY IRRITANT ECZEMA

Substances which cause this type of eczema may be divided into two classes:

(1) *Strong* These are usually caustic substances with which patients come into contact at work, such as strong acids or alkalis, or chemical solvents. These are likely to produce eczema after only one or two exposures, usually as a result of inadequate protective precautions at work or, if the exposure occurred at home, ignorance of the possible hazard. The most common sites are the hands or face. It is not practical to give a comprehensive list of these strong caustic substances; the patient's occupation or hobbies will usually offer confirmatory evidence if such a diagnosis is suspected.

(2) *Weak* These substances are not caustic or directly damaging to the skin but, after prolonged or repeated exposures, they will induce eczema (Figure 3.4). Into this category falls the common skin complaint of 'housewife's eczema', caused by continual exposure to detergents, having the hands in water too frequently with inadequate drying, and exposure to cold windy conditions. Various oils, greases and other hydrocarbons, which may be encountered in the patient's occupation, can also cause this type of eczema. Other factors, such as humidity, trauma, dryness of the skin, sweating and secondary infection may all also play a part. Once again, the most common site is the hands. In the mild form the skin is dry and scaling with slight erythema but, in the more severe and chronic forms, there is thickening of the skin (hyperkeratosis) and splits or fissures. The backs and palms of the hands tend to be equally affected.

Bubble-bath preparations also contain detergents, which is why they bubble. These preparations have a degreasing effect on the stratum corneum, and will eventually lead to cracking of this layer and develop-

ment of an irritant eczema. Atopic individuals and those with generally dry skins are most susceptible to this effect of bubble-baths.

ALLERGIC CONTACT ECZEMA

Numerous chemical substances with which we come into contact in our everyday life are capable of sensi-

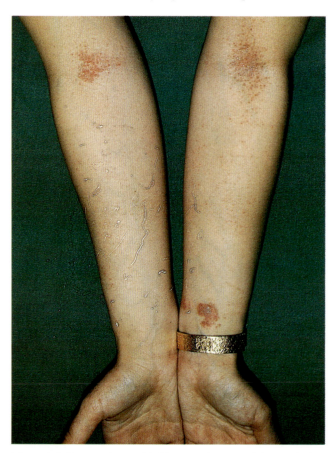

Figure 3.3 *Eczema due to nickel in a watch strap, with spread of the eczema to the antecubital fossae*

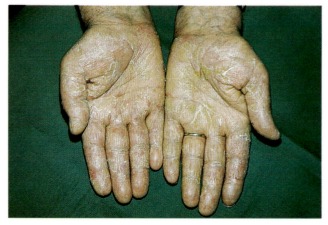

Figure 3.4 *Eczema on the palms due to long exposure to irritants*

tizing the skin so that eczema occurs. Why some patients develop an allergy to chemicals and others do not is as yet unknown. The number of known skin allergens is now so large that mention will only be made of the more common substances likely to cause contact eczema.

Rubber and elasticized garments

Rubber gloves (Figure 3.5) and suspenders frequently cause eczema, but any article of clothing containing rubber or elastic can have a similar effect (Figure 3.6).

Metals

Nickel is the most common metal to cause sensitivity and is most frequently found in suspenders, jewellery clips, brassière clips, zip fasteners and in the metal buttons on jeans (Figure 3.7).

Dyes

Dyes in clothing, shoes and hairnets can all cause contact eczema. Hair dyes are also a common cause of the condition (Figure 3.1).

Cosmetics

There are various organic chemicals in cosmetics which can sensitize patients. Substances in lipstick, eye shadow and nail varnish can all cause contact eczema. It should be appreciated that eczema due to nail varnish does not present on the fingers, but on the neck (Figure 3.8) and face where the skin has been touched by the nail varnish. The nail itself is not affected.

Perfumes

These substances are now more widely used as men as well as women are targeted by the cosmetic industry. Perfumes are now one of the most common causes of allergic contact eczema.

In addition to being applied to the skin, perfumes are now found in air-fresheners and household polishes. Perfumes released in these aerosols will cause contact eczema on the exposed areas, particularly on the face around the eyes and possibly on the neck under collars. Perfumes are also added to hand and face creams produced by the cosmetic industry.

Leather

Chemicals present in leather or used in the tanning process can sensitize patients, and this may present as eczema due to a hatband, shoes (Figure 3.9) or watch strap.

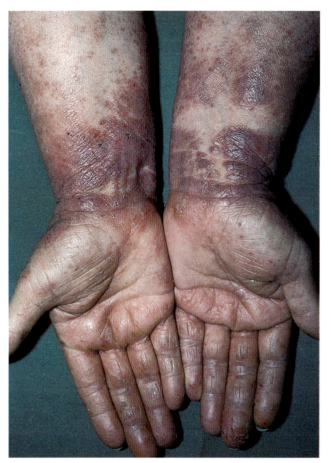

Figure 3.5 Eczema from rubber gloves. There is sparing on the wrist due to protection from a watch. There is less involvement on the palms than the wrists because skin is thicker on the palms

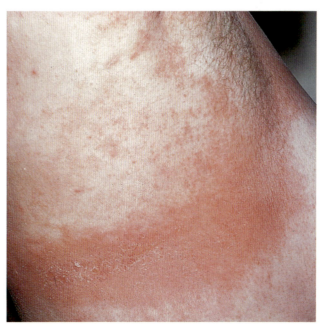

Figure 3.6 Eczema due to the elasticated part of a brassière

Plants

Sensitivity to plants may be seen in florists and gardeners and is usually present on the hands, face and neck. Occasional linear lesions can be produced by simply brushing against plants (Figure 3.10) to which the patient may be acutely sensitive.

Therapeutic preparations

Topical local anesthetics

Local anesthetics are not infrequently found in creams and ointments prescribed by doctors for irritating conditions, particularly pruritus ani and hemorrhoids. It should be remembered that these substances are potent sensitizers and, if eczematous changes occur,

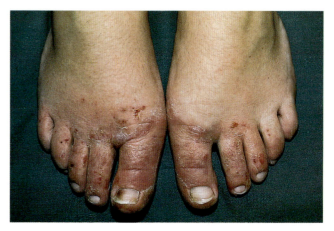

Figure 3.9 Eczema from leather shoes

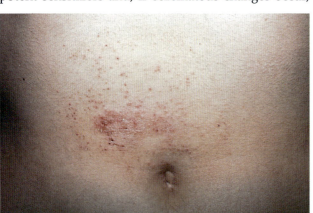

Figure 3.7 Eczema from a metal button (nickel) on jeans

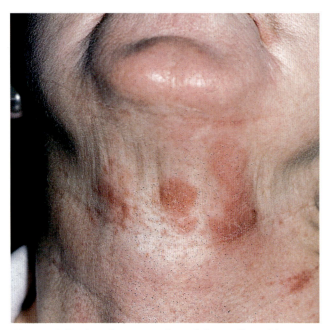

Figure 3.8 Patches of eczema on the neck from nail varnish

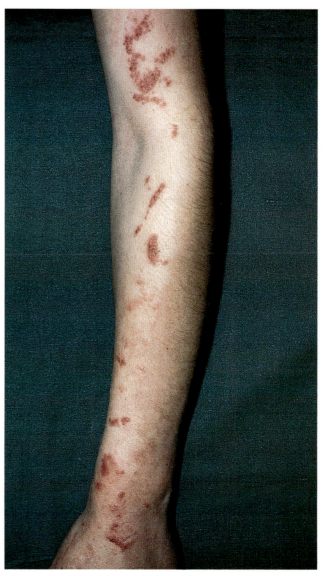

Figure 3.10 Linear lesions which may be seen in contact eczema to plants

contact eczema to these substances should be excluded by stopping their use and/or by patch tests.

Topical antihistamines

Although these substances are widely used and easily obtainable from a chemist without prescription, there are many dermatologists who consider that there are no indications for their use. Antihistamines applied topically cause a high incidence of sensitization, and occurrence of acute eczema (Figure 3.11) after their use or exacerbation of an existing skin condition suggests sensitivity.

Topical antibiotics and antiseptics

Neomycin and soframycin are probably the most common topical antibiotics to cause sensitization (Figure 3.12). Hydroxyquinolines are antiseptics that are frequently combined with a topical steroid in proprietary preparations and, like antibiotics, are common sensitizers. When antiseptics and antibiotics are combined with a topical steroid, the diagnosis of a contact eczema may be difficult as the steroid suppresses the response to sensitization. If eczema is proving particularly chronic or shows exacerbation after the use of these substances, patch tests to the antibiotics and antiseptics should be carried out. Acriflavin, still a commonly used antiseptic, often causes contact eczema.

Ointment and cream bases and preservatives

Patients may become sensitive to ointment or cream bases, or to the preservatives added to the them. Lanolin, which was a common ointment base, is now used less often in the pharmaceutical industry because of the risk of sensitization. However, it is still used in hand creams and cosmetics.

The diagnosis of sensitivity to the base or preservatives is suggested by exacerbation or persistence of an eczematous condition or by the appearance of eczema in addition to the condition being treated with the ointment.

Topical steroids

Although rare, topical steroids may themselves act as antigens which sensitize T lymphocytes and induce contact eczema. However, the anti-inflammatory effect of the steroid may partially inhibit the eczema. In cases of no response to a topical steroid as expected or of worsening, the possibility that the patient is allergic to the steroid has to be considered.

Adhesive tape

Many patients are allergic to adhesive tape and this is due either to the colophony or rubber antioxidants in the adhesive.

Diagnosis

An adequate patient history and the distribution of the eczema will frequently suggest the diagnosis. However, in cases which are not clear-cut, the application of suspected materials to a small area of skin in the

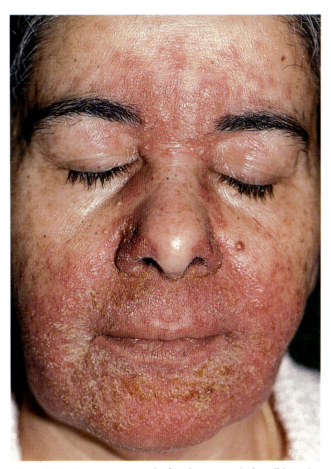

Figure 3.11 Acute eczema on the face due to a topical antihistamine preparation

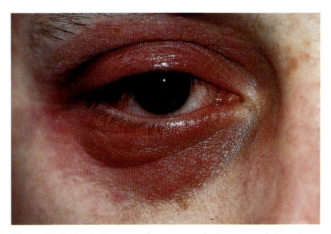

Figure 3.12 Contact eczema from neomycin in an eye ointment

form of a *patch test* is helpful. The test is not without risks and is therefore best carried out by experienced practitioners. The suspected substance is applied to the skin and usually occluded for 24 h. The tests are read at 48 and 96 h. If positive, a small patch of eczema develops at the site of application (Figure 3.13).

Treatment and management

The most important point in the management of contact eczema is the prevention of further exposure of the skin to the substance responsible for the reaction. If this is achieved, no further treatment may be required. If further exposure is not prevented, then there is no treatment which will keep the patient free of eczema.

Topical therapy
Only bland and non-sensitizing substances should be used. Topical antihistamines and local anesthetics should be avoided.

In the acute vesicular or weeping stages, compresses, soaks and lotions are indicated. If the hands or feet are involved, then the limb should be soaked in 1:8000 potassium permanganate made up in warm water. The area should be immersed for 10–15 min three or four times a day. If the part cannot be soaked in a basin or bucket, compresses using physiological saline can be used. The compress should be kept moist by replenishment of the solution and held in position for 15–30 min.

After soaking or the use of compresses, a corticosteroid preparation should be applied. In the acute

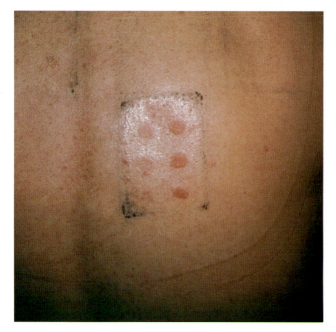

Figure 3.13 *Positive patch tests. Eczema developing at the site of application of chemicals applied to skin for 48 h*

stages, a lotion is indicated as the vehicle and, initially, 1% hydrocortisone lotion should be applied at half-hour intervals. In the acute stages, creams and ointments should be avoided.

When the eczema becomes less moist, and scales and scabs begin to form, the compresses and soaks should be stopped and topical corticosteroid cream applied three or four times a day. One per cent hydrocortisone cream is usually effective but, if the healing is slow, a more potent corticosteroid preparation may be used. If the area of skin involved is extensive, it is important that a sufficient amount of topical preparation be given to the patient. A useful rule of thumb is that it takes approximately 30 g of cream to cover the total skin surface of an adult in one application.

Dressings
In the acute stages, clean linen dressings are probably best. Gauze should be avoided as it tends to stick. After the acute stages, tube gauze dressings can be used.

Blisters
Only the large blisters need to be pricked as these increase irritation and general discomfort.

Systemic therapy
Corticosteroids
These are required, and justifiable, only in a small number of patients with contact eczema in whom the eruption is very extensive and acute. The initial dose should be approximately 30 mg of prednisone daily, which should be reduced by 5 mg daily as soon as the condition begins to improve.

Antibiotics
Not infrequently, acute eczema becomes secondarily infected. The infecting organism is most commonly a staphylococcus and/or streptococcus, and an appropriate systemic antibiotic should be given. If there is no response within 1 or 2 days, a swab should be taken for culture and sensitivity testing. If the eczema becomes impetiginized (i.e. a superficial bacterial infection occurs), topical antibiotics in an appropriate base will also be helpful. The antibiotic of choice is probably fusidic acid because of the low incidence of resistance of staphylococci and streptococci to this antibiotic. Ideally, swabs should be taken for culture and sensitivity.

Antihistamines and sedatives
An acute eczema is very irritating and causes a great deal of discomfort. Oral antihistamines such as promethazine 25–50 mg at night or trimeprazine 10 mg two or three times a day are helpful because of their antipruritic and hypnotic action. If the patient is agitated, diazepam 5 mg three times daily is helpful.

4

Atopic eczema

Eczema in infancy is most commonly atopic and thus the term *infantile eczema* is used by some authorities synonymously with atopic eczema. It is also referred to as *flexural eczema* as the flexor aspects of the limbs are commonly affected. It should, however, be remembered that atopic eczema can occur in adults and involve any part of the skin, so 'atopic' is used in preference to 'infantile' and 'flexural' to describe this form of eczema.

The term 'atopic' was originally used to mean 'strange' but, because this type of eczema is associated with asthma and/or hay fever, the name was subsequently used to imply 'allergic' eczema. 'Atopen' has been used in the past to mean allergen or antibody.

The pathogenesis of atopic eczema is poorly understood and the role of external allergens is still to be determined. Dietary proteins and house-dust mite antigens have been incriminated as a cause of atopic eczema, but the evidence supporting a role for these antigens is not conclusive.

It has recently been shown that atopic individuals have a different immune response to some external antigens compared with non-atopic subjects. Thus, external antigens may not be the primary cause of the disease; rather, the abnormal immunological response may trigger the eczema.

Recent studies have shown that T lymphocytes play an important role in atopic eczema. This observation has already led to new treatments and is likely to influence the development of future therapies.

AGE INCIDENCE

Atopic eczema is not present at birth and usually does not occur before the age of 3 months. The most common time of onset is during the first and second years of life, although it may present for the first time later in childhood and, rarely, in adults.

DISTRIBUTION

The most frequent sites are the popliteal fossa (Figure 4.1) and the antecubital fossa (Figure 4.2), but the face (Figure 4.3), neck, wrists and hands are also frequently involved. The eruption is usually symmetrical and, if a unilateral or a solitary lesion presents, then alternative diagnoses must be considered. Occasionally, the eczema may spread from the usual sites and large areas of the skin become affected, particularly the arms and legs (Figure 4.4). Very rarely, the condition becomes generalized.

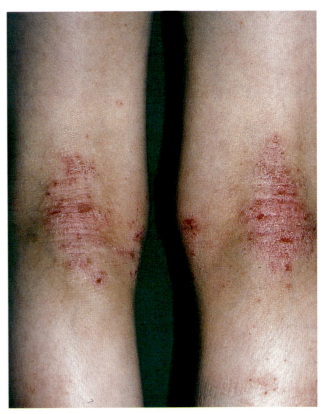

Figure 4.1 *Atopic eczema in the popliteal fossae. The skin is red, excoriated and lichenified*

TYPE OF LESION

The typical physical signs are erythema, scaling and thickening of the skin (lichenification; Figures 4.1 and 4.4). The features of acute eczema, i.e. crusting and weeping, are not common but may occur; blisters are rare. Atopic eczema is a very irritating condition and excoriations with bleeding are frequently seen (Figures 4.1 and 4.5). Lichenification is thought to be a response of the skin to continual scratching.

Alterations in pigmentation of the skin, either hypo- or hyperpigmentation (Figure 4.6), may occur, particularly in black children, who may also present with small (1–2 mm) fine papules on the trunk in addition to the more typical lesions described above.

Because of the excoriations and since, as in most skin disorders, the protective function of the skin is lost, secondary bacterial infection is not uncommon. Such infection may present as pustules or purulent crusted areas.

A physical sign sometimes seen in atopic eczema is white dermographism. If the red eczematous skin is firmly stroked with a blunt instrument, a white line appears within 30–45 seconds (Figure 4.7).

NATURAL HISTORY

Atopic eczema is a very common disorder. The results of various surveys have shown that between 1 – 10% of the population may be expected to have some degree of atopic eczema during childhood. In the majority of those affected the eczema is mild and usually clears permanently before the child is 5 years old. This type of eczema is subject to exacerbations, and the child may be clear for many months between flare-ups. The causes of the exacerbations are usually not obvious, but climatic

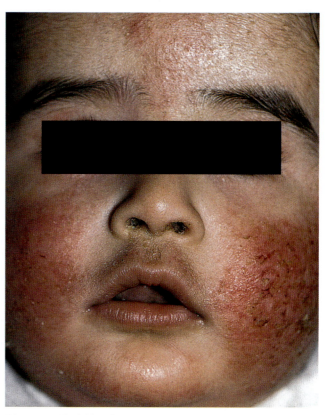

Figure 4.3 Facial involvement in atopic eczema

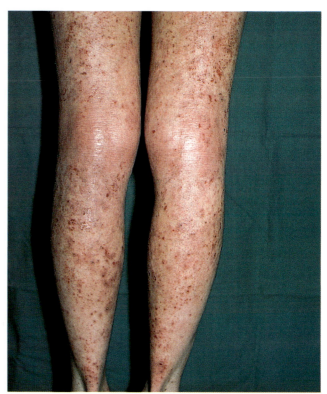

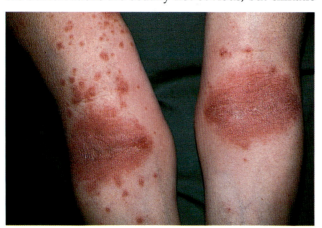

Figure 4.2 Acute atopic eczema in the antecubital fossae

Figure 4.4 Widespread atopic eczema

and emotional factors can sometimes be incriminated. Atopic eczema usually improves in a climate which is warm but with a low humidity, and is aggravated by cold and wind. The eczema is frequently made worse by emotional problems and stress.

In the vast majority of children, perhaps 95%, the eczema will clear permanently in childhood but, in a small number, it will persist into adult life. It is not possible to give the parents an exact age when the condition will resolve as subsequent outbreaks may occur even after months or years. This should always be mentioned at the first interview.

FAMILY HISTORY AND ASSOCIATED CONDITIONS

Atopic eczema is associated with asthma and hay fever. The three disorders together are referred to as the atopic syndrome, but it should be stressed that the majority of atopic subjects only develop one of the three disorders. The atopic syndrome is genetically conferred and there is frequently a positive family history of one of the three complaints when a child with atopic eczema is seen for the first time. The exact mode of inheritance is as yet unknown, but it appears to be a dominant trait.

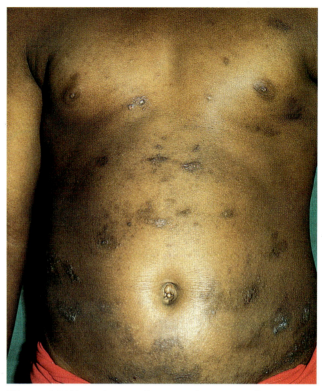

Figure 4.6 Hyperpigmentation secondary to atopic eczema, a common feature in black patients

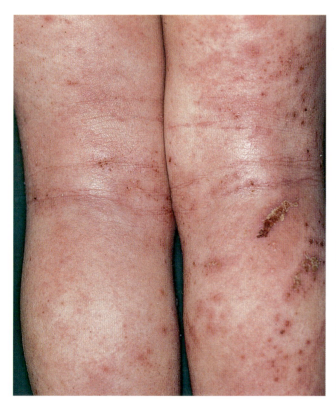

Figure 4.5 Severe atopic eczema. The eruption is confluent and excoriations are a common feature

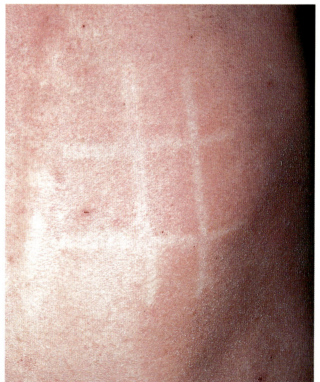

Figure 4.7 White dermographism in atopic eczema

Only a small number of patients with atopic eczema will develop asthmas or hay fever in later life, probably as teenagers or in early adult life; by then the eczema has usually cleared.

MANAGEMENT AND TREATMENT

Once the diagnosis of atopic eczema has been made, it is important to explain the natural history of the complaint to the parents; otherwise, the parents will be disappointed and will tend to lose confidence in the doctor every time there is a flare-up or reappearance of the eczema.

Topical treatment

As atopic eczema is, like other eczemas, an inflammatory condition of the skin, the basis of treatment is to counteract the inflammation with anti-inflammatory substances.

In the *acute* phase, when there may be weeping or oozing, drying lotions and compresses are indicated. For the hands and feet, potassium permanganate at a strength of 1:8000 made up in warm water is suitable. Physiological saline is an effective alternative and has the advantage of not staining the skin brown. One per cent hydrocortisone lotion or cream should be applied following the soaks or compresses and the area covered with clean linen.

In the most common form of atopic eczema, the skin is red, dry and scaly. The basis of treatment is topical corticosteroid preparations. However, it must be stressed to the parents (and patients, if old enough) that topical corticosteroids are not 'curative' but suppressive, but will invariably control the eczema if used correctly. However, because of the publicity given to the potentially adverse effects of topical steroids, many patients will not use these preparations and thus deny the beneficial effects to the child.

The factors influencing side effects of topical steroids are dealt with in detail in Chapter 25 and they are particularly relevant to the management of atopic eczema. Ideally, the strength of the topical steroid should be the weakest that will control the eczema. If the eczema is mild, weak (Group I) topical steroids may be effective but, if severe, they almost certainly will not. In clinical practice, it has been found that, if the eczema can be completely cleared, the child often remains clear and in remission for a considerable time, during which time no corticosteroids are required. It appears that once the eczema becomes severe, it becomes self-perpetuating and the phenomenon of autosensitization, well recognized in all types of eczema, may be responsible.

Thus, in practice, it is more sensible to use a strong (Group III) or very strong (Group IV) topical steroid for a short duration to clear the eczema completely than to use one that is weak or moderate strength continuously, which will only partially suppress the eczema. In the end the quantity of steroid used (measured in units of steroid activity) may well be less by using a potent steroid for a short duration rather than a weak or moderate steroid for a long time. In addition, once severe eczema has been cleared, it is often possible to deal with any subsequent recurrence using a steroid of weak or moderate strength.

A number of generalizations in the treatment of atopic eczema with topical steroids can be made:

(1) Use a steroid of the weakest possible strength to clear the eczema;

(2) It is often better to use a strong steroid for a short time than a weak or moderate one for a long time;

(3) *In infants* below the age of 1 year, only weak topical steroids should be used and are usually effective;

(4) *The face* – only weak (Group I) topical steroids should be used as the skin is very thin on the face (*see* Chapter 25);

(5) *Extensive and persistent eczema* – in this situation, a short course (not more than 2 weeks) of a strong (Group III) or very strong (Group IV) topical steroid may be used. If there is a recurrence, it can often be controlled with a weaker topical steroid;

(6) *Lichenified eczema* – a short course (2–3 weeks) of a very strong topical steroid will probably be necessary to clear the eczema;

(7) *Quantity* – patients are often given insufficient quantities of topical steroid preparations. As a general rule, an adult requires approximately 30 g to cover the total skin surface. With this information, it should be possible to prescribe the amount required for a given period of use;

(8) *Base* – as a general rule, if the eczema is dry and scaly, an ointment should be used and, if exudative, a cream is better;

(9) Topical steroids should not be given on repeat prescription without first seeing the patient. Although this rule might be relaxed for weak steroids, it should not be so for stronger ones.

Coal tar
This has anti-eczema properties and, although it has largely been replaced by topical steroids, it appears to be helpful in counteracting dry skin, a feature of eczema, if combined with emulsifying ointment BP for washing. A 15% liquid coal tar in emulsifying ointment is applied to

the affected skin prior to bathing and the patient should stay in the bath for approximately 15 min before washing the excess ointment off with water.

Systemic therapy

Antihistamines

Atopic eczema is a very irritating condition that sometimes interferes with sleep and, thus, antihistamines such as promethazine hydrochloride and trimeprazine tartrate are particularly helpful at night-time. They should be given approximately 1 h before the child is due to go to bed.

Antibiotics

Atopic eczema is frequently infected by staphylococcal and streptococcal organisms. Some dermatologists have even suggested that bacterial organisms play a role in the cause of the eczema in genetically susceptible individuals. In some patients, long-term antibiotic treatment is helpful in controlling the eczema, particularly in those who have recurrent clinical infection. As a rule, systemic antibiotics should be given if there is clinical infection, as evidenced by excessive crusting, pus formation, lymphangitis and/or lymphadenopathy. If the eczema is severe, then it is acceptable to continue topical steroid therapy with the antibiotic treatment, but weak topical steroids should be used rather than potent ones. In addition, there are topical preparations which combine antibiotics (fusidic acid) with corticosteroids.

Systemic steroids

The majority of cases of atopic eczema are controllable with topical steroids. If the disease is extensive and not responding to topical measures, this may be an indication for systemic steroids, particularly in adults. Fortunately, such cases are becoming extremely rare with the advent of newer topical steroid preparations.

PUVA (see Chapter 25)

In severe atopic eczema in adults not satisfactorily controlled by topical measures, PUVA can be helpful in controlling the disease. It can be considered an alternative to systemic steroids.

Cyclosporine

As atopic eczema is almost certainly a T lymphocyte-mediated disease, cyclosporine is effective and can be considered an alternative to PUVA and/or systemic steroids. There are potentially serious side effects and strict patient monitoring is essential (see Chapter 25).

Diet

As already mentioned, the role of dietary proteins in the etiology of atopic eczema has yet to be determined.

Over 100 different foods have been reported to cause or aggravate atopic eczema. It is likely that there is an inability in atopic individuals to deal appropriately with foreign antigens and that no particular antigen is the cause of atopic eczema. It appears that while some foods may aggravate eczema in a given individual, other foods are responsible in others. Unfortunately, there are no specific tests to predict which foods might be responsible for aggravating the disease. The only way to determine the role of a dietary substance is avoidance (for a month) and subsequent challenge.

The argument against foreign dietary antigens being the cause of atopic eczema is the fact that the disease may first appear when the child is still being breast-fed. In practical terms, the difficulties with elimination diets may far outweigh the benefits obtained. In addition, children may be at risk of nutritional deficiencies from unsupervised diets that are too strict.

ECZEMA HERPETICUM

Occasionally, a widespread vesicular eruption is seen in patients with atopic eczema caused by the herpes simplex virus or, rarely, Coxsackie virus. The eruption is most common on the face (Figure 4.8) and is thought to occur at the time of primary infection. The diagnosis can be confirmed by appropriate culture of the blister fluid. If eczema herpeticum is suspected, treatment with acyclovir should be commenced.

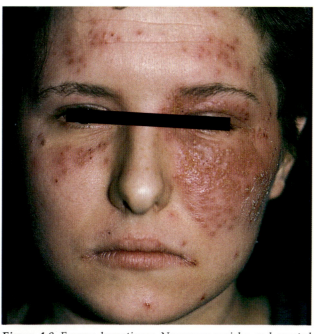

Figure 4.8 *Eczema herpeticum. Numerous vesicles and crusted lesions on the face*

5

Varicose eczema and asteatotic eczema

Eczema of the lower leg, usually above the medial malleolus in the middle-aged and elderly, has in the past been referred to as varicose, hypostatic or gravitational eczema. As the etiology of this pattern of eczema is still under dispute, none of these terms is ideal. However, until the underlying pathogenetic mechanisms of this pattern of eczema are established, the term 'varicose eczema' will be retained because there is no better term.

It has been assumed that varicose eczema is associated with increased venous pressure in the lower leg which, in turn, may lead to edema, fibrin cuffs around the capillaries and subsequent anoxia of the tissues. Repeated trauma from rubbing and scratching the leg have also been implicated in the pathogenesis.

SITE

The most common site for varicose eczema and ulceration is the medial side of the leg just above the malleolus (Figure 5.1). The eczema may spread to the lateral side of the leg and/or to the dorsum of the foot and involve the whole leg (Figures 5.2 and 5.3). Like any other eczema, autosensitization may occur and the condition may affect any area of the skin and become widespread; occasionally, this is the presenting feature in varicose eczema.

APPEARANCES

The eczema usually first begins as a red patch which may be associated with slight edema of the ankle (Figures 5.1 and 5.3). Subsequently, the area becomes scaly and, in the chronic state, the scales become pigmented and have a greasy appearance. Varicose eczema is often purpuric and, in the chronic state, the skin surrounding the eczema is often pigmented (Figure 5.2). This may be due to melanin, hemosiderin or both. Lichenification and vesiculation are usually not seen. The eczema may be persistent for many years without

showing much alteration, or the skin may break down and ulceration develop (Figure 5.4). Occasionally, a patient with no previous eczema on the legs may sustain a slight injury to the lower leg which subsequently develops into a varicose or hypostatic ulcer with little or no surrounding eczema (Figure 5.5). In such patients, there must be an underlying venous stasis. Because of the chronicity of these ulcers and their poor venous drainage, there is often secondary bacterial infection with crusts and/or pus formation. However, if there is no varicose eczema of the legs, it must be seri-

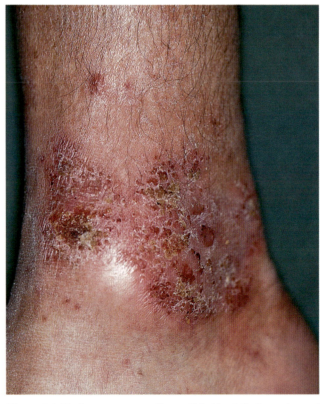

Figure 5.1 *Varicose eczema on the medial side of the lower leg and ankle, the most common site*

ously considered whether the ulcers are due to an underlying condition such as peripheral arterial disease, blood dyscrasias, nodular vasculitis or poly-arteritis nodosa, or a manifestation of a drug eruption.

A physical sign sometimes seen in association with long-standing hypostasis is atrophy blanche (Figure 5.6). The whiteness of the skin is due to atrophy and scar formation, and telangiectasia is present in this type of skin lesion.

TREATMENT

Apart from the direct treatment of the eczema and ulcers, measures to counteract the hypostasis are of paramount importance.

Postural drainage

Elevation of the feet when sitting should be encouraged. Raising the foot of the bed by approximately 23 cm frequently helps to heal varicose ulcers which have otherwise proved resistant to treatment. If possible, the patient should also lie on the raised bed for half an hour during the day, particularly if there is a tendency for fluid to accumulate in the lower leg.

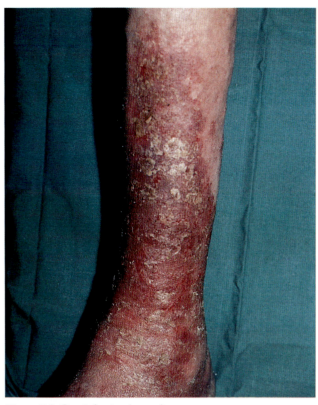

Figure 5.3 *Crusted extensive varicose eczema*

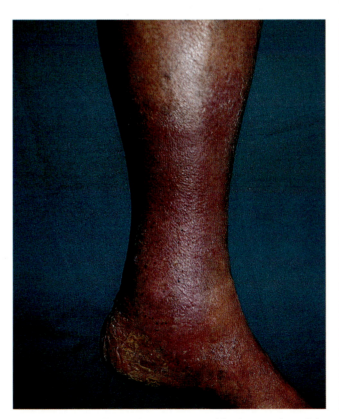

Figure 5.2 *Extensive varicose eczema, with pigmentation of the affected area*

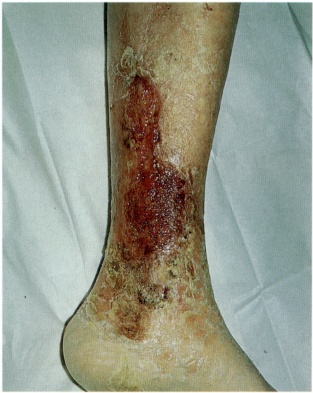

Figure 5.4 *Ulceration and associated eczema on the medial side of the leg*

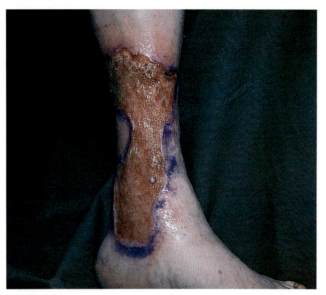

Figure 5.5 *Extensive ulceration with no associated eczema*

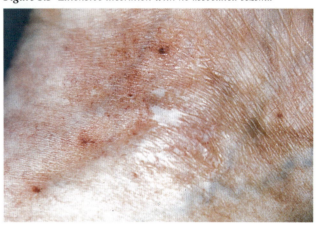

Figure 5.6 *Atrophy blanche. Small white 'scars' sometimes found in association with varicose eczema*

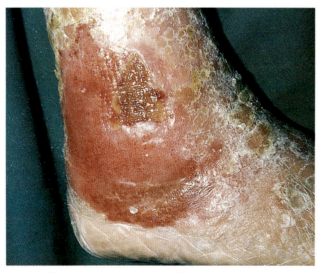

Figure 5.7 *Acute erythema surrounding an ulcer due to sensitivity to a preservative in a topical preparation*

Standing

Avoidance of prolonged periods of standing is important in the treatment and further prevention of varicose eczema and ulcers. Walking is far less harmful as the muscle activity increases venous return.

Support stockings and bandages

Elastic stockings are recommended in the early stages of mild developing edema, or when the eczema and ulcers have healed, to prevent further progress of the condition. In the definitive treatment of the eczema and/or ulcers, more elaborate support measures are required. If there is no superadded infection of the ulcers and/or eczema, bandages impregnated with tar or zinc paste can be applied directly to the leg. The paste bandage is then covered with a firm elastic bandage, and may be left in place for 1–2 weeks.

It is important that they are applied correctly. The bandaging should be carried out by the district nurse at home or as an out-patient. The bandages have a healing action due to the zinc or tar and also provide support. It should be stressed that bandages must be applied from just proximal to the toes to just below the knee.

If daily or even twice-daily topical treatment to the ulcer or eczema is required, then paste bandages are not suitable. In these circumstances, an elastocrepe bandage can be applied from the ball of the foot to just below the knee over the dressings used in the treatment of the eczema and ulcers. If stronger support is required and can be tolerated by the patient, a Bisgaard or blue-lined bandage can be applied.

Topical treatment for eczema

In the *acute* stages the patient should rest in bed for a short time, with the leg elevated and protected by a cradle. The eczema is treated with compresses of potassium permanganate 1:10 000, and clean linen dressings should be used. As the eczema settles and becomes subacute, 1% hydrocortisone cream can be applied to the skin twice daily and the leg covered with tube gauze and a firm support bandage, e.g. elastocrepe. In the later stages, more powerful topical steroid preparations are sometimes helpful but these should be used with caution for, if ulceration develops, the steroids will delay healing and often enlarge the ulcer. The cream is applied once or twice a day and covered with the tube gauze and support bandage. Alternatively, in the chronic forms of varicose eczema even without ulceration, the occlusive tar or zinc paste bandages may be used as described above.

Topical measures for ulcers

Most varicose ulcers seen for the first time are secondarily infected. A swab should be taken for culture and the ulcer cleaned with normal saline. If there is a considerable amount of debris and pus, the ulcer should be cleaned twice a day. The ulcer should be covered with a non-adhesive dressing followed by an elastocrepe or blue-lined bandage. There are over 100 various types of dressings on the market for the treatment of varicose (or gravitational) ulcers. Claims are made that they absorb the exudate, remove slough, control infection and promote granulation tissue. None of these claims appears to be justified, and if the simple measures of postural drainage and correct bandaging are not followed, then these expensive dressings will prove useless. To increase the chances of healing, it is helpful to apply pressure to the ulcer with a sorbo-rubber pad over the dressing and bandaging over the pad.

If it is not possible to clear the infection by the above measures, i.e. cleaning with saline and postural drainage, then topical antiseptics should be used. (Topical antibiotics should be avoided because of the high risk of contact eczema). Gentian violet and brilliant green are highly effective because of their persistent activity even in the presence of considerable exudate. Recently, gentian violet, which has been widely used for decades, has lost favor because of claims that it is carcinogenic in animals. However, there is no evidence of ill-effects when applied to the skin or wounds in humans. The informed advice of the British Association of Dermatologists Therapy Group is that restriction is only necessary in mucous membranes. Gentian violet is now becoming more difficult to obtain and brilliant green may have to be used instead. Systemic antibiotics may occasionally be required but should only be used after culture and the sensitivity of the organisms are known. Once the ulcer is clean and no longer infected, and the patient is ambulant, then occlusive paste bandages are helpful in the management. The bandages may be applied as described above, and need only be changed weekly or every 2 weeks.

If the ulcers prove resistant to treatment, bed rest with the feet elevated often promotes healing.

Apart from sensitization to topical antibiotics, there is a high degree of sensitization in varicose eczema to other substances such as lanolin, found in ointment bases, and ointment preservatives (Figure 5.7). This should always be considered if the eczema shows no improvement or deteriorates, and particularly if the eczema spreads to other parts of the body. If sensitization to any local medicaments is suspected, patch tests should be carried out.

Surgery

On the rare occasions that an ulcer shows no signs of healing, grafting may be considered. As varicose eczema is not thought to be due to varicose veins, treating them will not help the problem.

ASTEATOTIC ECZEMA

Asteatotic means without sebaceous secretion. However, this is probably not the cause of asteatotic eczema. Although the skin is dry and lacks 'grease', the basic fault appears to be in the stratum corneum, which is partly composed of fat. Thus, factors which affect the strength and integrity of the stratum corneum predispose to asteatotic eczema. The aging process, lack of humidity, cold weather, excessive use of degreasing agents (soaps and detergents in bubble-bath preparations) and a predisposition to dry skin, such as atopic individuals and those with ichthyosis, are all factors that may play a part in the etiology of asteatotic eczema.

Age incidence

As mentioned above, asteatotic eczema is most common in the elderly. It may be seen in younger individuals if other causative factors are operative.

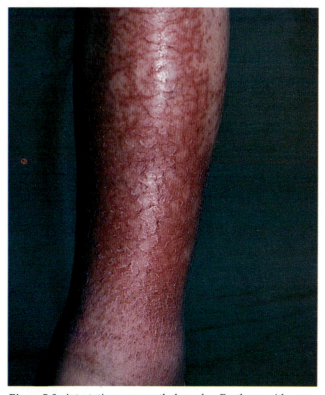

Figure 5.8 *Asteatotic eczema on the lower leg. Erythema with superficial fissuring of the skin*

Site

Asteatotic eczema is most commonly seen on the legs (Figures 5.8 and 5.9). It may subsequently occur on the thighs (Figure 5.10), extensor surfaces of the arms and the back. It is uncommon for asteatotic eczema to become widespread.

Morphology

Asteatotic eczema in its mildest form presents as dry scaly skin (Figure 5.9), but progresses to superficial fissures of the stratum corneum which interconnect, giving the characteristic crazy-paving appearance (Figures 5.8 and 5.10). The fissures give the appearance of cracking skin, hence the term 'craquelé'. The fissures have a red base (Figure 5.10) and, if the condition is not treated, it may progress to a more florid eczematous process with red discoid patches. Initially, these patches are scaly but, if the process is acute, there may be exudation leading to a crusted appearance.

Treatment

It is important to make enquiries as to the patient's bathing habits and make sure that they are not adding detergents (e.g. bubble-bath preparations), soda or bath salts to the water. Mild soaps or an emollient cleanser should be used. The bath water should not be too hot as this also aggravates the problem. Some individuals bathe or shower too frequently, and should be encouraged to change this habit.

If the inflammatory component to the eczema is mild, a Group I topical steroid in a greasy ointment base should be recommended twice a day. If the eczema is more acute, then a Group II topical steroid should be used.

It should be stressed that ointments and not creams should be used. Once the eczema has cleared, and if the patient is considered at risk of developing asteatotic eczema again, then a 'greasy' emollient should be applied to the skin after bathing.

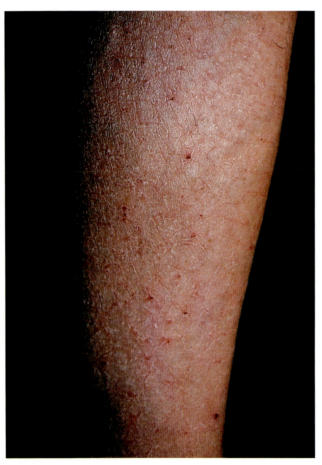

Figure 5.9 *Asteatotic eczema. Dryness and scaling of the lower leg with some superficial fissuring*

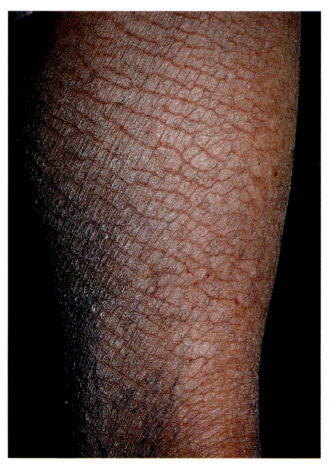

Figure 5.10 *Eczema craquelé. Chronic asteatotic eczema, dryness and red fissures of the skin*

6

Seborrheic eczema

Two distinct types of eczema may be considered under the heading of seborrheic eczema. One is the adult form, most commonly seen in young and middle-aged adults; the other is the infantile variety, which may begin as early as the age of 6 weeks, and is usually only present in infants under the age of 18 months.

ADULT SEBORRHEIC ECZEMA

Seborrheic eczema is one of the endogenous eczemas and the subdivision is based solely on clinical grounds. The term 'seborrheic' is somewhat misleading because seborrhoea is not always present and is not required to make the diagnosis. However, the sites commonly involved in this type of eczema are those areas of the skin which have relatively more sebaceous glands per unit surface area, i.e. face, scalp and upper trunk. However, eczema occurring where two skin surfaces are in contact, e.g. groins, axillae, perianal region, is considered a variant of seborrheic eczema and, at these sites, there is no increase in sebaceous glands per unit surface area.

As with other endogenous eczemas, the cause of seborrheic eczema is unknown, but there is often a positive family history. In the past, pyococcal infection of the skin was implicated as a possible cause, but the bacteria, if present, are now thought to colonize the skin as a secondary manifestation of the disorder. The term 'seborrheic diathesis' has also been used in the past to imply that subjects were prone to develop this type of eczema, but that it may occur at different sites at different times in their lives. The term has now been dropped as it has little meaning and does not contribute to our understanding of the disorder.

Sites

There are three main distributional subtypes of seborrheic eczema. All or only one may be present:

(1) The head and neck. Possibly the most common site is the scalp (in its mildest form, it is referred to as dandruff). On the face, seborrheic eczema usually begins in the nasolabial fold (Figure 6.1) and at the sides of the nose (Figure 6.2), and frequently spreads to the medial sides of the cheeks (Figure 6.2) and chin (Figure 6.3). Other common sites include the eyelids (Figure 6.4), ear (Figure 6.5) and skin behind the ear (Figure 6.6);

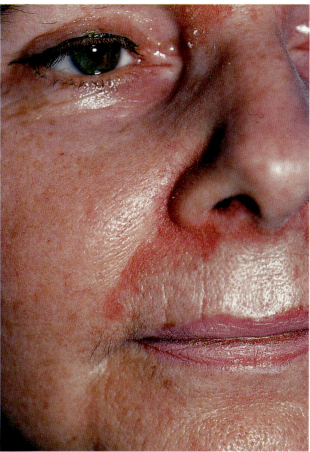

Figure 6.1 *The nasolabial fold is a common site for seborrheic eczema*

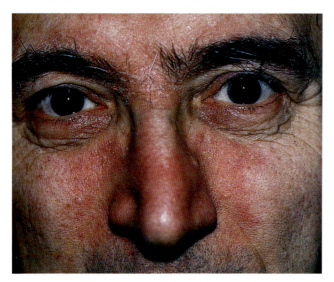

Figure 6.2 *Seborrheic eczema on the medial cheeks and between the eyebrows, both common sites*

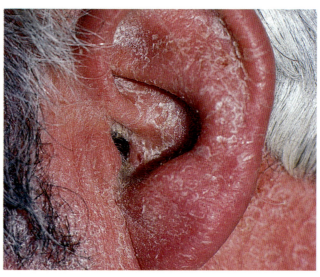

Figure 6.5 *Confluent seborrheic eczema on the pinna and surrounding skin*

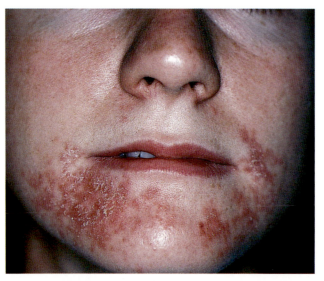

Figure 6.3 *Redness and scaling on the chin and nasolabial fold*

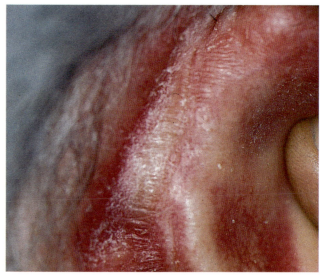

Figure 6.6 *Seborrheic eczema behind the ear, a common site*

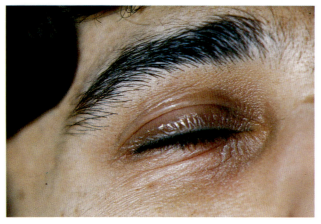

Figure 6.4 *Seborrheic eczema on the eyelid*

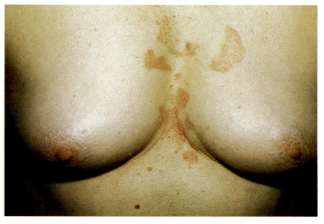

Figure 6.7 *Seborrheic eczema over the sternal area*

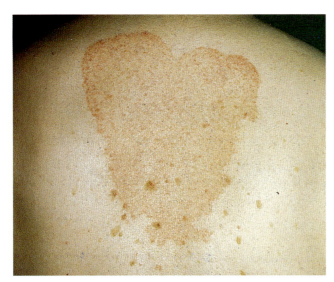

Figure 6.8 Seborrheic eczema between the shoulder blades

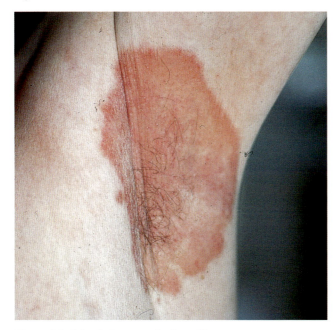

Figure 6.9 Seborrheic eczema in the axilla

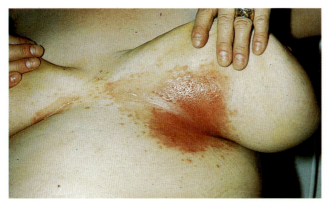

Figure 6.10 Intertriginous seborrheic eczema under the breasts

(2) Presternal and interscapular areas of the trunk (Figures 6.7 and 6.8); and

(3) Intertrigo. This term refers to seborrheic eczema where two skin surfaces are in contact. The common factor appears to be perspiration which is unable to evaporate, keeping the area continuously moist. The common sites for this type of eczema are the axillae (Figure 6.9), groins, submammary region in obese women (Figure 6.10), umbilicus and abdominal

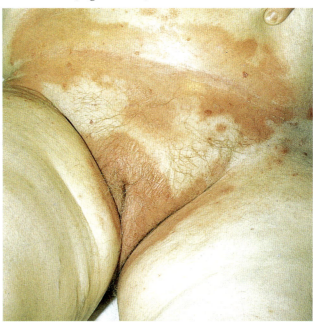

Figure 6.11 Seborrheic eczema in an abdominal fold in an obese individual

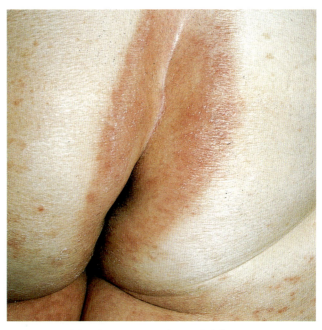

Figure 6.12 Seborrheic eczema in the natal cleft

folds in obese persons (Figure 6.11), natal cleft and perianal skin (Figure 6.12), and the glans penis and undersurface of the foreskin in men (Figure 6.13).

Morphology of lesions

On the scalp, the mildest seborrheic eczema is manifested by a diffuse scaling *(dandruff)*. In more severe forms, the scaling becomes thicker and at times may be difficult to distinguish from psoriasis of the scalp. In the

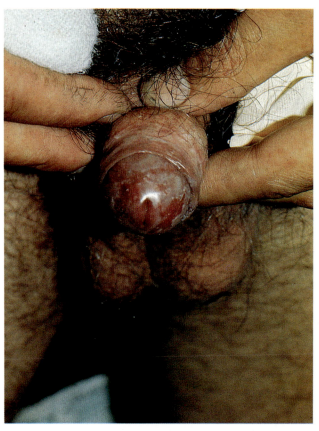

Figure 6.13 *Seborrheic eczema on the glans penis and foreskin*

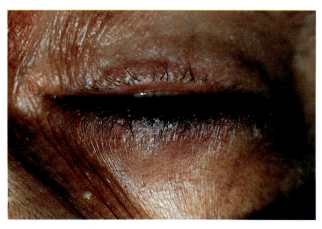

Figure 6.14 *Blepharitis. Seborrheic eczema on the edges of the eyelids*

most severe forms, there is erythema, crusting and even exudation. Seborrheic eczema *per se* is not a cause of hair loss, although the continual scratching may cause a reversible loss of hair.

When seborrheic eczema involves the pinnae or nasolabial folds, it usually presents as redness and scaling (Figures 6.3 and 6.5). In the later stages, there may be fissuring above, below or behind the pinna. On the trunk, seborrheic eczema occurs predominantly in the presternal and interscapular regions, and the lesions are red and scaly (Figures 6.7 and 6.8). They may appear as small discs or annular lesions. Occasionally, the eczema predominantly affects the hair follicles and presents as a follicular papular eruption.

Intertrigo

When the eczema affects the intertriginous areas (Figures 6.9–6.13; axillae, groins, submammary regions and umbilicus), the skin is red and sometimes macerated. In the natal cleft, particularly posteriorly, the skin may be fissured. In seborrheic eczema, the blistering and lichenification (thickening) present in other types of eczema of the skin are not seen, and this may be a useful point in establishing the diagnosis.

Infection with ringworm fungi is common in the groins and with *Candida albicans* in all intertriginous areas. A rash in the groins or perianal area spreading away from the intertriginous fold suggests possible infection with ringworm fungi. Ideally, specimens should be taken for myocological examination. If satellite papules (Figure 6.10) and pustules are present, this suggests secondary infection with *C. albicans*.

Associated conditions

Blepharitis (Figure 6.14) and otitis externa are often considered to be seborrheic eczema at specific sites and may occur without eczema elsewhere. There is reportedly a higher incidence of acne and rosacea in patients who have or subsequently develop seborrheic eczema. However, there is no evidence as yet that one disorder causes the other.

Natural history

Seborrheic eczema may be chronic and persistent or periodic. The exact cause is unknown, but it is sometimes precipitated by overwork, lack of sleep and tension.

Treatment

Scalp
In the mild forms of seborrheic eczema, frequent shampooing may be all that is required. Patients should be

reassured that frequent shampooing does not damage the hair or lead to baldness. The hair can be washed every 2–3 days. There are numerous shampoos for the treatment of 'dandruff', but no specific shampoo which appears to reverse the process. The hair is often greasy in seborrheic eczema and, frequently, all that is required is a simple detergent shampoo.

Strongly perfumed shampoos should not be used as they may act as irritants. Shampoos containing tar products may be helpful as the latter tend to suppress eczema. If the condition is more severe with irritation, erythema and scaling of the scalp, a topical corticosteroid preparation will often reverse the eczematous process. There are now a number of corticosteroid scalp lotions specially designed for the scalp, and they are pleasanter to use than creams or ointments.

In the more severe and chronic forms of scalp involvement with thick adherent scales, a preparation containing keratolytics is required. A suitable preparation is 2% salicylic acid and 2% sulfur in aqueous cream BP. This should be applied two or three times a week at night and shampooed off the following morning. On the other nights, a topical corticosteroid preparation as mentioned above should be used.

Face, pinnae and trunk

At these sites, topical corticosteroid preparations are the most effective treatment. Because the eczema tends to be moist, and in exposed and visible areas, creams are often better and more acceptable than ointments. They should be applied at least twice a day. Weak topical steroids are generally effective, and should only be used for eczema on the face. The eczema is often recurrent and, as the skin is very thin on the face, local side effects due to collagen damage may easily occur as a result of prolonged use of potent topical steroids. In addition, the complication of perioral dermatitis (*see* Chapter 25) may occur, particularly in women, following the application of potent steroids even for a short duration. On the trunk and pinnae, moderate-strength topical steroid creams may be used if weak ones are ineffective.

It has been suggested that fungal organisms may have a role as the cause of seborrheic eczema, and topical antifungal preparations, particularly the imidazoles, have been reported to he helpful in suppressing seborrheic eczema of the face. Recently, it has been claimed that lithium succinate (combined with zinc sulfate) in a cream base is useful in controlling eczema on the face. It should be stressed that neither topical antifungal nor lithium succinate creams appear to be superior to weak topical steroids.

If the seborrheic eczema, particularly when involving the face, is severe and difficult to control, then the possibility of AIDS should be borne in mind in patients thought to be at risk.

Intertrigo

The two main aims of management are:

(1) To keep the area as dry as possible; and

(2) To counteract the eczema specifically.

As the skin is moist and macerated, there is often secondary infection with bacteria and/or fungi; to counteract this, one should aim to keep the skin as dry as possible. Although not cosmetically acceptable, the time-honored *pigmenta magenta* is highly effective in keeping intertriginous areas dry and counteracting secondary infection. The preparation should be applied once a day, usually in the morning and, at night, a corticosteroid cream or lotion should be applied. Ointments are best avoided in intertriginous areas. As the absorption of drugs is greatly enhanced in intertriginous areas due to the moisture, Group IV topical steroids should not be used at these sites. Initially, Group I steroids should be tried and only if these prove ineffective should Group II ones be used. Very occasionally, Group III steroids may be necessary, but these should only be used for short periods (1–2 weeks) and not frequently.

The obese are more prone to intertrigo because opposing skin surfaces are more likely to be in contact. Thus, in recurrent intertrigo, weight loss is advisable.

If the intertrigo fails to clear, specimens should be taken for mycological and bacteriological examination to exclude infection with ringworm fungi, *C. albicans* or *Corynebacterium minutissimum*. Hailey–Hailey disease or so-called benign familial chronic pemphigus (*see* Chapter 14) should be considered in cases of persistent eruptions in the intertriginous areas.

Systemic steroids

As in other forms of endogenous eczema, systemic steroids should be reserved for very severe or widespread disease which do not respond to topical measures. Fortunately, such cases are extremely rare.

SEBORRHEIC ECZEMA OF INFANCY

This includes a number of clinical entities. The term seborrheic eczema is used because the sites of involvement are the scalp and intertriginous areas. The disorder appears to be self-limiting and usually disappears by the age of 2 years. There does not appear to be a higher incidence of adult seborrheic eczema in later life.

Cradle cap

This may appear for the first time in infants 1 month old. In its mildest form, it presents as yellow-brown greasy scaling on the scalp. The disorder is very common and tends to be self-limiting, clearing after 6 months. In its more severe forms, the scales become thicker and heaped up, presenting as thick, yellowish lumps (Figure 6.15). In generalized seborrheic eczema of infancy, the scalp may be red and scaly.

Corticosteroids are rarely required for treating seborrheic eczema of the scalp; mild keratolytics are usually all that is required. One per cent sulfur and 1% salicylic acid in aqueous cream BP applied at night and shampooed out the next morning with a simple detergent shampoo is a simple and effective regimen. In the more severe cases with thicker scales, the strength of the keratolytics may be increased to up to 5% sulfur and 5% salicylic acid.

Diaper rash

This is a very common disorder. It is arguable whether this should be considered an exogenous eczema due to ammonia in the urine or a seborrheic eczema similar to the intertrigo seen in adults due to continual moisture of the skin. It appears that some infants have a predisposition to eczema in the diaper area and this constitutional factor is probably the most important one.

The eruption is usually confined to the diaper area (Figure 6.16) but, like other eczemas, there may be spread of the rash to other areas (*see below*). The diagnosis usually presents no difficulties. The rash in its mildest form is simply erythema. In the more severe forms, there is exudation and even fissuring. A rare manifestation of diaper eczema is a papular and vesicular eruption on the genitalia.

Although diagnosis presents no difficulties, management does. As the disorder is due to moisture or ammonia, or both, on the skin, the most appropriate treatment is to leave the diapers off. Most mothers, however, do not consider this advice practical but find it impossible. A compromise may have to be reached in which the diaper is left off for short periods during the day and changed at least once during the night. Diaper liners, which tend to keep the skin drier than does the diaper, should be used.

If these simple measures fail, then the eczema should be treated with Group I steroid creams. As a rule, potent topical steroids (Groups III or IV) should not be used because of the increased absorption of steroid into the skin due to moisture and occlusion. *Candida albicans* is frequently found in diaper eczema probably as a secondary invader, although there are those who consider that it plays a role in the production of the eruption. Occasionally, better results can be obtained by combining nystatin with the Group I steroid cream.

Generalized seborrheic eczema of infancy

This eruption usually begins as a diaper eczema which then appears in areas outside of the diaper. This eruption may appear as one of two forms or as a combination

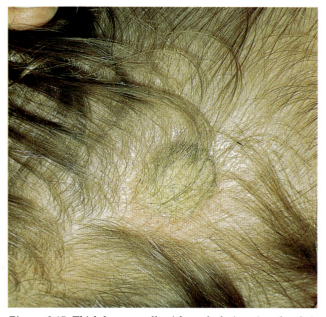

Figure 6.15 *Thick lumpy, yellowish, scaly lesions in seborrheic eczema of the scalp*

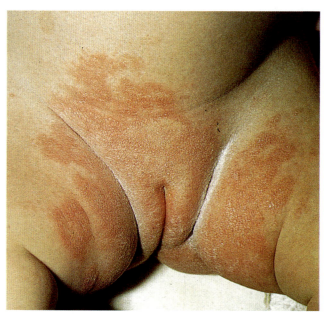

Figure 6.16 *Diaper rash is confined to the diaper area*

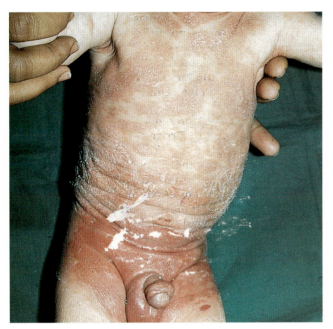

Figure 6.17 Severe seborrheic eczema of infancy with confluent patches on the trunk

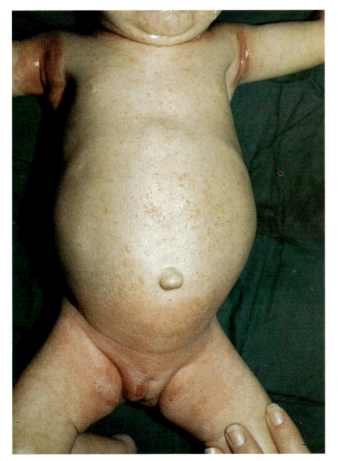

Figure 6.18 Spread of seborrheic eczema of infancy to the axillae

of both. There is extension of eczema from the diaper area onto the trunk (Figures 6.17 and 6.18) and down the thighs. This may spread as a confluent erythema (Figure 6.17) or as small red patches (Figure 6.18).

Not infrequently, these lesions develop a white scaly surface as seen in psoriasis (Figure 6.17), and the term 'diaper psoriasis' has been used to describe this eruption. However, this term is probably best avoided as there is no evidence that these infants have a higher incidence of psoriasis in later life.

The prognosis for generalized seborrheic eczema of infancy is excellent. The rash clears permanently once the infants are out of diapers. The second type of spread seen in generalized seborrheic eczema of infancy is confluent erythema in other intertriginous areas, e.g. the axillae (Figure 6.18) and neck (Figure 6.19). The face (Figure 6.19) is frequently involved and may in fact be the first site affected.

The cause of the spread of the eczema in generalized seborrheic eczema is not known. As in diaper eczema, *C. albicans* infection has been implicated, but there is no conclusive evidence that this organism is the sole cause.

The treatment of generalized seborrheic eczema of infancy is similar to that of diaper eczema. Weak (Group I) topical steroid creams such as 1% hydrocortisone, possibly combined with nystatin, should be applied three times a day. If there is no satisfactory response, then the strength of steroid cream may be cautiously increased, but this should probably be left to a specialist.

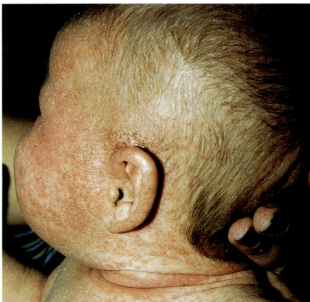

Figure 6.19 The face is a common site for seborrheic eczema of infancy

7

Discoid eczema and pompholyx eczema

DISCOID ECZEMA

This pattern of endogenous eczema is sometimes referred to as nummular eczema. There are no known definite etiological factors and, like many other skin disorders, the name is based solely on descriptive grounds.

Morphology of lesions

The lesions of discoid eczema occur mainly on the extensor surfaces of the limbs. The eruption tends to be subacute, and the lesions exhibit crusts and exudation (Figures 7.1 and 7.2). The lesions may coalesce to form large confluent areas of eczema (Figure 7.3) or small satellite lesions may develop around the initial lesion (Figure 7.2).

Distribution

The lesions of discoid eczema occur mainly on the extensor surfaces of the limbs and tend to be distributed symmetrically (Figures 7.3 and 7.4). Certain localized areas may be involved, such as the nipples or the backs of the hands (Figure 7.3). The number of patches when these sites are involved can vary from a few to many. Like other patterns of eczema, discoid eczema may occasionally become extensive and generalized, possibly due to autosensitization.

Age incidence and natural history

Discoid eczema seldom affects people under 20 years of age. It appears to be particularly common in young and middle-aged adults, but it does occur in the elderly, particularly those with dry skins. The eczema usually lasts for a period of several months, but tends to clear eventually. The relapse rate does not appear to be as high as in other types of endogenous eczema, e.g. atopic or seborrheic.

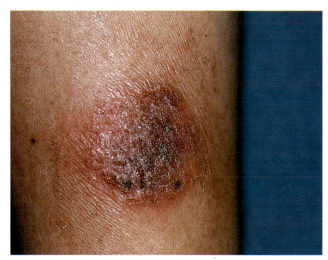

Figure 7.1 *Crusted lesion in discoid eczema*

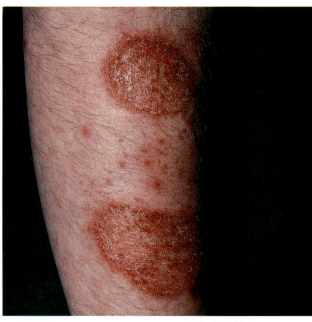

Figure 7.2 *Satellite lesions developing in discoid eczema*

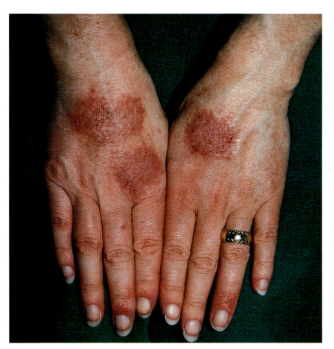

Figure 7.3 *Symmetrical eruption on the backs of the hands in discoid eczema*

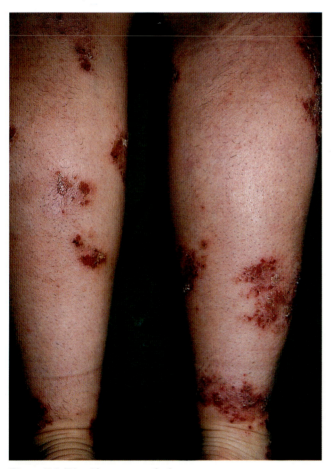

Figure 7.4 *Discoid eczema on the legs*

Management and treatment

In the acute stages of discoid eczema with exudation, lotions and compresses should be applied and the affected areas covered with clean linen dressings. Potassium permanganate soaks 1:10 000 or physiological saline should be used initially. As the lesions become drier, a topical steroid cream should be used, specifically, one that is moderately potent (Group II or III). The cream should be applied at least twice a day, and the affected areas subsequently covered by tube gauze dressings, or cotton gloves for the hands.

In the more chronic phase, a steroid ointment should be used. Discoid eczema usually requires a strong (Group III) topical steroid, which will usually clear the eczema within 2 weeks. If recurrence is rapid, this should be treated in the early stages with a Group II steroid. If the bouts of eczema are infrequent, Group III steroids may be used.

Antibiotics

Like other eczemas, there is always a possibility of secondary infection with pathogenic organisms. The lesions may become frankly purulent or impetiginized, i.e. have yellow crusts. A short course of a systemic antibiotic, such as erythromycin, apparently leads to better results than the use of topical antibiotics. Bacteriological tests should be carried out if there is no response to treatment.

Systemic steroids

Fortunately, these are only rarely required to control this type of eczema, and should never be used as a first measure.

PUVA

PUVA is an effective treatment for resistant discoid eczema but should be reserved for patients whose discoid eczema cannot be controlled by topical steroids.

Baths

Discoid eczema has sometimes been attributed to too-frequent bathing, particularly with antiseptics and toilet preparations added to the bath water. Such added substances should therefore be avoided and a mild emollient, such as aqueous cream BP, applied after bathing.

POMPHOLYX ECZEMA

This type of eczema occurs on the hands and feet. The name is taken from the Greek word *pompholyx*, which means 'bubble' as the disorder is characterized by numerous blisters. If the eczema is confined to the hands, it is sometimes referred to as cheiropompholyx and, if confined to the feet, as podopompholyx. Another term sometimes applied to this form of eczema is 'dyshidrotic' as the eczema appears to be aggravated by excessive sweating of the palms and soles.

Distribution

Pompholyx eczema affects the hands (Figure 7.5) and feet (Figure 7.6) either together or separately. The hands are more commonly involved. The eczema tends to affect those areas involved by emotional sweating, i.e. on the hands – the palms, sides of fingers, and dorsal aspects of the fingers over the distal two phalanges – and on the feet – the soles and sides of the toes.

As with the fingers, the dorsal surface of the toes over the distal phalanges may be involved. The eruption tends to be symmetrical (Figures 7.5 and 7.6), whether the hands or feet are affected. Pompholyx eczema, like other forms of eczema, may spread from the palms and soles to affect other areas of the body. Initially the eczema spreads to the backs of the hands and then up the arms (Figure 7.7), and may even give rise to a generalized eruption.

Type of lesion

The characteristic lesion is the blister, which varies in size from 1 mm to 1 cm or even larger (Figures 7.8 and 7.9). The small blisters are more common. There may be only a few blisters or they may be numerous and involve the entire palm and sides of the fingers. Because the keratin layer is so thick on the palm and sole, the blisters (although epidermal) do not rupture immediately and appear as small firm vesicles (Figures 7.8 and 7.9). The blisters may eventually rupture; the skin breaks down and presents an exuding or crusted surface (Figure 7.10) or the blisters may resolve slowly, the fluid being reabsorbed into the circulation with no break in the skin surface.

The blisters frequently occur in groups on the palms, although the whole palm is not necessarily involved. Occasionally, only the sides of the fingers and not the palms are affected. If only the dorsal aspects of the fingers are involved, the condition may be confused with other types of eczema.

In the more chronic forms of the disorder, no blisters may be seen, but the eczema will present as scaling and fissuring on the palms (Figure 7.11) and soles (Figure 7.12), which may be difficult to heal.

Natural history and precipitating factors

The disorder is rare in early childhood, but can occur at any age. The eczema tends to occur as attacks and runs a self-limiting 2- to 4-week course. Occasionally, the disorder becomes chronic and new blisters appear as the old ones clear. Alternatively, the patient may have one or many episodes during the year, and then may be free of attacks for a number of years. Frequently, the attacks are precipitated by warm weather and helped by cooler weather.

The other known precipitating factor is emotional stress, thought to induce the attacks by increasing perspiration on the palms and soles.

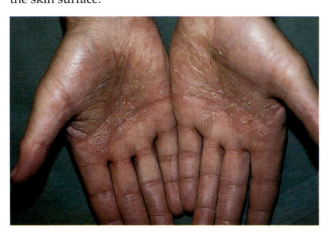

Figure 7.5 Symmetrical pompholyx eczema on the hands

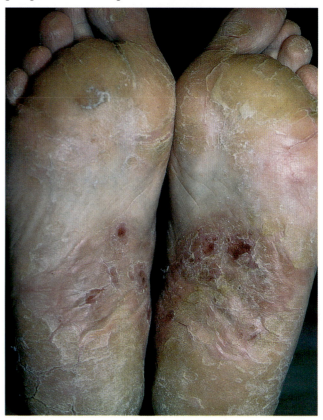

Figure 7.6 Symmetrical pompholyx eczema on the feet

Management and treatment

In the early stages when the blisters first appear, there is usually intense irritation, and antipruritics such as promethazine or trimeprazine are helpful. Both of these drugs tend to cause drowsiness of which patients must be warned although, because of this side effect, they are very good for use at night as they tend to promote sleep.

Soaks

If the blisters are rupturing and there is exudation, warm potassium permanganate soaks 1:8000 should be given for 10–15 min four times a day. Potassium permanganate is probably the most effective solution in which to soak the affected parts, but it has the slight disadvantage of staining the skin and nails brown.

Corticosteroids

In the acute stages, a Group I steroid cream is probably all that is required. This should be applied after the potassium permanganate soaks.

In the subacute and chronic stages, the more powerful topical corticosteroid preparations, such as Groups III and IV, should be used. Ointment bases are necessary in the chronic stages when the skin is dry and fissured.

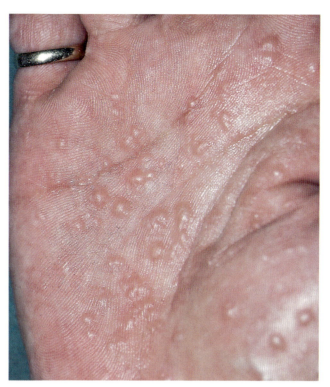

Figure 7.8 Blisters on the palm in pompholyx eczema

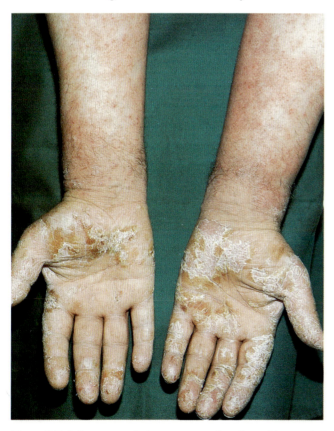

Figure 7.7 Subacute pompholyx eczema on the palms with spread of the eczema to the forearms

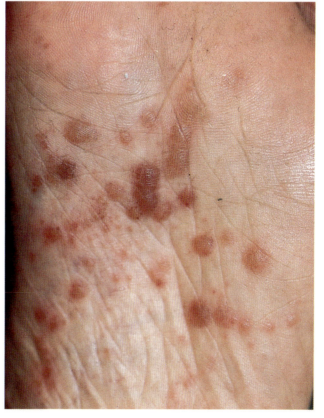

Figure 7.9 Blisters on the sole in pompholyx eczema

Unfortunately, topical corticosteroids do not appear to be helpful in preventing further attacks, and play no part in prophylaxis. Systemic corticosteroids may shorten an attack of pompholyx eczema but, as most attacks are self-limiting, their use is probably not justified. In the chronic forms of the disease, there is usually relapse when the steroids are withdrawn, so they are probably best avoided in the first place.

PUVA
If the eczema is persistent and not controlled by the more potent topical steroids, improvement may be obtained by PUVA treatment.

Antibiotics
Pompholyx eczema not infrequently becomes infected and may present as pustules rather than blisters. In these instances, there may be lymphangitis or cellulitis if the affecting organism is a *Streptococcus*. If the organism is a *Staphylococcus*, yellow crusts are present.

A course of erythromycin or flucloxacillin should be given. If possible, swabs should be taken for culture and sensitivity testing, and the appropriate antibiotic given if there is no response to the original antibiotic.

Dressings
In the acute stages, the affected hands and feet should be covered with clean linen dressings and the limb rested. In the subacute and chronic stages, cotton gloves or socks should be used.

General advice
There is no certain way to prevent further attacks. If the attacks are precipitated by emotional problems, these should be dealt with. The patient may benefit from the appropriate psychotropic drugs. If the attacks are precipitated by heat, this should be avoided if possible and, if the feet are affected, cotton socks are to be used.

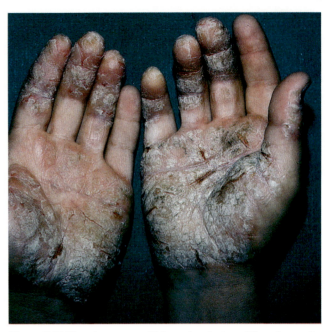

Figure 7.11 Chronic eczema with hyperkeratosis and fissuring on the palms

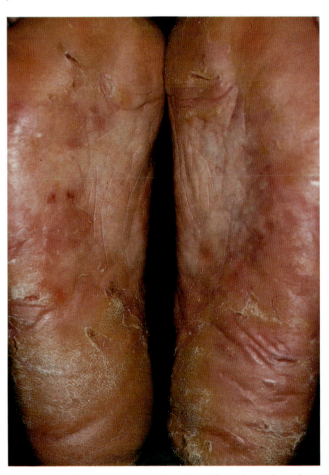

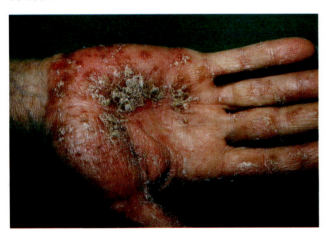

Figure 7.10 Crusts and blisters in subacute pompholyx eczema

Figure 7.12 Chronic eczema on the soles with erythema, hyperkeratotic scaling and fissures

8
Psoriasis

Psoriasis is a common skin disorder estimated to affect approximately 2% of the white population at some stage of their lives.

ETIOLOGY

The exact cause of psoriasis in unknown. One-third of patients with this complaint give a history of psoriasis in a blood relative. It is thought that there is a specific inherited defect in the skin which allows psoriasis to develop under certain circumstances.

Psoriasis is characterized by proliferation of the epidermal keratinocytes and a failure of maturation of these cells into normal keratin. There is now firm evidence that this proliferation of keratinocytes is mediated by activated T lymphocytes. The antigen which may trigger the lymphocytes may be bacterial or viral and, eventually, a self-antigen.

Accumulating experimental work as well as clinical observations have indicated that streptococcal antigens may initiate psoriasis, at least in a proportion of individuals. Subsequently, self antigens may maintain the psoriatic process because of possible cross-reactivity between bacterial and self antigens. The inherited defect may affect antigen presentation, T lymphocytes or keratinocyte response to cytokines.

In the majority of patients, there is no obvious precipitating factor. However, a number of factors are known to precipitate or aggravate psoriasis:

(1) Streptococcal infections. Psoriasis sometimes first appears 2–3 weeks after a streptococcal infection. The mechanism is unknown;

(2) Mental stress. Psoriasis is not *caused* by mental stress but, in persons with the probably inherited defect in the skin, worry may precipitate the psoriasis initially, or aggravate it in those who already have the disease;

(3) Trauma. Trauma to the skin can induce lesions in some patients with psoriasis; and

(4) Drugs. Chloroquine and lithium can sometimes precipitate or aggravate psoriasis.

AGE INCIDENCE

Psoriasis is extremely rare in those under 5 years of age. It is uncommon between the ages of 5 and 10 but does occur. The most common age at which it first appears is between 15 and 30 years. The incidence of first attack then falls progressively with advancing years, although psoriasis may appear for the first time in the eighth and ninth decades of life.

NATURAL HISTORY

Psoriasis tends to be a chronic disorder. The extent and chronicity of lesions vary greatly from patient to patient. In a survey of over 2000 patients, 38.5% reported a remission in their disease at some stage, including spontaneous remissions and those induced by treatment. The length of time remissions last is variable. Those induced by therapy vary according to the inherent activity of the disease. It seems that this inherent activity of the disease varies not only between patients, but also in the same patient at different times, and this latter variation probably accounts for the spontaneous remissions as well as exacerbation of the disease. What factors control disease activity are not yet known.

As a general prognostic rule, if no new plaques are developing but old ones persist, the psoriasis is considered to be stable and often a remission can be obtained with treatment. The formation of many new lesions is a poor prognostic sign and relapse is likely when treatment is stopped. In addition, the more widespread the disease, even if stable, the poorer the prognosis.

CLINICAL PRESENTATION

Psoriasis is usually easy to diagnose on clinical grounds but, occasionally, the diagnosis can be extremely difficult because of varied presentations.

Distribution and morphology

The classical lesion of psoriasis is a raised, scaly, circular or oval plaque whose edges are sharply demarcated (Figure 8.1). Occasionally, it has a geographical pattern. The *scaling* tends to be silvery or white (Figure 8.1). Sometimes, this type of scaling is not present and the lesion presents as a red plaque. If the diagnosis of psoriasis is suspected, the lesion should be gently excoriated with a wooden spatula; if it is psoriasis, the white silvery scale will appear (Figure 8.2). Further confirmation can be obtained if all the scale is removed to reveal a red, smooth, slightly moist area with capillary bleeding points (Figure 8.3). The most common sites involved in psoriasis are the knees (Figure 8.4) and elbows (Figure 8.5), followed by the sacral area (Figure 8.6) and the scalp behind the ears. It is important to examine all sites if a diagnosis of psoriasis is suspected.

Trunk and limbs
Psoriasis on the trunk and limbs may present in a number of ways. It may appear as discoid or oval patches (Figures 8.7 and 8.8), which can vary in size from 1 to 10 cm with completely normal-looking skin in between. In the more severe forms, the plaques become more numerous and larger (Figure 8.8), and eventually

confluent (Figure 8.9). Very occasionally, the whole of the skin surface may become involved in so-called *erythrodermic psoriasis.* In this form of the disease, the skin may not have the typical white silvery scales of psoriasis, but presents as a generalized erythema with superficial scaling (Figure 8.9), which may be indistin-

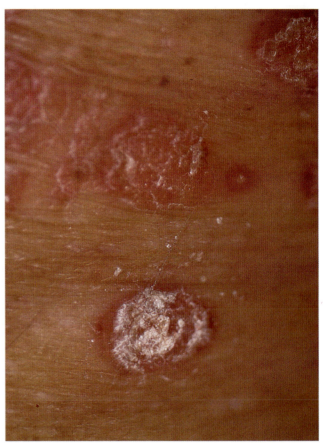

Figure 8.2 *Two psoriatic lesions. The upper lesion is a red plaque with minimal scaling; the lower had a similar appearance, but after excoriation the typical white scale was produced*

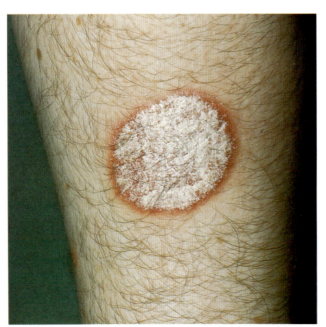

Figure 8.1 *Typical lesion of psoriasis. There is a clear line of demarcation between involved and uninvolved skin*

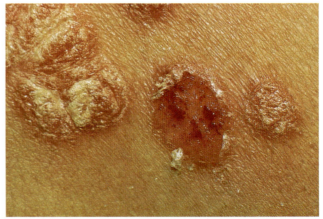

Figure 8.3 *Capillary bleeding points in a psoriatic lesion after removal of the scales*

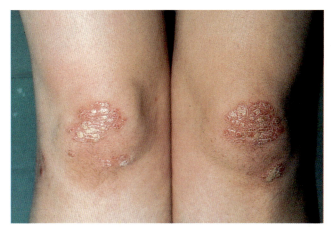

Figure 8.4 *Symmetrical plaques of psoriasis on the knees, one of the common sites*

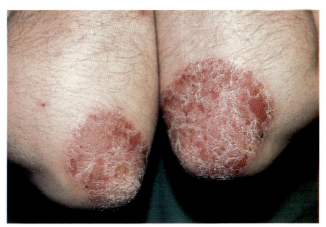

Figure 8.5 *Symmetrical lesions of psoriasis on the elbows, a common site*

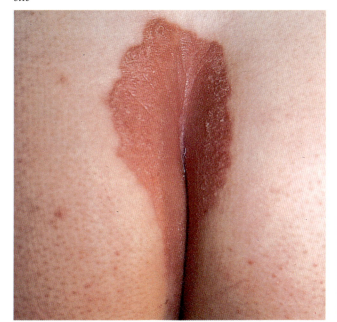

Figure 8.6 *Psoriasis in the sacral area*

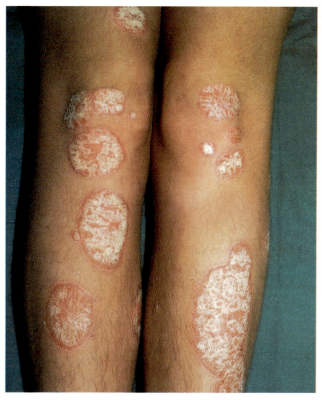

Figure 8.7 *Numerous oval and discoid plaques of psoriasis on the legs*

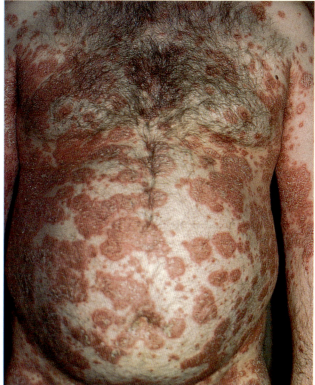

Figure 8.8 *Active psoriasis with numerous large plaques*

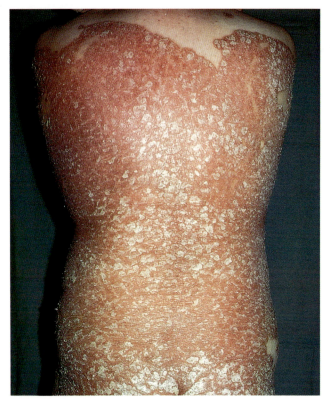

Figure 8.9 Confluent psoriasis. This may progress to erythrodermic psoriasis with total skin involvement

guishable from erythroderma due to eczema. Another presentation is numerous small red papules which still have the classical scale if excoriated. These appear suddenly on trunk and limbs. This presentation is sometimes referred to as *guttate psoriasis* (Figure 8.10). This is the usual pattern that appears after a streptococcal infection. Guttate psoriasis tends to have a good prognosis and often clears spontaneously within 3 months.

Scalp

Involvement of the scalp is fairly common. It may occur with the disease affecting the skin at other sites, but occasionally affects *only* the scalp; the diagnosis may then be difficult on clinical grounds alone. As with the skin elsewhere, psoriasis may involve the whole of the scalp or only small areas. The scales on the scalp lesions

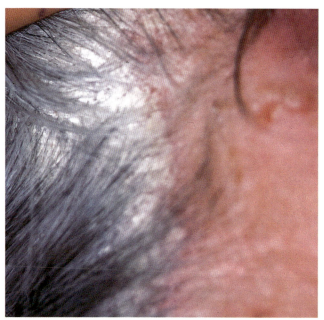

Figure 8.11 Thick white plaques of psoriasis on the scalp

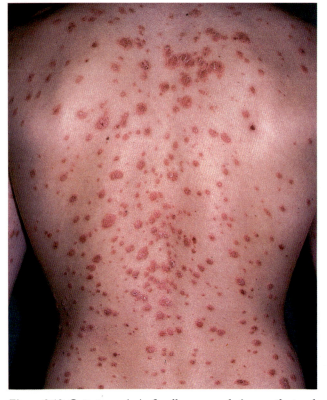

Figure 8.10 Guttate psoriasis. Small numerous lesions on the trunk

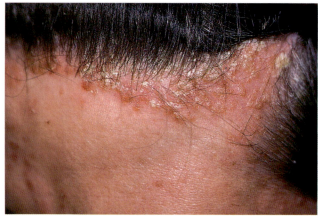

Figure 8.12 Psoriasis on the scalp. It is uncommon for the disease to extend beyond the hairline

tend to be heaped up so that they feel lumpy and irregular (sometimes referred to as 'rocks'), and often the diagnosis is made by palpation as well as inspection. Psoriasis of the scalp usually stops at the hairline and does not spread to the neck or face in the majority of patients (Figures 8.11 and 8.12).

Intertriginous areas

If psoriasis affects the skin in the groins, axillae (Figure 8.13), perianal region, between the toes, under the breasts (Figure 8.14) or in the umbilicus, the appearances will differ from the classical raised red plaque with silvery white scales. Where the skin surfaces are in apposition and the areas are moist, there is no dry scale and the lesions present as smooth confluent red plaques, which may or may not be raised. Occasionally,

particularly between the toes, the scale which is present has a macerated appearance in what used to be called 'white' psoriasis.

Genitalia

Psoriasis may occur on the penis and vulva as red patches. Some scaling is usually present, but it is not thick as in psoriasis elsewhere. Occasionally, it presents as red shiny patches. In children, the genitalia are a common site for psoriasis (Figure 8.15).

Palms and soles

There are two different types of psoriasis affecting the palms and soles. Neither has the classical appearances of psoriasis and, if localized only to these sites, may give rise to difficulty in diagnosis. It may present as localized

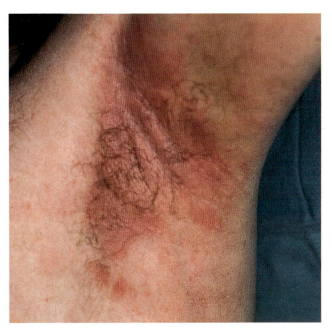

Figure 8.13 *Intertriginous psoriasis in the axilla*

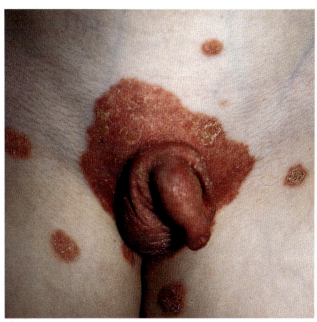

Figure 8.15 *Psoriasis on the genitalia in a child. This is a common site in children*

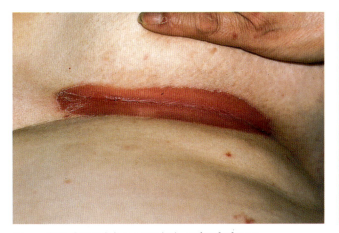

Figure 8.14 *Intertriginous psoriasis under the breast*

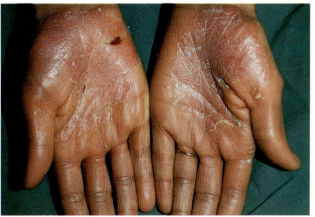

Figure 8.16 *Symmetrical erythema, scaling and fissuring on the palms in psoriasis*

confluent areas of erythema, scaling and fissuring, tending to be symmetrical (Figures 8.16 and 8.17). Like psoriasis elsewhere, there is often a sharp line of demarcation between the affected and unaffected skin (Figure 8.16). The appearances are sometimes difficult to distinguish from chronic eczema of the palms and soles.

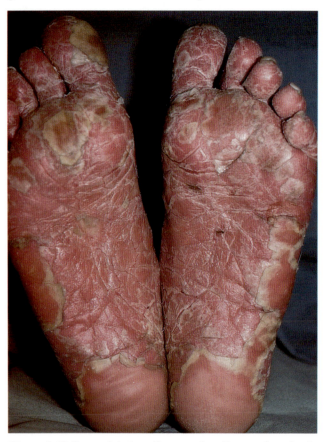

Figure 8.17 *Symmetrical erythema and scaling on the soles in psoriasis*

Another manifestation of psoriasis affecting the palms and soles is termed *pustular psoriasis,* although it is not certain whether this disorder is true psoriasis or representative of a separate disease entity. The other terms sometimes used for this condition are persistent palmar and plantar pustulosis or recalcitrant eruption of the palms and soles. Pustular psoriasis presents as discrete red scaly areas on the palms and soles, and small sterile pustules may be present (Figure 8.18). The disorder may be symmetrical or, occasionally, only affecting one palm or sole. As some of the terms applied to this condition imply, the disorder tends to be very persistent and may last for years. Typical psoriatic lesions elsewhere on the skin present in less than 20% of patients with pustular psoriasis.

Nails

The nails are frequently involved in psoriasis and may be helpful in establishing the diagnosis if the nature of the skin eruption is in doubt. The nails are involved in a number of ways:

(1) The nails show small pits (Figure 8.19) with wide variation in the number of pits present;

(2) The terminal part of the nail plate separates from the nail bed (onycholysis) so that the distal part of the nail appears white (Figure 8.20). Occasionally the area under the nail plate proves a suitable place to harbor chromogenic bacteria, and the patient may present with black or green nails;

(3) The nail-plate becomes thickened and there is a thick scale (hyperkeratosis) under the nail plate (Figure 8.21); and

(4) Brown translucent areas appear under the nail plate, sometimes referred to as 'oil-drops'. The lesions are due to small areas of psoriasis on the nail bed.

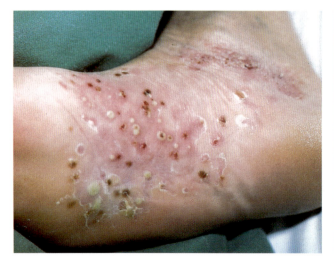

Figure 8.18 *Localized pustular psoriasis on the sole*

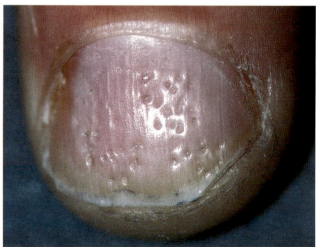

Figure 8.19 *Pits in the nail in psoriasis*

Occasionally, psoriasis affects only the nails and there are no skin lesions. In these circumstances, the diagnosis can be extremely difficult to establish and particularly difficult to distinguish from a fungal infection if the involvement causes thickening of the nail-plate with subungual hyperkeratosis. Occasionally, but not always, in psoriasis, all of the nails are involved but, in a fungal infection, only a few (at least at the onset) are involved. To establish the diagnosis, specimens of the nail should be taken for culture and microscopy carried out to determine whether fungus is present.

Arthritis

Approximately 5% of patients with psoriasis develop an arthritis, which is distinguished from rheumatoid arthritis by the absence of the rheumatoid factor in the serum. Psoriatic arthritis is therefore sometimes referred to as 'seronegative arthritis'. The joints of the hand are frequently affected but, unlike rheumatoid arthritis, the terminal interphalangeal joint may be involved (Figure 8.22) as well as the other joints of the fingers and hand (Figure 8.22). The knee and ankle joints are also commonly affected. Occasionally, 'psoriatic arthropathy' occurs without the skin lesions of psoriasis. Under these circumstances the diagnosis will have to be made by the clinical features, the absence of rheumatoid factor in the serum, exclusion of other causes of arthropathy such as gout and systemic lupus erythematosus, and possibly a family history of psoriasis.

The treatment of psoriatic arthritis is similar to that of rheumatoid arthritis. Salicylates and NSAIDs are useful whereas systemic steroids should be avoided as they make control of the skin lesions more difficult; when the dose of steroid is reduced, there is frequently a flare-up of the lesions. Methotrexate, cyclosporine or salazopyrin may be used with good results in severe cases.

Treatment and management

Once the diagnosis of psoriasis has been made, it is most important that certain features of the disorder are explained to the patient before embarking on any form of treatment. First, the patient must be reassured that the disorder is not contagious and that it is not a sign of internal disease. It should be explained that psoriasis does not, in itself, have any serious systemic effects.

Patients will often ask about the cause of psoriasis, and they must be given an explanation of their disease. With our present knowledge, patients can be told that they have a (probably hereditary) defect of the skin which, under certain circumstances, will cause the skin to develop a psoriatic lesion. However, they should also be reassured that just as psoriasis may appear for the

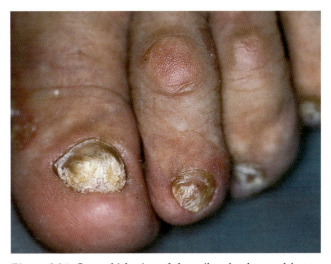

Figure 8.21 *Gross thickening of the nail and subungual hyperkeratosis in psoriasis*

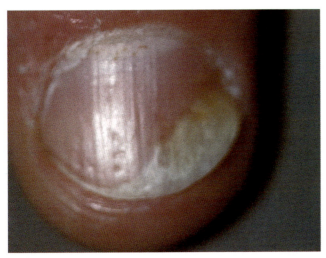

Figure 8.20 *Onycholysis. Separation of the nail plate from the nail bed*

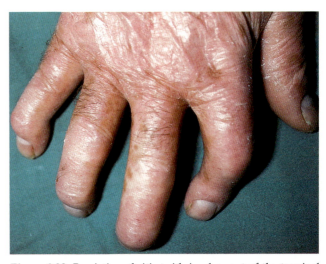

Figure 8.22 *Psoriatic arthritis, with involvement of the terminal interphalangeal joint*

first time after 30 or 40 years of life, so it may well disappear for no apparent reason. They should also be told that when psoriasis clears, there are no marks or scars and the skin returns to a normal appearance. It is, however, only fair to tell patients that, at present, there is no known *permanent* cure for the disorder, but something can always be done to improve the condition, even if the effects are not long-lasting. Patients should also be told that the psoriasis can always be cleared by intensive therapy but that, when the lesions do clear either spontaneously or as a result of treatment, then the duration of remission cannot be foretold, although it could be permanent.

Finally, each patient must be regarded individually. Some patients who have minimal psoriasis, and who have had the nature of the condition explained, will be perfectly satisfied to receive no treatment, but others with the same involvement will demand vigorous treatment to try to clear the condition.

Whatever course is finally adopted, the physician must be sure that the treatment being given is not worse than the disease being treated, which may often be the case with psoriatic patients. Psoriasis is a benign condition, and the treatments most commonly employed are topical measures rather than systemic therapy. However, even topical treatments are not without side effects which must be taken fully into consideration.

INTERTRIGINOUS PSORIASIS

Corticosteroids are the drugs of choice for psoriasis at these sites. Group I steroids are not always effective and thus Group II steroids are usually necessary. Not infrequently, Group III corticosteroids may have to be used for a short period (i.e. 1–2 weeks) to clear the lesions, but not more frequently than every 2 months. As a general rule, Group IV steroids should not be used in the intertriginous areas and the steroid preparations used in these areas should have a cream base.

GUTTATE PSORIASIS

It is important to remember that, in the majority of patients, guttate psoriasis is a self-limiting disorder. The disorder can be considered to be an active form of the disease and it is important not to use preparations such as dithranol, which may irritate the uninvolved skin as otherwise psoriasis may develop at these sites. If the disorder is not causing any symptoms, and the condition and natural history have been explained to the patient, no treatment is necessary. If the lesions are causing discomfort or irritation, this may be relieved by a Group II corticosteroid.

PLAQUE PSORIASIS

This is the most common form of psoriasis.

Topical treatment

Steroids

If the disease is not extensive and no new lesions are appearing, topical steroids may be used. Ideally, the aim should be to clear the lesions within 2–3 weeks and then stop treatment. Group I and II steroids are usually ineffective in clearing plaque psoriasis. It may be justified to use a Group IV preparation as the stronger the steroid, the better the clinical effect. However, if there is no clearing within 3 weeks, it is unlikely to occur and treatment with this particular topical preparation should be stopped. If there is a rapid reappearance of the psoriasis when treatment is stopped, it is inadvisable to use these preparations again.

The phenomenon of tachyphylaxis occurs with topical steroids when used in the treatment of psoriasis; thus, although there may be initial improvement, if the same strength steroid is continued, it will subsequently prove ineffective. A break in treatment or change of treatment then becomes necessary. If Group IV topical steroids are helpful, they should not be used for longer than 3 weeks and another course should not be used for another 3 months. If topical steroids are used as a palliative to alleviate soreness or irritation, only Group II steroids in an ointment base should be employed. However, it is inadvisable to use even these preparations on a long-term basis and a change of treatment should be made after a few months.

The advantages of topical steroids are that, compared to tar and dithranol preparations, they are pleasanter to use. The disadvantage is that, if they are Group IV or even Group III, there is a risk of local side effects to normal skin if used for long periods, as may occur in psoriasis. Very occasionally, if the psoriasis is active, there may be a rebound of the psoriasis after the use of Group IV topical steroids.

Dithranol

This is a highly effective treatment for psoriasis. However, dithranol has two main disadvantages. The first is that it will produce a purple stain on clothing and the bedclothes, and on the uninvolved skin surrounding the psoriatic lesions. Second, dithranol is an irritant to uninvolved skin and, if used at too great a strength, will produce soreness, erythema and blister formation. Because of these side effects, dithranol should be used with caution.

Two methods of use have been devised, depending on whether it is used in a hospital setting (as an in-patient or on a daily basis in special out-patient centers) or at home by the patient. In hospital, dithranol is made up in Lassar's paste to stop the preparation spreading to the surrounding skin. It is usual to start with 0.1% concentration of dithranol and increase the concentration every few days, to 0.25%, 0.5% and 1%, providing there is no burning of the surrounding skin. Psoriasis tends to clear first from the upper trunk and last from the legs, so it is not uncommon to use stronger concentrations of dithranol on the legs, while weaker ones will suffice for the upper trunk. It usually takes 3–4 weeks to clear plaque psoriasis with dithranol.

When patients use dithranol at home, it should be as the 'short-contact dithranol' regimen. The dithranol should only be applied for 15–30 min and then washed off. However, to be effective, the strength of dithranol has to be considerably greater than that used in a hospital setting. Thus, a 2% dithranol preparation should be used.

When treatment is commenced, the dithranol should be washed off after 15 min. The time may be increased to up to 30 min providing there is no burning or soreness. The advantage of short-contact dithranol is that it is convenient for home use, as patients can wear old pyjamas while the dithranol is on the skin, but they can still go to work and lead a normal life. Patients should be warned that dithranol may stain the bath and therefore as much of the preparation should be wiped off before getting into the bath.

If the short-contact dithranol regimen is going to be effective, results show within 4 weeks. It is probably not worth continuing with dithranol for longer periods.

Dithranol should not be used on the face, genitalia or intertriginous areas, where it may produce severe reactions due to its irritant properties.

Coal tar

Coal-tar preparations have been used for many years in the treatment of psoriasis, but are now used much less frequently with the advent of topical steroids and dithranol. Crude coal tar is more effective than the purified products, although the latter are pleasanter to use. In the treatment of chronic plaque psoriasis, 5% crude coal tar in Lassar's paste or a suitable ointment base is applied daily. These preparations should be washed off in a bath to which 30 ml coal-tar solution has been added. Afterwards, patients should receive a suberythema dose of ultraviolet light. With this regimen, it usually takes 3–4 weeks to clear psoriasis.

The disadvantages of this regimen are that coal-tar preparations have a strong smell and are also fairly messy, and have to be covered with tube gauze dressings. Patients having this treatment will either have to attend hospital on a daily basis or be in-patients.

Calcipotriol

Calcipotriol is a vitamin D analog recently introduced for the treatment of psoriasis following the observation that oral vitamin D was helpful in clearing the rash. Vitamin D, whether taken orally or applied topically, will have a deleterious effect on calcium metabolism if used in a dose sufficient to have an antipsoriatic effect and taken for any length of time. Analogs of vitamin D have therefore been developed which retain the antipsoriatic effect but have a considerably reduced effect on calcium metabolism.

The advantages of calcipotriol over other topical preparations currently available are that it is pleasant to use (unlike tar and dithranol) and does not have any effect on dermal collagen, as may occur with the long-term use of potent topical steroids. However, although calcipotriol has antipsoriatic properties, as with other topical preparations used on an out-patient basis, it does not totally clear the lesions, and some patients do not appear to derive much benefit.

Phototherapy

It has long been known that the sun often helps psoriasis, and it has been shown that the middle-range ultraviolet rays (UVB) are the beneficial ones. Many patients require considerable amounts of UVB to clear their psoriasis and high-intensity lamps may be necessary for clearance to be obtained. It often takes 4–8 weeks to clear patients. Considerable care has to be taken not to burn patients with this treatment, and it probably should be left to specialists.

The disadvantage of this treatment is that it is time-consuming and patients will probably have to attend special centers.

PUVA (see Chapter 25)

This treatment is highly effective in clearing psoriasis but should be reserved for extensive plaque psoriasis or that which relapses readily after topical treatments. The time taken for PUVA to clear psoriasis usually ranges from 4–6 weeks, treatment being carried out three times a week. Maintenance treatment carried out once a week or once every 2 weeks is often sufficient to prevent a relapse.

Climatic therapy

Many patients find that sunlight improves their psoriasis and take their holidays in warm sunny climates in an attempt to clear their disease. However, there is a small proportion of patients whose disease is made worse by sunlight, and patients should always be warned not to overdo the exposure because, if they develop a sunburn reaction, they may develop psoriasis at those sites (the Koebner phenomenon).

The problem of sunburn is overcome at the Dead Sea where a special treatment center for psoriasis has been established. Because of the unique geographical features of the Dead Sea, the majority of the burning rays (UVB) are filtered out by the aerosol which forms above the sea and surrounding beaches. The Dead Sea is the lowest point on earth and surrounded by mountains. The sea evaporates and the moisture is trapped by the surrounding mountains. Thus, patients can remain on the beach for the whole day without becoming sunburnt. The combination of the UVA and small amounts of UVB clear the psoriasis after 3–4 weeks. The salts from the Dead Sea also appear to have a beneficial effect on clearing of the disease.

Systemic drugs

Systemic drugs should only be used for psoriasis if the disease is severe, i.e. extensive and/or incapacitating, such as when it affects the palms and fingers, thereby limiting their use, or the soles, where it interferes with walking. All the currently effective systemic drugs for psoriasis have potential side effects, some of which are serious. As a general rule, patients who are considered for systemic treatment will have failed to respond satisfactorily to topical preparations and ultraviolet light treatment, including PUVA (if it is available).

Retinoids
Acitretin is a retinoid shown to have a beneficial effect on psoriasis. The daily dose is 0.5–1.0 mg/kg/day. Oral retinoids are invariably accompanied by side effects that are mild in the majority of patients (*see* Chapter 25). Prior to treatment for psoriasis with retinoids, which is likely to be long term, it is important that serum fasting lipids and liver function tests are performed to check for abnormalities.

Methotrexate
This is a very effective drug for clearing psoriasis. The dose is usually 10–30 mg weekly. A proportion of patients develop a feeling of nausea and lethargy for 48 h after taking the drug. Side effects include gastrointestinal ulceration and bone marrow depression. Unfortunately, methotrexate is hepatotoxic and may cause liver fibrosis, particularly after long-term treatment. Regular monitoring of liver function is necessary and liver biopsy may be required.

Cyclosporine (see *Chapter 25*)
Cyclosporine is the first drug used for psoriasis based on the known pathogenesis of the disease rather than empirically. It has a selective action on the activated T lymphocytes and inhibits cytokine production.

Cyclosporine is highly effective in clearing psoriasis. The initial dose should be 3 mg/kg/day. The maintenance dose usually varies from 2–5 mg/kg/day and should not exceed 5 mg/kg/day. Cyclosporine has few subjective side effects and is well tolerated. The most serious side effects include hypertension and nephrotoxicity and, thus, careful monitoring, particularly of renal function, is essential (*see* Chapter 25).

Choice of systemic drug
Methotrexate and cyclosporine are equally effective in clearing psoriasis in the majority of patients, but some respond better to one drug and some to the other. Both methotrexate and cyclosporine tend to be more effective than retinoids. Which drug is chosen often depends on the personal choice of the physician, although cyclosporine has the least subjective side effects. The supervision of systemic treatment with retinoids, methotrexate or cyclosporine should be by a hospital-based physician who has experience of these drugs.

ERYTHRODERMIC PSORIASIS

When psoriasis is generalized, it indicates very active disease and treatment in a dermatology unit will be necessary. Topically, only Grade II steroid ointments should be used and only for symptomatic relief to control any irritation and 'cracking' of the skin.

Patients with erythrodermic psoriasis are at risk of developing hypothermia because of excessive heat loss due to increased blood flow to the skin. Often, patients improve when admitted to hospital and with the application of moderate-strength steroid ointments. However, if this is not the case, treatment with systemic drugs will be necessary. Oral steroids may be necessary if the patient is severely ill. However, as the dose is reduced, other oral treatment will be necessary as there may be a rebound of the psoriasis with worsening of the condition.

PUSTULAR PSORIASIS

This form of psoriasis is usually resistant to the topical drugs currently available for treatment of psoriasis. It does, however, respond to PUVA, retinoids and cyclosporine. Pustular psoriasis also responds to triamcinolone 4 mg twice daily. Triamcinolone compared to other oral steroids appears to be unique in this respect. There is no rebound phenomenon when the dose of triamcinolone is reduced.

PSORIASIS OF THE SCALP

Psoriasis at this site is often persistent. It is also difficult to apply ointments and creams which are not water-miscible as they are difficult to wash from the hair. Thus, different vehicles for the drugs have been formulated.

There are a number of steroid lotions available for treating psoriasis of the scalp but, unfortunately, they are frequently not effective. Sometimes, keratolytics in a simple cream base applied at night will remove the excessive scaling, and make the disorder less obvious and more acceptable to the patient. Five per cent salicylic acid and 5% sulfur in aqueous cream BP is one such preparation.

If the above treatments are not successful, the following time-honored preparation should be tried: solution of coal tar 10%; salicylic acid 5%; sulfur 5%; coconut oil 40%; emulsifying ointment 40%. It is not very pleasant to use, and an out-patient should probably use it only 2–3 times per week at night, shampooed out of the scalp the following morning.

PUVA will not be effective in treating psoriasis of the scalp because the hair filters out the light, but acitretin, cyclosporine and methotrexate are effective.

General measures

Diet
Patients often ask whether they should avoid any particular food or include any extra vitamins or minerals in their diet.

At present, there is no evidence that any dietary restrictions or additions make any difference to psoriasis.

Sunlight
Natural sunlight frequently helps psoriasis, but it can also make it worse, particularly if patients overexpose themselves and become sunburnt. Patients should be warned of such an occurrence.

Psychiatric treatment
There is no conclusive evidence that patients with psoriasis are more neurotic than controls without psoriasis. However, it is not surprising that many patients with such a disfiguring condition may become depressed.

It must be admitted that, in certain individuals, emotional problems will precipitate or aggravate the condition. These problems should be dealt with appropriately.

Psoriasis Association

A Psoriasis Association has been founded in Great Britain and one of its aims is to help those who have this condition. It is well worthwhile for patients with psoriasis to be put in touch with this group if their disorder is causing social problems.

9

Pityriasis rosea and lichen planus

PITYRIASIS ROSEA

Pityriasis rosea is one of the so-called papulosquamous eruptions. The term 'pityriasis' is derived from a Greek word meaning 'bran-like'. Pityriasis rosea is a common dermatosis of unknown etiology, but with characteristic lesions and a good prognosis. The disorder tends to affect males and females equally. It is rare in infancy and old age, and affects mainly young adults. It occurs more commonly in a temperate climate and appears predominantly in the spring and autumn.

Pityriasis rosea usually begins with a solitary lesion, the herald patch (Figure 9.1). This lesion is nearly always on the trunk and never on the face. It is an annular scaly patch with a slightly raised edge and is reddish-brown in color. At this stage, the lesion may be mistaken for tinea corporis. On direct questioning, the patient may admit to a mild sore throat and malaise. Within 1–2 weeks, other lesions that are usually smaller than the herald patch begin to appear. They occur mostly on the trunk (Figure 9.2), but may also involve the neck and upper parts of the limbs whereas the face, hands and feet are rarely affected. The lesions tend to be oval (Figure 9.3) with their long axes lying along the lines of cleavage of the skin (Figure 9.4). Another characteristic and diagnostically helpful feature that may be visible is centripetal scaling of the lesions (Figures 9.3 and 9.5). Occasionally, they may have a different appearance and present as small papules 3–4 mm in diameter with a slightly scaly surface. This is sometimes referred to as papular pityriasis rosea.

The severity of pityriasis rosea varies a great deal; the lesions may be so numerous that practically all of the skin of the trunk is affected, or there may be only a few scattered on the limbs and trunk. Apart from the appearances, the disease is frequently symptomless, although sometimes there is occasional irritation. The disorder runs a self-limiting course and clears within 2–3 months of onset.

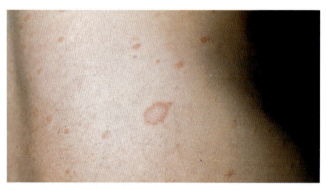

Figure 9.1 *Herald patch in pityriasis rosea. The lesion is often annular and larger than the other lesions*

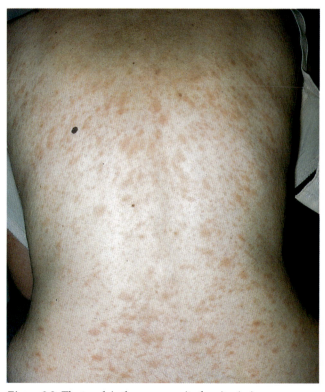

Figure 9.2 *The trunk is the common site for pityriasis rosea*

It is extremely uncommon for patients to develop a further attack of pityriasis rosea and, because of this, an infectious etiology with subsequent immunity has been suggested, but not proven.

The differential diagnosis of pityriasis rosea includes secondary syphilis, some forms of eczema, psoriasis and tinea corporis.

Treatment

Once the patient has been reassured that the condition is benign with a self-limiting course, no active treatment is usually required. Suppression or partial suppression of the lesions may be obtained with intermediate-strength corticosteroid (Groups II or III) preparations. If there is associated irritation, then topical corticosteroids as described above should be used twice daily. Systemic antihistamines, such as trimeprazine 10 mg thrice daily, should also be prescribed.

LICHEN PLANUS

Lichen planus is another papulosquamous eruption of unknown etiology. It is not as common a dermatosis as psoriasis, but it does account for 1% of all new cases seen in a skin clinic, compared with 5% for psoriasis.

The term 'lichen planus' means a flat-topped papule, and this is the most common form of presentation of the disorder. Lichen planus affects mainly young and middle-aged adults, and men and women are equally affected.

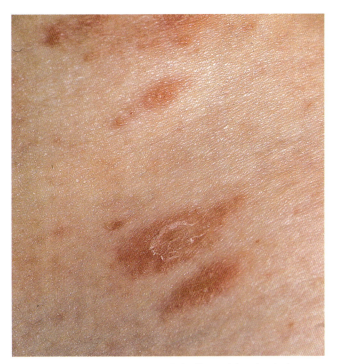

Figure 9.3 Lesions are characteristically oval in pityriasis rosea. Centripetal scaling can be seen on some of the lesions

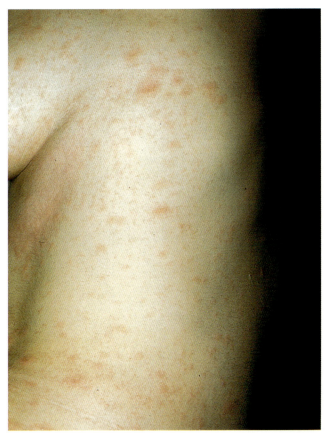

Figure 9.4 Oval lesions with their long axes along the lines of cleavage of the skin in pityriasis rosea

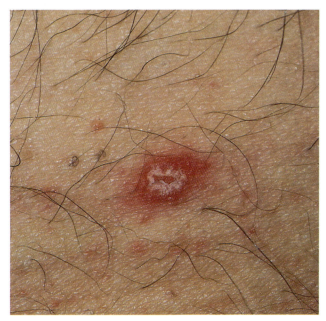

Figure 9.5 Centripetal scaling in pityriasis rosea

Morphology and distribution

The appearances of the lesions vary with the site of involvement. The most common and typical lesion is the flat-topped papule, which often has a shiny surface (Figures 9.6 and 9.7). The lesions are usually small, approximately 5 mm in diameter. They are either red or violaceous in color (Figures 9.6–9.8), and occasionally white steaks (Wickham's striae) can be seen on the surface of the lesions (Figure 9.9). There may be a slight central umbilication of the lesion (Figure 9.7). The papules may affect any part of the skin, but the most common site is the wrists (Figure 9.6). The severity of the disease may vary from the presence of a few scattered papules to the whole skin being covered with numerous papules (Figures 9.8 and 9.10).

Occasionally, the lesions fuse to form plaques with a similar violaceous color, and white streaks may be discernible. Lichen planus, like psoriasis, shows the Koebner phenomenon, i.e. the lesions will appear in a linear pattern along a scratch or any trauma to the skin (Figure 9.11).

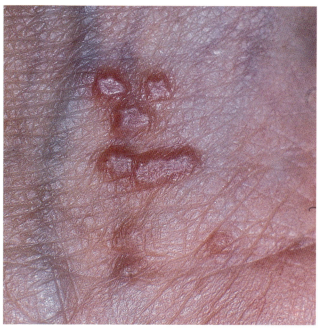

Figure 9.7 Flat-topped papules in lichen planus

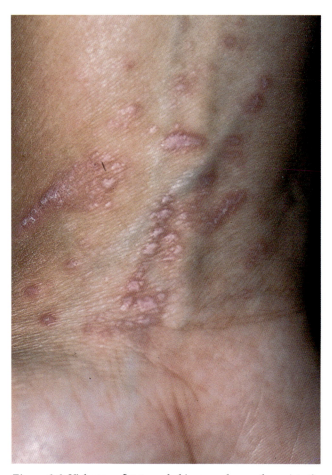

Figure 9.6 Violaceous flat-topped shiny papules on the wrist, the most common site for lichen planus

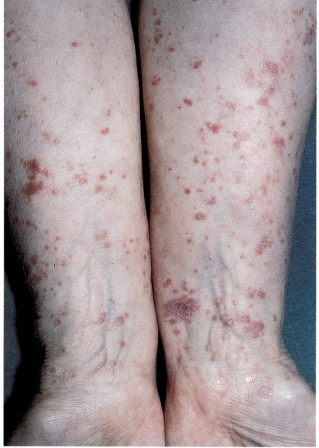

Figure 9.8 Numerous papules of lichen planus on the arms

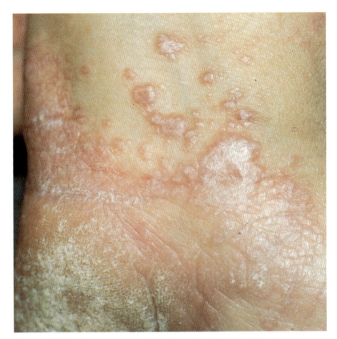

Figure 9.9 Lesions on the wrists showing Wickham's striae

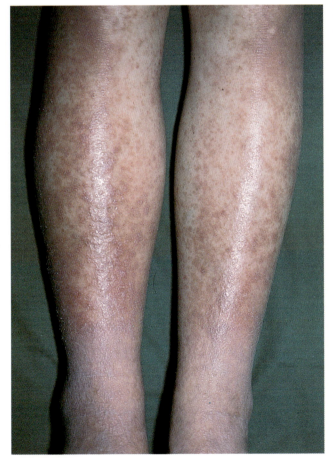

Figure 9.10 Red papules and plaques in extensive lichen planus

Lichen planus on the legs and occasionally on the arms may take the form of what is termed 'hypertrophic lichen planus' (Figure 9.12). In this instance, the lesions are plaque-like and have a thick warty (hyperkeratotic) surface. This type of lichen planus may be difficult to distinguish from patches of chronic eczema if there are no classical lesions of lichen planus at other sites. In very acute cases of lichen planus, the lesions may form blisters.

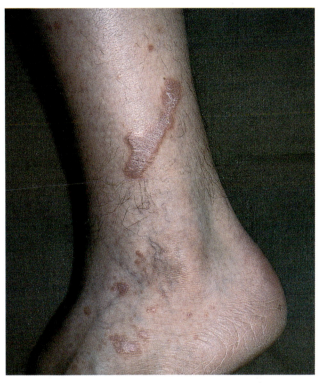

Figure 9.11 Linear lesion of lichen planus at the site of trauma (Koebner phenomenon)

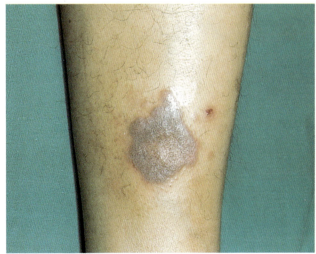

Figure 9.12 Hypertrophic lichen planus on the leg

Lichen planus is associated with increased pigmentation (Figure 9.13) and, when the lesions clear, there is often residual hyperpigmentation for many weeks or months. In blacks, lichen planus presents as hyperpigmented papules.

Scalp
This is not a common site of involvement, but the important fact is that, on the scalp, lichen planus may

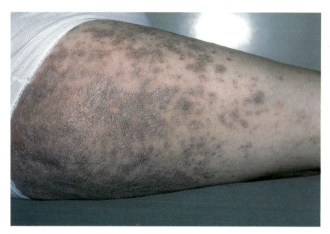

Figure 9.13 *Hyperpigmentation seen with resolving lichen planus*

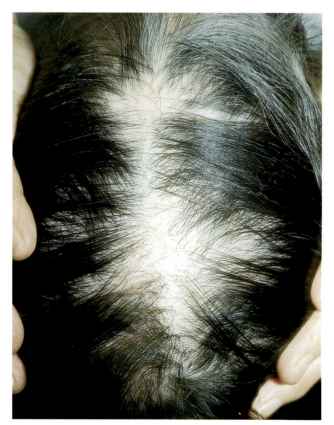

Figure 9.14 *Patchy hair loss after lichen planus of scalp*

produce atrophy of the skin with subsequent loss of hair (Figure 9.14). The hair loss tends to be patchy, but is permanent.

Nails
The disease process can also affect the nail matrix. Usually the involvement of the nails is minimal and presents as longitudinal ridging which eventually clears. Occasionally, there is severe involvement of the nails with pterygium formation (the cuticle grows forward and attaches itself to the nail plate), and there may be permanent loss of the nail plate (Figure 9.15).

Palms and soles
Because of the thick keratin at these sites, the appearances of the disorder are modified. Although the lesions may present as small papules, they do not have the flat-topped appearance with white streaks but often

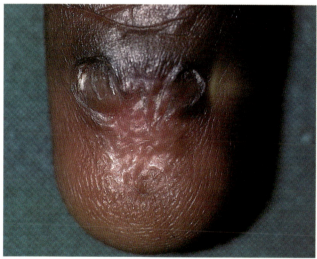

Figure 9.15 *Lichen planus showing loss of the nail plate and pterygium formation*

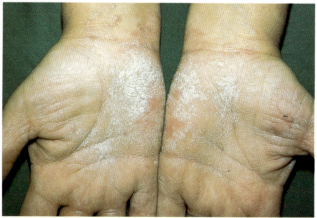

Figure 9.16 *Hyperkeratotic scaly plaques on the palms in lichen planus*

present as hyperkeratotic brownish papules. If the lesions merge together, hyperkeratotic plaques (Figure 9.16) are formed which become fissured, and the appearances are then similar to psoriasis at this site or chronic eczema.

Mucous membranes and genitalia

The buccal mucosa is the most common site of involvement (present in about 50% of cases). In the early stages, there are small white papules which subsequently fuse to form a white lacy pattern (Figure 9.17). It is important to remember to examine the buccal mucosa when lichen planus is suspected from lesions on the skin; if it is involved, it will establish the diagnosis. The lips, gums and tongue may also be similarly affected, as may be the vulval and vaginal mucosa. On the glans penis, the white streaks often join to form annular lesions (Figure 9.18). Occasionally, only the oral cavity and genitalia are

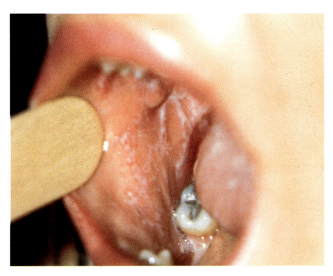

Figure 9.17 White linear lesions on the buccal mucosa in lichen planus

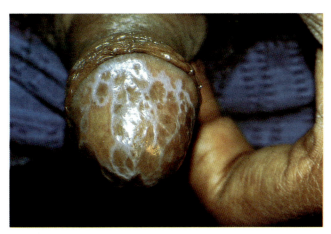

Figure 9.18 Annular white lesions on the penis in lichen planus

involved. There are reports of lichen planus of the mucosal surfaces progressing to leukoplakia and even carcinoma, but this is a very rare complication. The vast majority of the lesions at these sites will undergo spontaneous resolution.

Erosive lichen planus

Occasionally the lesions on the mucosal surfaces, particularly the gums and tongue, may present as erosions rather than the white plaque-like lesions.

Duration and recurrence

If untreated, lichen planus will usually last for several months and then tend to disappear. The hypertrophic forms of the disorder tend to be persistent and may last for many years. Similarly, erosive lichen planus of the mouth and genitalia tends to be persistent. Approximately 20% of patients will have a relapse of the condition after a first episode.

Etiology

The cause of lichen planus is unknown and, although a viral or other infective agent has been considered, these hypotheses have not been confirmed. A number of drugs, notably mepacrine, chloroquine, gold and para-aminosalicylic acid, may induce an eruption which clinically may be indistinguishable from lichen planus.

Treatment

If the condition consists of only a few lesions, no treatment may be required. However, the lesions are frequently associated with irritation and this in itself leads to the patient seeking help.

Intermediate-strength (Group II or III) topical steroids are helpful in alleviating irritation and may partially clear some lesions. Group IV steroids are more effective in clearing lesions, but should only be used for short periods, i.e. 2–3 weeks. If the disease is widespread and causing irritation, systemic steroids or PUVA will probably clear the rash.

If systemic steroids are used, the initial dose should be 30 mg prednisone daily for 2 weeks. The drug should then be tailed off over the next 2 weeks. If the disease process is active, there will be a recurrence when the systemic steroids or PUVA are stopped; in practice, this affects around 25% of patients with lichen planus.

Maintenance treatment with PUVA or steroids may be required, but is probably only justified in a small proportion of patients.

Cyclosporine (*see* Chapter 25) is also highly effective in clearing lichen planus, and may be considered an alternative to PUVA and systemic steroids in widespread or severe disease with mucous membrane involvement.

The lesions on the mucous membranes of the mouth usually require no treatment if confined to the buccal mucosae. However, if severe, they may respond to topical steroids. The current most effective way of using steroids in the oral cavity is to spray the affected areas with a steroid inhaler such as used for asthma.

In severe erosive lichen planus, systemic steroids or cyclosporine may be necessary to control the disease. Involvement of the mucous membranes of the genitalia should be treated with Group II or III topical steroids.

The hypertrophic form of lichen planus on the limbs responds well to intralesional triamcinolone injections.

10

Fungal infections

Disorders of the skin, hair and nails caused by fungus are still common in dermatological practice, and the importance of establishing the correct diagnosis has become greater for two reasons.

First, with the development of more effective anti-fungal preparations, it is now possible to successfully treat fungal infections of the skin, hair and nails.

Second, the powerful topical corticosteroids are used to treat many fungal infections because the disease has been incorrectly diagnosed or just considered to be another 'rash' which will clear with this modern panacea. Unless this is realized, these disorders, which are easily treatable, become unnecessarily chronic and troublesome complaints.

There are many thousands of species of fungi but, like bacteria, only a minority are pathogenic to humans. These may be arbitrarily divided into those affecting the skin and those capable of deep invasion and causing systemic disease.

A few species such as *Candida albicans*, may affect the skin and also cause systemic disease. The fungi causing skin disease generally live in keratin and do not affect the deeper and viable parts of the skin. However, possibly when the immune mechanisms of the host are upset, fungi will invade the dermis, albeit rarely, thereby resulting in the production of abscesses or granulomatous nodules.

RINGWORM

This is a lay term for fungal infections which has arisen because a number of fungal infections of the skin begin as small inflammatory lesions but subsequently spread out to form annular or ring lesions. The disorders the fungus cause are referred to as *tinea* (a Latin word meaning 'gnawing worm'), usually with a qualifying noun according to the part of the body affected, e.g.

tinea capitis. The fungus actually lives in the keratin, producing enzymes which break up keratin, giving rise to a clinical lesion affecting the skin, hair or nails.

There are three genera of ringworm fungi – *Trichophyton*, *Microsporum* and *Epidermophyton* – and all are referred to as dermatophytes. A few of these species produce characteristic lesions at certain sites of the body but often the clinical manifestations of the different species are similar, and require culture for specific mycological diagnosis.

Some species of fungi are pathogenic only to humans while others are pathogenic to animals and humans. The species which affect only humans produce persistent non-inflammatory lesions whereas ringworm contracted from animals tends to be inflammatory and short-lived.

Ringworm infections are not as contagious as is generally believed by the general public. It seems that many individuals, although repeatedly exposed to ringworm fungi – such as in a family where one member is affected – have keratin with properties which do not permit the fungus to grow and produce clinical lesions.

Diagnosis

Examining scrapings of the skin or specimens of nail and hair in 10% potassium hydroxide is an easy and simple way of establishing the diagnosis. The potassium hydroxide dissolves the keratin and the fungi are then easily seen by microscopy (Figure 10.1).

An alternative or additional method is to culture the infected keratin in Sabouraud's medium. This is necessary to establish the species, but it takes 2–3 weeks for the fungus to grow and, with the advent of griseofulvin and terbinafine, which are active against the majority of superficial ringworm species, culturing will not usually be required in the clinical management of the disorder.

Management

Many new antifungal drugs have been developed over the last few years and have improved the treatment of fungal infection of the skin and nails. These antifungal drugs may be classified into the following groups:

Azoles

These comprise two groups: the imidazoles and the triazoles.

The imidazoles include miconazole nitrate and clotrimazole, which are only used topically as they are not absorbed from the gastrointestinal tract. The imidazoles have a broad spectrum of antifungal activity and are effective against ringworm fungi (dermatophytes), *Candida* organisms and *Pityrosporum* yeasts (one of which causes pityriasis versicolor). The imidazole ketoconazole is absorbed from the gastrointestinal tract and is effective against a similar range of organisms, but its use is not recommended as it may cause severe liver damage.

The triazoles include the two orally active preparations itraconazole and fluconazole. Itraconazole is effective against ringworm fungi and *Pityrosporum orbiculare* (the fungus which causes pityriasis versicolor). Fluconazole is effective against ringworm fungi and *C. albicans*.

Allylamines

The drug which has gained wide acceptance in this group is terbinafine. It may be used orally or topically. When used orally, it appears to be effective only against the ringworm fungi but, used topically, it is also effective against *P. orbiculare*.

Polyenes

These are an older group of antifungals. The two main polyenes in clinical use are nystatin and amphotericin B.

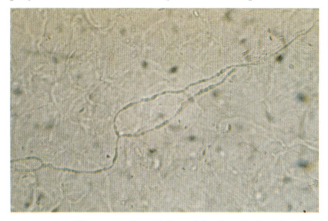

Figure 10.1 *Demonstration of fungal hyphae in keratin. Skin scrapings have been soaked in 10% potassium hydroxide for 20 min and the hyphae are now easily seen on microscopy*

They are not effective against dermatophytes, but are active against superficial *Candida* infections.

Morpholines

This is a relatively new group of antifungal preparations. The only member of this group used in clinical practice is amorolfine. This is effective against dermatophytes and *Candida* infections. It is available only as a topical preparation.

Miscellaneous

Griseofulvin was for many years the only oral preparation for treating dermatophyte infections of the skin, hair and nails. It is an effective drug except for toenail infections, where it has been replaced by terbinafine and the triazoles. Whitfield's ointment (6% benzoic acid and 3% salicylic acid) is the oldest topical preparation against dermatophyte and *P. orbiculare* infections. It is just as effective as the newer preparations, but not as pleasant to use.

Choice of antifungal preparation
Oral treatment

This will depend to a certain extent on which site is to be treated. If it is an extensive skin infection, then the choice is among griseofulvin, terbinafine, itraconazole and fluconazole. Griseofulvin has to be taken for 4 weeks, itraconazole and fluconazole for 1–4 weeks, and terbinafine for 2–4 weeks (depending on the site of infection). Griseofulvin is considerably more economical than terbinafine or itraconazole.

Infections of the hair respond well to griseofulvin and this is probably still the drug of choice. Fingernail infections respond well to griseofulvin (taken daily for 6 months), terbinafine (taken daily for 6 weeks), and itraconazole and fluconazole (taken weekly for 9 months). Toenail infections do not respond well to griseofulvin, but there are high cure rates with terbinafine (taken daily for 3 months), and itraconazole and fluconazole (taken weekly for 9 months).

Topical treatment

The response to topical preparations appears to be similar. The well-established preparations are Whitfield's ointment, miconazole nitrate and clotrimazole. The new preparations terbinafine and amorolfine will have to show a higher cure rate if they are to gain widespread acceptance.

Ringworm of the feet (tinea pedis)

The feet are the most common site for fungal infections. This is probably due to the fact that fungus grows better in moist rather than dry areas, and the close fit of the toes and footwear fashions are both contributory factors in encouraging the growth of fungus.

Fungal infection of the feet tends to be a disease of young and middle-aged adults, and is more common in males than females. It is rare in children. The exact mode of transmission is not certain and, although swimming pools, showers, etc. are implicated as the usual source, host susceptibility is clearly an important factor as familial cross-infections are rarely seen.

Clinical presentation

In the majority of patients, tinea pedis is manifested by peeling and slight maceration of the skin between the toes (Figure 10.2). The peeling usually extends to the plantar surface of the toes, and this clinical point is useful in distinguishing tinea pedis from eczema or psoriasis between the toes (Figure 10.3). The peeling and scaling may involve any of the interdigital spaces, although it is rarely seen between the first and second toes. The disorder is frequently confined to the interdigital spaces and gives rise to only slight irritation. However, the disease may become more extensive and involve the sole. If the infecting fungus is *Trichophyton rubrum*, the disease is manifested as diffuse scaling and hyperkeratosis. If the organism is *T. mentagrophytes*, then the disorder may be represented by blisters and acute exudative dermatitis (Figure 10.4) either on the soles or extending from the interdigital spaces to the dorsum of the foot.

Differential diagnosis

It is important that not all scaly skin between and around the toes is attributed to fungus, as other conditions can also cause this appearance and the treatment will be different. Simple maceration of the skin due to excess sweating is probably the most common differential diagnosis, but psoriasis and eczema may also affect only the distal half of the foot.

Treatment

In mild tinea pedis between the toes, topical antifungal preparations should be used. If there is no improvement and maceration is present, then an astringent lotion such as magenta paint BP used daily for a few days is helpful.

If the infection extends to the sole and/or dorsum of the foot, topical preparations may be used for 2–3 weeks to see if there is significant clearance; however, a course of an oral antifungal agent (*see above*) is frequently necessary. Tinea pedis has a high rate of recurrence even after courses of oral treatment.

Acute inflammatory fungal infections of the feet

In the early stages, these should be treated like an eczema. Potassium permanganate soaks 1:8000 four times daily for 10 min on each occasion and clean linen dressings should be used. One per cent hydrocortisone lotion may help to settle the inflammation. As it settles,

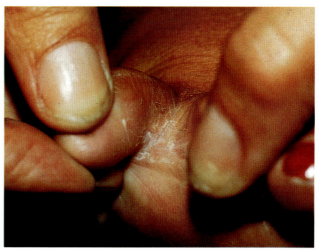

Figure 10.2 Scaling and erythema between the toes, the most common site for fungal infections

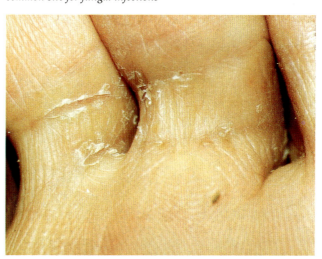

Figure 10.3 Scaling extending from between the toes to the plantar surface in a fungal infection. This helps to distinguish it from psoriasis and eczema

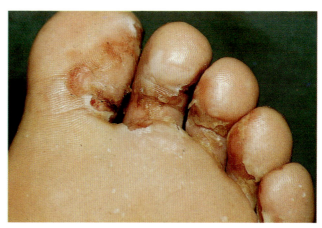

Figure 10.4 An acute exudative eruption which may be seen in fungal infection

the irritation may be relieved by 1% hydrocortisone cream. The condition may subside with these simple measures. In addition to the above treatment, a course of an oral antifungal drug should be given.

Ringworm of the hands

This is very much rarer than that of the feet. It is usually caused by *T. rubrum* and presents as a slight erythema and diffuse scaling of the palmar surface of the hands (Figure 10.5). The diagnosis should be established by demonstrating the fungus, and treatment is with an oral antifungal drug.

Ringworm of the groins (tinea cruris)

This is the second most common site to be involved after the feet. It is more commonly seen in males than in females. The infection usually begins in the crural fold as erythema and slight maceration. It spreads out in an annular pattern with a raised red scaly margin (Figure 10.6). It may spread down the thigh or sometimes backwards up to the buttock. The disorder in the early stages has to be distinguished from intertrigo (seborrheic eczema) and intertriginous psoriasis.

Treatment
In mild infection confined to the groin, a topical antifungal preparation may be effective in clearing the eruption. If there is extensive spread down the medial thighs or posteriorly to the buttocks, oral treatment is indicated. If there is acute inflammation, which sometimes occurs with fungal infection in the groins in warm climates, then sitz baths with potassium permanganate 1:8000 or the daily application of magenta paint BP will be helpful.

As with fungal infection of the feet, there is a high relapse rate of infection in the groins. Tight clothing should be avoided.

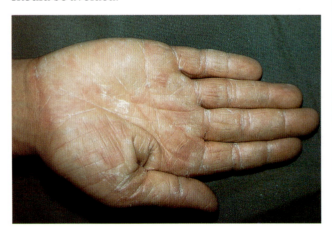

Figure 10.5 *Diffuse scaling on the palm due to a fungal infection*

Ringworm of the body (tinea corporis)

Annular lesions
This is the characteristic type of lesion which even lay people are familiar with as being due to a fungus. The lesion usually begins as a small red papule which then advances to form a ring (Figure 10.7). Occasionally, however, there is no clearing in the center and an oval or discoid red scaly plaque is the presenting feature. Topical preparations may be tried if the lesion is solitary; otherwise, oral medication should be used.

Tinea granuloma
This may take one of two forms. It can be a discrete infiltrating granuloma of the skin, which should be distinguished from other skin granulomata. This type of lesion is usually caused by a fungus from an animal source. Although the lesions are usually self-involuting,

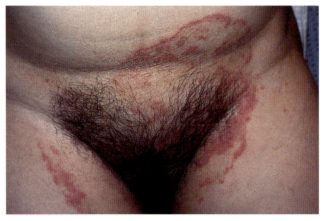

Figure 10.6 *Fungal infection in the groins extending to the medial thighs and abdomen*

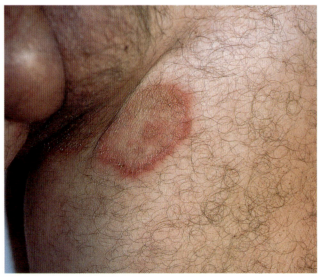

Figure 10.7 *A typical annular lesion of ringworm*

griseofulvin 500 mg daily should be given for 4–6 weeks.

The other type of granuloma is found on the hairy parts of the limbs as it is an infection around the hair follicles; often, small papules (Figure 10.8) and pustules are present. The diagnosis is frequently missed. It should be thought of if there is a chronic unilateral inflammatory process on an arm or leg. The disorder responds well to oral antifungal treatment.

Ringworm of the scalp (tinea capitis)

Tinea capitis is due to fungus affecting the hair (which is a form of keratin) and the keratin of the scalp. Fungal infections of the scalp due to organisms which cause fluorescence of the hairs when viewed by ultraviolet irradiation, 330–360 nm (Wood's light), are confined

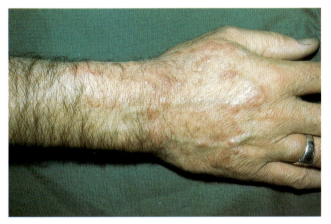

Figure 10.8 *Granulomatous fungal infection on the back of the hand and arm*

almost entirely to children. Non-fluorescent ringworm of the scalp occurs both in children and adults. The fungi which produce such fluorescence are *Microsporum audouinii* and *M. canis,* the latter derived from animals, usually cats. The most common organism to cause ringworm of the scalp is *M. audouinii.* The condition is contagious and minor epidemics may often be found in schools.

Clinical features

The disease usually presents as a small oval or discoid patch on any part of the scalp. The predominant feature is loss of hair (Figure 10.9). If the lesion is carefully examined, it will be seen that the hairs are broken off near to the skin surface and there is incomplete or non-uniform loss of hair. The skin is usually scaly and nearly always affected in addition to the hair keratin (Figure 10.9). These two features of a scaly base and broken hairs of varying lengths rather than complete loss of hair are important physical signs in distinguishing the condition from alopecia areata (although occasionally in the latter, there may not be complete baldness but a diffuse loss). Involvement of the scalp with fungus may occur as a solitary lesion or multiple lesions with sometimes nearly the whole of the scalp involved. In addition to the scalp lesions, there are often scaly discoid patches on the neck just below the hairline.

As the infection with the fungus persists, signs of inflammation will appear. In addition to the skin being scaly, erythema and pustules develop (Figure 10.10). If there is progression of the inflammation, then the whole of the area shows signs of an acute inflammatory process with swelling, redness of the tissues, pustule formation and, occasionally, superficial ulceration. This type of lesion is known as a kerion (Figure 10.11). It is

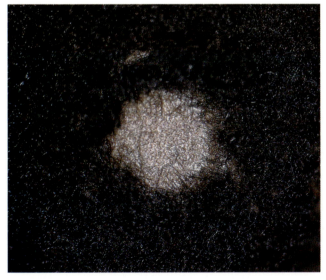

Figure 10.9 *A bald scaly patch due to fungal infection of the scalp. The scaling should distinguish the condition from alopecia areata*

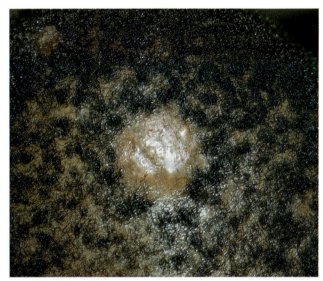

Figure 10.10 *Inflammatory changes, erythema and pustules which may be seen in fungal infections*

thought to be due to the tissues developing an inflammatory immune response to the fungi and, therefore, is ultimately self-healing. Despite the rather alarming appearance, it will eventually subside without specific treatment, and does not usually lead to scarring and permanent hair loss. Tinea capitis due to the fungus contracted from animals (*M. canis*) tends to produce an inflammatory response more frequently than that caused by *M. audouinii*.

The fungi which may affect the hair and scalp keratin but do not cause fluorescence of the hairs under ultraviolet irradiation do not always produce the same classical clinical appearances as those caused by *M. audouinii* and *M. canis*. Usually the only constant sign is the hairs breaking off at the scalp surface, producing an area with the appearance of black dots. This type of lesion has to be distinguished from the hair being broken due to trauma (trichotillomania) in which the hairs are not usually broken so close to the surface of the scalp. If there are associated inflammatory changes, the condition has to be distinguished from excoriated seborrheic eczema or psoriasis.

Diagnosis

The diagnosis of tinea capitis depends on the demonstration of the fungus. In the disorder due to *M. audouinii* or *M. canis*, this can be done simply by Wood's light examination, when the affected hairs will show a green fluorescence. Ideally, specimens of the hair and scale from the scalp surface should also be taken for microscopic examination and cultured to confirm the diagnosis. In cases of non-fluorescent tinea capitis, the diagnosis has to be made by microscopy of the hair and scales, and subsequent culture.

If a child of school age has tinea capitis, it is the usual practice to screen other children with whom the child comes into contact at school. Since the majority of cases are due to fungi which cause the hairs to fluoresce, screening can be done by Wood's light examination. Other methods that are not employed but reported to give a higher incidence of positive identification include brushing the hair thoroughly and then putting the brush under a Wood's light, or placing the brush in a plate of culture medium to ascertain whether there is subsequent growth of the fungus.

All children who have tinea capitis will have to be kept away from school until they are clear of fungus, as judged by the clinical appearance and Wood's light examination (if positive initially).

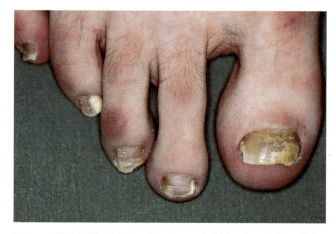

Figure 10.12 *Yellowish discoloration and thickening of the nail due to a fungal infection. The infection tends to start at the side of the nail*

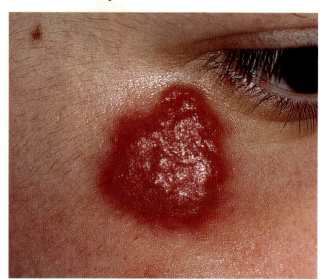

Figure 10.11 *A kerion. An infiltrated swelling with pustules due to a fungal infection. The head is the most common site for this type of response to a fungal infection*

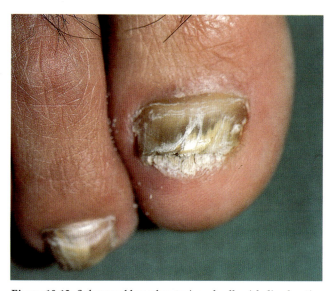

Figure 10.13 *Subungual hyperkeratosis and yellowish discoloration due to a fungal infection*

Treatment

Treatment of tinea capitis is with oral antifungal preparations. Griseofulvin is highly effective in clearing the infection but should be given for at least 6 weeks. As most of the infections occur in young children, a suspension of griseofulvin should be prescribed. The other oral antifungal preparations – terbinafine, itraconazole and fluconazole – are also likely to be effective, but experience with these preparations in children is still limited.

Ringworm of the nails (tinea unguium)

Both the toenails and fingernails can be involved, although the toenails are more commonly affected. The disorder may be caused by species of *Trichophyton* and *Epidermophyton* but not *Microsporum*.

Clinical features

Ringworm fungi usually begin to invade the nail by first affecting the lateral nail grooves, where there is soft keratin. The infection then spreads into the lateral portions of the nail plate, and usually causes a yellowish discoloration (Figure 10.12). Infection then usually spreads to involve the nail bed and may cause considerable hyperkeratosis (Figure 10.13). The process may stop at any stage or may continue to involve eventually the whole of the nail bed and nail plate, although the nail matrix is not affected. Apart from the subungual hyperkeratosis, involvement of the nail plate may produce considerable distortion of this structure (Figure 10.14).

Ringworm of the nails usually involves only one or two nails initially, and this may be confined to one hand or foot. The involvement of the nails in a hand or foot is often variable (Figure 10.15), unlike psoriasis in which the dystrophy tends to be uniform. Subsequently, other nails may become involved until all the nails of both feet or hands are affected. Why the nails are affected by fungi in some persons who have skin involvement (particularly feet) but not in others is unknown. Many persons have ringworm infection between the toes for many years and never have involvement of the nails.

Diagnosis

Since any treatment undertaken will be continued for a considerable length of time, it is important to establish the correct diagnosis before commencing therapy. Specimens of the affected nail plate and the hyperkeratotic material from the nail bed should be examined by microscopy and cultured for fungus.

The most common differential diagnosis of a fungal infection of the nails is probably psoriasis, particularly when the latter presents as subungual hyperkeratosis. Dystrophy of the nails caused by *C. albicans* is often diagnosed prior to hospital attendance as a ringworm infection. The important distinguishing feature is that, with a candidal infection, there is a chronic paronychia whereas, with ringworm fungus, the nail fold usually has a normal appearance. Both eczema and lichen planus may cause nail dystrophies by involvement of the nail matrix in the disease process. It is important to realize that diseases other than ringworm can cause dystrophies which, on clinical grounds, may sometimes be difficult to diagnose. Thus, before embarking on treatment for ringworm of the nails, it is important that the diagnosis has been established by demonstrating the presence of the fungus.

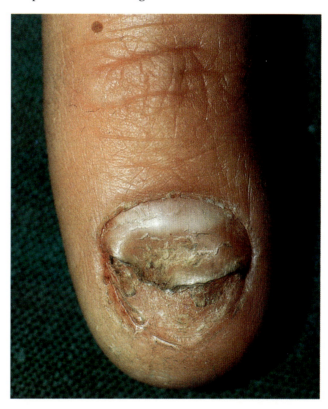

Figure 10.14 *Deformity of a fingernail due to a fungal infection*

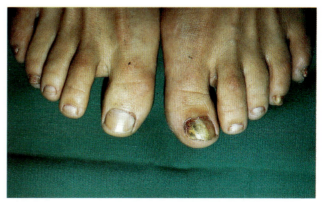

Figure 10.15 *Asymmetrical involvement of the nails due to a fungal infection*

Treatment

Fingernails

Treatment is highly effective with oral preparations. Griseofulvin 500 mg daily has to be taken for 6 months, as this is the time taken by the nail to grow and become impregnated with the drug. However, terbinafine 250 mg daily only has to be taken for 6 weeks as it is absorbed from the nail bed into the nail plate. Regimens with weekly doses of itraconazole and fluconazole have been reported to be successful when taken for up to 9 months. However, further studies are probably necessary before these drugs are advocated for routine use in the treatment of fingernail infections.

Toenails

Terbinafine 250 mg daily is a highly effective treatment with an approximately 80% success rate. It should be stressed that at the end of the 3 months, the nails may still appear dystrophic but, as the fungus should have been killed after this time, the nails should grow normally. This may take up to a year as this is the approximate time taken by toenails to be replaced.

Griseofulvin has a poor success rate in clearing toenail infections and therefore should not be used. As with fingernails, itraconazole and fluconazole have been reported to clear toenail infection with weekly doses for up to 9 months. The exact regimen for these drugs is still to be determined.

Topical treatment

In the past, topical antifungal preparations have not proved effective in clearing toenail infections due to lack of penetration. Recently, two topical preparations have become available for which success has been claimed. The first is the imidazole tioconazole, which is made up in a solution and applied twice daily for 6–12 months. The success rate, however, is relatively low at no higher than 20%. Amorolfine used in a lacquer and applied once a week, for 6 months for fingernails and 12 months for toenails, has produced cure rates approaching 40%.

TINEA VERSICOLOR

This condition is also known as pityriasis versicolor. The term 'versicolor' means change of color and is an apt description of the disorder. Tinea versicolor is caused by the fungus *P. orbiculare*, which affects only the stratum corneum.

Clinical features

The typical lesion is a fawn-colored macular patch of varying shape and size (Figure 10.16) but, often, patches may coalesce to form confluent areas on the upper trunk. The surface is sometimes scaly and scale can easily be produced from a lesion by gentle scraping with a scalpel. If the patient is exposed to sunlight, then the areas of the skin affected by the fungus do *not* pigment, but appear as white patches against a tanned skin (Figure 10.17). This is frequently the presenting manifestation after the patient has been on holiday.

The most common site to be affected is the upper trunk, although the neck and upper arms may also be involved.

Diagnosis

The diagnosis is easily made on clinical grounds alone, but can be confirmed by examining skin scrapings by microscopy after dissolving the keratin with 10% potassium hydroxide. The microscopic appearance is diagnostic. The hyphae are short, and numerous clusters of spores are seen.

Treatment

Topical preparations are effective in clearing pityriasis versicolor. However, because large areas of the trunk have to be treated, lotions are preferred by some rather

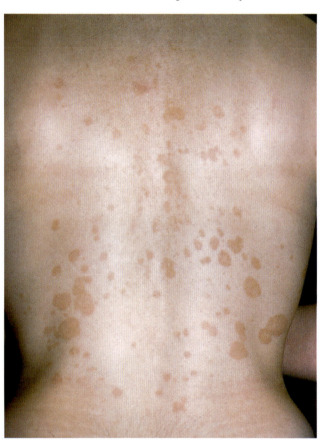

Figure 10.16 *Pale brown, slightly scaly, patches on the trunk in pityriasis versicolor*

than creams and ointments. The standard preparations are 2.5% selenium sulfide in a detergent base (Selsun shampoo) and 25% aqueous sodium thiosulfate. The preparations have to be left on overnight and are not particularly pleasant to use. The duration of treatment is usually over a period of 1–2 weeks, but cures have been reported with single applications.

Topical cream preparations of clotrimazole, miconazole nitrate and terbinafine are effective in clearing pityriasis versicolor. However, as these preparations should be applied to all skin of the infected area and not only to the clinically apparent lesions, large quantities of cream are usually required. Treatment should be continued for at least 2 weeks on a daily basis, and better results are obtained if the preparations are used for 4 weeks. Thus, large quantities of cream, possibly up to 200 g, may be required for a course of treatment. Whitfield's ointment (diluted to half-strength) is also effective and considerably cheaper than the azole and allylamine preparations, but is not pleasant to use.

The only oral preparation currently recommended for pityriasis versicolor is itraconazole (griseofulvin and terbinafine are not effective, and ketoconazole is not advised because of its potential hepatotoxicity). The dose is 200 mg daily for a week, and the success rate is approximately 80%. Itraconazole should be used when the disease is very extensive or when there has been failure to clear the fungus with topical preparations.

Whatever treatment is recommended, patients with hypopigmented areas should be warned that it may be months before the skin returns to its normal color and that failure to repigment at the end of treatment does not indicate failure of treatment. Whatever treatment is employed, there is a high recurrence rate in pityriasis versicolor.

ERYTHRASMA

This is usually considered together with fungal diseases, although the causative organism has now been shown to be a bacterium, *Corynebacterium minutissimum*.

Clinical features

The areas affected are intertriginous, namely, the groins, axillae, between the toes, and under the breasts. The

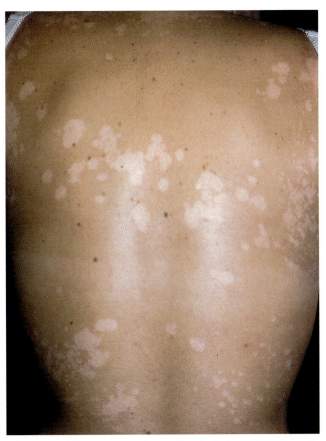

Figure 10.17 *Hypopigmented areas in pityriasis versicolor usually seen after exposure to sunlight. The normal skin tans, but not the areas affected by the fungus*

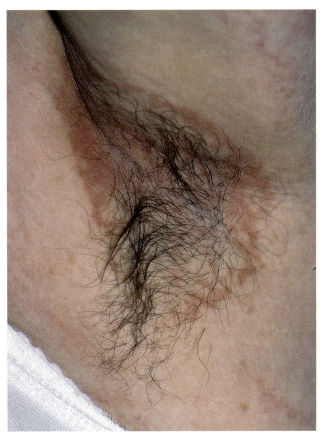

Figure 10.18 *Reddish-brown discoloration in the axilla due to erythrasma*

lesions are confluent, reddish-brown, scaly patches (Figure 10.18). There is no associated inflammation, which tends to distinguish the condition from seborrheic eczema. Under Wood's light, there is a pink fluorescence which helps in establishing the diagnosis. There have been reports that erythrasma may be responsible for persistent pruritus ani, and if this is appreciated and the condition correctly treated, this very distressing symptom may be cured.

Treatment

The topical azole preparations miconazole and clotrimazole are effective in clearing erythrasma, as is the topical antibiotic sodium fusidate. Erythromycin is the most effective oral preparation.

CANDIDOSIS

Candida albicans is a yeast-like parasite which differs from a true yeast in that it forms a pseudomycelium and does not reproduce by budding. This microorganism most commonly affects the skin and mucous membranes, but it can also cause systemic diseases such as gastroenteritis, endocarditis, septicemia and meningitis. It is important, however, to remember that it is most commonly present on the skin and mucous membranes and in the gastrointestinal tract without giving rise to pathological changes at these sites. In addition, isolation of the organism from diseased skin may not mean that *Candida* is the cause of the disorder, but may be merely coincidental. *Candida*, however, will seed itself in preexisting pathological conditions and, under these circumstances, is a secondary invader and may give rise to further pathological changes. The exact circumstances under which it becomes virulent and gives rise to disease are not known, but there is often an underlying condition, either local or systemic.

Cases of candidosis as seen by the dermatologist may be divided into those affecting the skin and those affecting the mucous membranes or mucocutaneous regions.

Like ringworm fungi, candidosis is frequently found in moist areas of the skin. In most instances, however, there is usually a predisposing cause for the infection.

Intertrigo

Candida intertrigo usually affects the groins, and submammary, perianal and perivulval skin. It presents as erythematous macerated skin in these areas and can be distinguished from simple seborrheic eczema because there are satellite lesions (Figures 10.19 and 10.20). The skin involvement may spread to the buttocks

or down the thighs (Figure 10.20). In candidal intertrigo at these sites, particularly in females, it is most important to test the urine for sugar as candidal vulvitis is one of the common presenting features of diabetes mellitus.

A fairly common site of infection of the skin by *Candida* is the space between two fingers, but not usually on the feet, as with ringworm. The condition presents as erythema, peeling and maceration of the skin on the sides of the two adjacent fingers. It can be distinguished from eczema of the hands since the lesion is frequently solitary and unilateral.

Treatment
Ideally, the diagnosis should be established by demonstrating the organism either by microscopy or culture. If there is any underlying cause for the skin involvement, such as diabetes, it must be treated, as otherwise local treatment will not be successful. Topical preparations are usually effective in clearing *C. albicans* infections of the skin. Nystatin is well established as an effective topical drug, but miconazole and clotrimazole are also

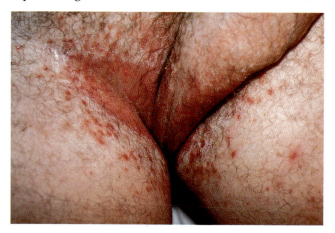

Figure 10.19 *Candidal intertrigo in the groins, characterized by satellite lesions*

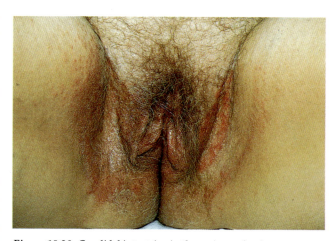

Figure 10.20 *Candidal intertrigo in the groins and vulva, a common site*

effective. There are proprietary preparations of nystatin and miconazole which, when combined with a Group I topical steroid, are often able to counteract the inflammation that is usually present. As in other types of intertrigo, the areas affected should be kept as dry as possible. Daily painting with magenta paint BP is often helpful as, in addition to its astringent properties, it has weak antibacterial and antifungal activity.

Oral preparations against *Candida* infections include fluconazole and itraconazole. However, topical preparations are usually effective in clearing candidal skin infections.

Candidal paronychia

This disorder, sometimes referred to as 'barmaids' disease', occurs predominantly in people who have their hands in and out of water throughout the day, and it is therefore much more common in women than in men. The underlying cause is thought to be damage and breaks in the cuticle due to a chapping effect. The organisms then gain entry into the posterior nail fold.

The paronychia may be subacute initially, with pain, swelling and redness of the posterior nail fold from which a small quantity of pus may exude. Later, the paronychia tends to become chronic with swelling and slight redness of the posterior nail fold and loss of the cuticle (Figure 10.21), but the condition is not painful. If it persists, as it usually does, there will be secondary dystrophy of the nail plate.

The nail dystrophy usually appears first at the lateral margins of the nail plate with brownish-green discoloration (Figure 10.21). Subsequently, the whole of the nail plate may be involved. Initially, only one or two fingers will be affected, but others will become involved if preventive measures are not taken.

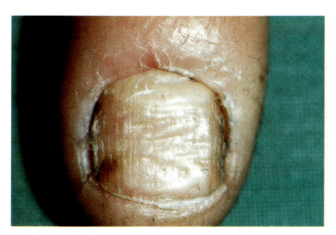

Figure 10.21 *Candidal paronychia. There is swelling of the posterior nail fold and loss of the cuticle*

Treatment

The most important measure is to keep the hands as dry as possible to prevent growth of the organism and allow healing of the nail fold. Patients must be instructed to wear cotton gloves within rubber gloves for all household duties and for their work if it involves having their hands in water. Topical measures are helpful but not curative if the fingers are continuously immersed in water.

Nystatin cream should be applied to the nail fold twice daily, but patients should be instructed not to push the cream under the nail fold as, otherwise, further damage to the reforming cuticle will occur. Painting with antifungal lotions is sometimes helpful and may be preferable to using creams.

Occasionally, bacteria are also present in chronic paronychia of the fingers and, if the organism can be isolated, a short course of the appropriate antibiotic applied topically or even given systemically may be helpful. The role of oral preparations in candidal paronychia is debatable. Itraconazole and fluconazole are effective in eradicating candidal organisms but, if the hands are continually wet and the cuticle fails to heal, reinfection will occur as soon as the oral preparations are stopped.

Oral mucocutaneous candidosis

Candidosis of the mouth is often referred to as thrush. The characteristic appearance is of creamy-white patches on the mucous membranes of the mouth. The patches are easily removed to reveal a red base. There may be only a few scattered patches on the tongue, cheeks, palate or gums but, in more severe instances, they may extend to involve the esophagus and upper respiratory tract. Occasionally, *Candida* infection is seen at the angles of the mouth as angular stomatitis (perlèche; Figure 10.22). However, not all cases of angular stomatitis are due to *Candida*. The presence of *Candida* is easily confirmed by examination of the material from the white patches.

Thrush is most commonly seen in infants. However, it does appear to be a complication of broad-spectrum oral antibiotics, the theory being that the alteration which occurs in the bacterial flora of the alimentary canal after administration of these antibiotics allows overgrowth with *Candida*. This may be too simple an explanation and host immunity is probably also an important point in the development of pathological lesions. Recently, underlying abnormal immune mechanisms and disorders of calcium and iron metabolism have been reported in persistent cases of oral mucocutaneous candidosis.

Treatment

In infants, nystatin suspension given as drops is usually effective. In older patients, oral nystatin pastilles may be used. Angular stomatitis usually responds well to topical nystatin combined with a weak topical steroid, e.g. hydrocortisone. Miconazole and clotrimazole creams are also effective. If oral candidoses persist, an underlying immunodeficiency, including AIDS, must be considered.

Candidal vulvovaginitis

The same general principles for oral thrush apply equally well for vaginal candidiasis. The organism is often present in the normal vagina, particularly during pregnancy, while taking the contraceptive pill or following antibiotic therapy. There is an increased incidence of *Candida* in women with pathological conditions of the cervix or vagina.

Candidosis of the vagina is characterized by a white or yellow curd-like discharge. This is associated with pruritus vulvae. The vulval area becomes red and swollen, and a white discharge is present. The condition may subsequently spread to give rise to a macerated eczema of the perineum, perivulval skin and groins.

Treatment with nystatin, clotrimazole or miconazole as pessaries or vaginal tablets is usually effective. Nystatin has to be used for a 2-week period and the newer preparations for shorter periods, which is an advantage. Oral treatment with itraconazole and fluconazole is also effective and sometimes preferred to local treatment. If the skin is also affected, this should be treated as described above for candidal intertrigo. The urine should be tested for sugar, and a search made for any predisposing gynecological conditions.

Chronic mucocutaneous candidosis

This syndrome includes persistent oral thrush, vulvovaginal candidosis, chronic candidal paronychia and skin involvement. The paronychia is usually accompanied by severe nail plate involvement, unlike that seen with the paronychia due to excessive moisture. The skin lesions usually involve the intertriginous areas, and the face (Figure 10.23) and hands; very occasionally, there is widespread involvement. The lesions are red and scaly (Figure 10.23), and there may be gross hyperkeratosis. The syndrome of chronic mucocutaneous candidosis usually begins in infancy and childhood, and is due to an underlying abnormality of immune mechanisms. Some of these abnormalities are severe, and are associated with other infections. One group of patients has a high incidence of endocrine disorders, particularly Addison's disease and hypoparathyroidism and, less often, diabetes and hypothyroidism.

Patients with chronic mucocutaneous candidosis should be investigated by a clinical immunologist and any immune defect corrected if possible. Endocrine disorders should be excluded. Itraconazole and fluconazole offer the best means of controlling the mucosal and skin lesions.

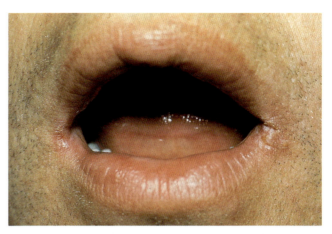

Figure 10.22 *Angular stomatitis. Secondary infection with* Candida *is common*

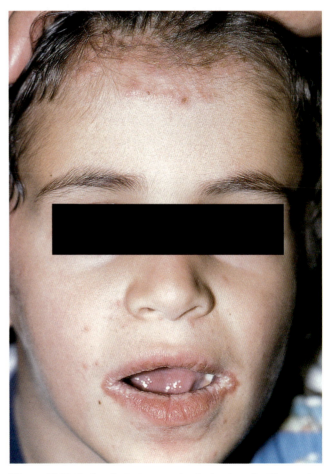

Figure 10.23 *Red scaly lesions on the forehead, and white patches and fissuring of the lips in chronic mucocutaneous candidosis*

11
Viral infections

WARTS

Warts represent a very common viral infection of the skin. They are caused by the human papillomavirus of which different types cause different clinical lesions.

The wart virus affects the epidermal cell, causing cellular proliferation and excess keratin production. Thus, the viral wart is a small tumor on the skin with a thickened rough surface (Figure 11.1). The appearance of the wart, however, varies depending on the site involved.

Histologically, warts are composed of finger-like processes of epidermis with dermal capillaries extending up between these processes. These capillaries come very close to the surface and are often a useful diagnostic point. If the surface of the wart is pared with a scalpel, bleeding points may be seen. On other occasions, the vessels are thrombosed and are seen as small black dots in the wart (Figure 11.2). This appearance has sometimes led to the mistaken diagnosis of a malignant melanoma.

Warts, being a viral disease, are contagious. However, apart from genital warts, they are not as contagious as is commonly supposed, and infection of several members of a family is not common. Immunity to the wart virus is probably important in determining whether the virus causes clinical lesions.

Before deciding on the treatment of warts, the natural history of the condition must be appreciated. The vast majority of warts undergo spontaneous resolution in the course of time. However, this period varies from a few months to a few years and, as yet, there is no way of predicting how long warts may last if left untreated.

As no drug is effective against the wart virus, treatment is empirical. Warts are epidermal structures and,

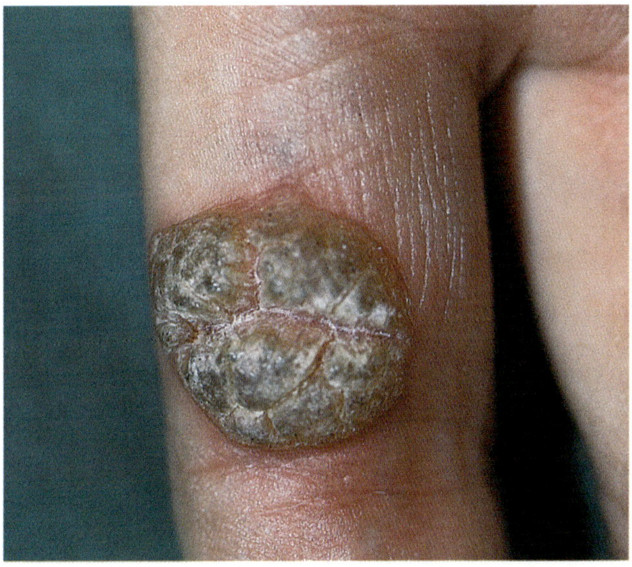

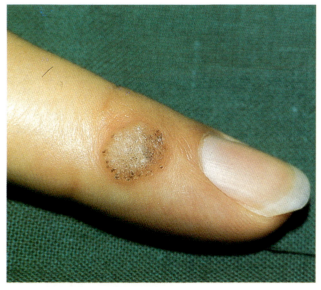

Figure 11.1 Viral wart, characterized by a hyperkeratotic surface with fissuring

Figure 11.2 A viral wart; the 'black dots' are enlarged thrombosed capillaries, a characteristic feature

therefore, if they undergo spontaneous remission, they will leave no scar or mark. Thus, treatment that is too radical and involves damaging the dermis should be avoided. Treatment may be either radical or palliative.

Radical treatment

All of the radical procedures described below are aimed at removing or destroying the tumor. None of the procedures has a 100% success rate, not even in the best hands. The results will depend on a number of factors; the two most important are:

(1) That the procedure is carried out properly; and

(2) The degree of host immunity that the patient has to the wart virus at the time of the procedure.

Curettage and cautery
This should be done under local anesthetic. The wart is scooped out with a small curette. The base and edges of the ulcer thus produced are cauterized to stop the bleeding and to destroy any cells containing wart virus that may be left behind.

Carbon dioxide snow or liquid nitrogen
These substances work on the principle that, when applied to the skin for the appropriate length of time, they produce a subepidermal blister and the epidermis (which contains the wart) will be shed. The length of time that they are applied to the skin will depend on the site and size of the lesion treated.

Podophyllin
This is a plant resin containing a number of cytotoxic compounds, the most active of which is podophyllotoxin. Both the crude resin and the purified podophyllotoxin are used in the treatment of warts. Podophyllin destroys epidermal cells and, like most cytotoxic agents, this effect is more pronounced on proliferating cells compared with unaffected cells. The strength of the podophyllin used and the medium in which it is used will depend on the site of the lesion.

Formalin
This is only suitable for the treatment of plantar warts.

Lasers
Carbon dioxide lasers can be used to destroy warts, but scarring may occur from damage to the dermis.

Miscellaneous
A variety of other modalities have been used in the treatment of resistant warts, including intralesional bleomycin, intralesional interferons and topical 5-fluorouracil. These treatments should only be used by a physician familiar with their use. The results of treatment with these agents are variable.

Escharotics
The most commonly employed are nitric acid and trichloracetic acid. However, the results are not predictable and there may be severe burning of the surrounding tissues.

Surgery excision and radiotherapy
These are mentioned only because they have been advocated in the past. Neither is justifiable for the treatment of such a benign and self-limiting disorder.

Palliative treatment

If the warts are numerous, as often occurs, none of the above measures is really suitable. Painting with salicylic acid, a keratolytic, in a suitable base will tend to break up the excess keratin on the surface of the lesion and make the wart less conspicuous. Simple occlusion with airtight adhesive tape (changed weekly) for 6–8 weeks tends to cause maceration of the epidermis, and may lead to destruction of the wart.

In some instances, placebo therapy is required and there are reports of its success. However, whether it is a true placebo effect or simply the natural history of the lesion which causes the disappearance of the wart is not ascertained.

Warts on the hand

This is one of the most common sites for warts. They may occur on the palms or backs of the hands, and they may be numerous (Figure 11.3) or solitary. The lesion usually presents as a small hyperkeratotic papule usually 2–5 mm in diameter (Figure 11.2). However, occasionally, they may be larger. If the warts occur on the skin around the nails, they may simply present as thickened and rough skin on the nail folds (Figure 11.4). On the backs of the hands, they may appear as small, brown, barely palpable lesions (sometimes referred to as plane or flat warts).

Treatment
Treatment for warts on the hands is usually sought for cosmetic reasons or because the lesion is at a site which interferes with the patient's work. In the first instance, simple painting with 10% salicylic acid in collodion should be tried. If the lesion does not show signs of spontaneous cure after 2–3 months and the patient continues to ask for further treatment, then this should be decided on the number of lesions present. If the wart is solitary or small in number, treatment with carbon dioxide snow, liquid nitrogen, or curettage and cautery will probably give the best result. If the warts are numerous, the patient will have to continue with palliative or placebo measures.

If the warts are periungual, curettage and cautery are best avoided, particularly if the warts are on the posterior nail fold, as permanent damage to the nail bed may follow. Periungual warts often respond to podophyllin applied under occlusive strapping. The podophyllin at this site is best used in an ointment base. The ointment is applied weekly and the tapes changed weekly. If the podophyllin cannot be tolerated, simple occlusive strapping should be tried for 6–8 weeks.

Cryotherapy with liquid nitrogen or carbon dioxide snow is suitable for periungual warts, although the treatment may have to be carried out more than once. The interval between treatments should be 2–3 weeks.

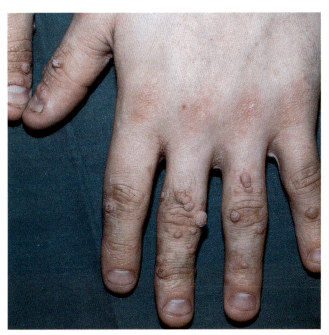

Figure 11.3 *Numerous warts on the hand*

Plantar warts

The sole of the foot is another common site for warts. These are often referred to as verrucas by the patient. The presentation of plantar warts to the doctor is usually as a result of a school inspection of the feet. The other reason for presenting is because the wart is on a weight-bearing part of the sole and is causing pain.

Warts on the soles of the feet do not present as small raised papules because the pressure on the sole forces the lesion into the dermis and thus causes pressure on the nerve endings, giving rise to pain. The typical plantar wart is a flat, circular hyperkeratotic lesion (Figure 11.5). There is often gross hyperkeratosis over the surface of the lesion, making it difficult to distinguish from a simple callosity. In these instances, the lesion should be pared with a scalpel. If it is a callosity, only uniformly thickened keratin will be found; if it is a wart, capillary bleeding points or the clefts between the finger-like processes of the structure will be seen.

Warts on the soles of the feet may be solitary or multiple. Occasionally, there may be a group of warts which involves a confluent area on the sole of the foot. These are sometimes referred to as 'mosiac warts' (Figure 11.6).

Treatment

If the warts are not causing any discomfort, the best advice may be to leave them alone and wait for spontaneous resolution. The average duration of untreated warts is 2–5 years. Warts tend to last for shorter periods in children and longer in adults. If topical preparations are used, then patients should be advised to remove as much keratin from the surface of the wart as possible by either pumice stone after bathing or paring with a suitable instrument. Removing the keratin will allow

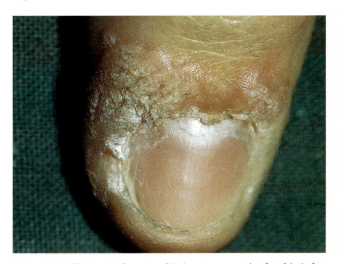

Figure 11.4 *Periungual warts; this is a common site for this infection. They present as rough scaly patches*

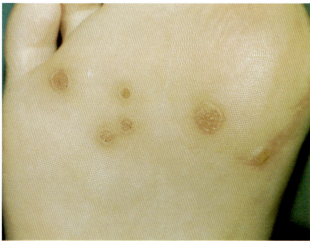

Figure 11.5 *Plantar warts are not usually raised above the surface because of the weight- bearing pressure on the sole*

greater penetration of the chemicals. Salicylic acid either alone or combined with podophyllin is the standard treatment and there are many proprietary preparations containing salicylic acid.

Formalin soaks are sometimes effective if carried out correctly. Five per cent formalin solution should be poured into a saucer or flat dish and the part of the sole with the wart(s) soaked in this lotion for 15 min daily. If the wart is near the toes and the formalin is likely to go between or under the toes, then these places should be protected by applying vaseline before soaking in formalin. If this is not done, the skin may become fissured and sore at these sites. The treatment should be continued for at least a month and the hyperkeratotic dry skin pared away before each soak to allow the lotion to penetrate to the deeper parts of the wart. If after a month of proper treatment there is no improvement, the strength of the formalin should be increased to 7% and subsequently, if necessary, to 10%. It is usually easy to see if the treatment is being carried out regularly because the skin in contact with the formalin will become dry and flaky.

If formalin therapy is not successful and the lesions are solitary or few, then curettage and cautery or cryotherapy may be used. If the lesions are on the toes, they should be treated as described above for periungual warts on the fingers. Mosaic warts appear to be particularly resistant to treatment, possibly because of the extent of the lesions. This implies little or no immunity to the wart virus and, thus, the lesions persist.

Warts on the face and trunk

The face and neck are the next most common sites for warts after the hands and soles of the feet. Warts on the face may present as either the typical rough scaly papule (Figure 11.7) or as flat plane warts (Figure 11.8) similar to those on the backs of the hands. In children, warts are frequently seen on the lips due to sucking of the fingers which have warts on them. On the lips the warts present as smooth white papules. On the neck and beard area, warts are usually seen as grouped papules, probably due to autoinoculation during shaving.

Treatment
Strong acids, podophyllin and formalin should not be used for the treatment of warts on the face. If the lesions

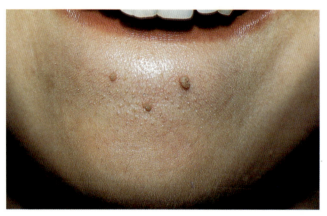

Figure 11.7 Typical warts on the chin

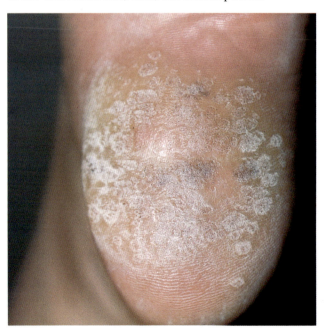

Figure 11.6 Mosaic wart on the sole of the foot

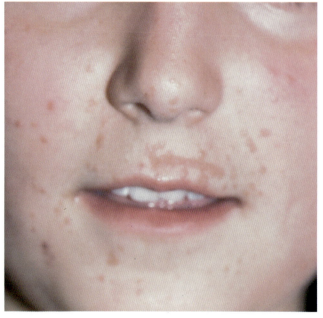

Figure 11.8 Flat warts on the face. There is a linear lesion on the upper lip and warts are arising at the site of previous trauma (Koebner phenomenon)

are unsightly or cause difficulty during shaving, then the treatment of choice is cauterization. Cryotherapy may also be used.

Perianal and genital warts

In these moist areas, the spread and growth of the warts may be very rapid (Figure 11.9), so it is extremely rare to find solitary or only a few lesions. The warts are raised above the skin.

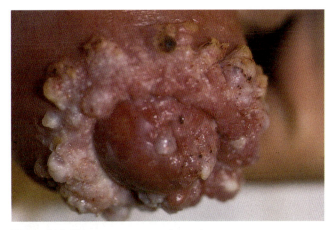

Figure 11.9 Numerous warts on the penis

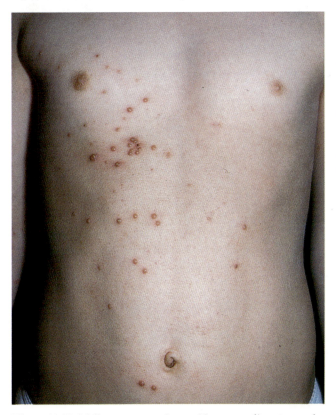

Figure 11.10 Molluscum contagiosum. Numerous discrete papules in an asymmetrical eruption

Treatment

Podophyllin preparations are often effective in clearing genital warts and therefore should be tried initially. Either 25% podophyllin resin in compound benzoin tincture or spirit, or 0.5% solution of podophyllotoxin may be used. If the podophyllin resin is used, it is advisable that a physician or trained nurse handles the preparation. The surrounding skin should be protected with vaseline and the patient instructed to wash off the podophyllin after 6–8 h. The treatment should be carried out weekly. In the majority of cases, the warts will disappear after a few applications but, in others, the lesions may prove resistant to treatment, although their size and number is controlled.

The podophyllotoxin preparation is designed for the use of patients with penile warts. It should be applied twice daily for 3 days and may be repeated after an interval of 7 days. Reinfection of the skin is common if the warts are also present in the anal canal or vagina. In such instances, it may be necessary to ask for the assistance of the appropriate surgeon to destroy the lesions by either cautery or lasers. Genital warts can also be treated by cauterization, lasers or cryotherapy. The latter, as a rule, will not require local anesthesia whereas cautery and lasers will require the use of either a local or general anesthetic.

MOLLUSCUM CONTAGIOSUM

This is another viral tumor of the skin which is most commonly seen in children, but does occur in adults. Autoinoculation is common, and the lesions are usually multiple and grouped on a particular part of the body (Figure 11.10). The individual lesion has a characteristic appearance: it is a small, bulbous, sessile papule, the surface of which is umbilicated (Figure 11.11). The lesion is pearly in color, but red when there is secondary

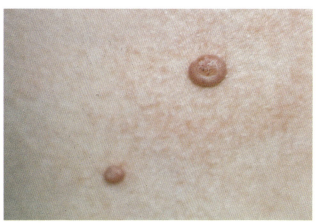

Figure 11.11 Molluscum contagiosum. A pearly papule with central umbilication

bacterial infection. Although autoinoculation is common, it is rare to find more than one member of a household with the complaint at any given time.

Treatment

Molluscum contagiosum lesions tend to be self-limiting, the average duration being 6–9 months, although in some instances the lesions may persist for 3–4 years. In the very young, it is often advisable to recommend no treatment as the effective ones tend to be painful. Any treatment which disrupts the architecture of the lesion induces resolution. The treatments most commonly used are cryotherapy, curettage and piercing of the lesions with a sharpened orange stick. The discomfort from these procedures can be lessened by using a topical anesthetic cream 1 h prior to treatment. Chemical preparations which have been used include podophyllin, salicylic acid and tretinoin (Retin A), and all are irritants at the concentrations required to clear the lesions and will therefore cause discomfort. As the lesions are due to epidermal proliferation, they will heal without scarring.

HERPES SIMPLEX

There are now two recognized types of herpes simplex virus: type I is responsible for the common lesions seen on the face; and type II causes genital herpes. The characteristic clinical lesions of the herpes simplex virus on the skin is a group of blisters on an erythematous base. The most common site for herpes simplex is on the lips or around the mouth (Figure 11.12), but the skin lesions may appear anywhere. Very rarely, the virus may affect the internal organs and cause systemic illness, or a generalized skin eruption in patients with atopic eczema.

The time of the initial infection with the herpes simplex virus is rarely determinable (unless the primary illness is severe), but almost all of the population will eventually become infected, as evidenced by the routine presence of neutralizing antibodies to the herpes simplex virus.

The most common site affected is the lips (herpes labialis). The appearance of the blisters is often preceded by a tingling or burning sensation, as it is thought that the virus lives in the nerve endings of the skin, which are then affected by the virus as it becomes active and migrates into the skin.

Herpes simplex infection of the lips may be precipitated by an illness with a high fever (herpes febrilis) or after exposure to the sun or wind. The first visible lesion is a group of small blisters (Figure 11.12). These may become pustular (Figure 11.13) after 2–3 days and then

rupture to form a crust (Figure 11.14) and finally a scab. Complete healing of the lesion usually takes 10–14 days after the appearance of the blisters. The lesions of herpes simplex may occur repeatedly, with the shortest interval between attacks being as little as 6 weeks. The lesions usually appear at the same site in recurrent herpes

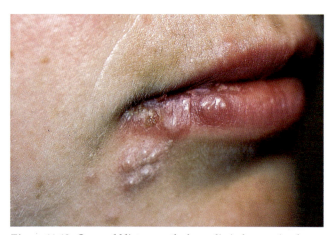

Figure 11.12 Grouped blisters on the lower lip in herpes simplex

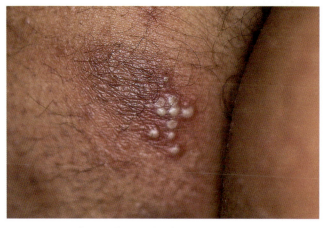

Figure 11.13 Grouped pustular lesions in herpes simplex. The buttock is a not uncommon site in this infection

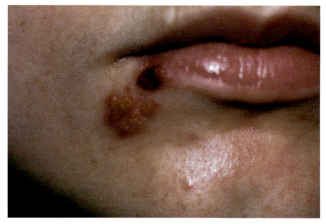

Figure 11.14 Crusting in a late stage of herpes simplex

simplex, which is attributed to the virus remaining in the skin or nerves innervating the particular area. However, the virus has never been demonstrated in the skin between episodes of clinical involvement, but can be shown to be present in the blisters.

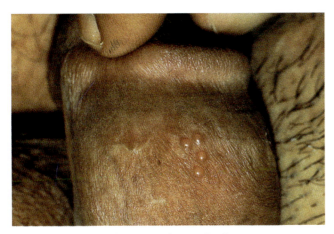

Figure 11.15 Grouped blisters in herpes simplex

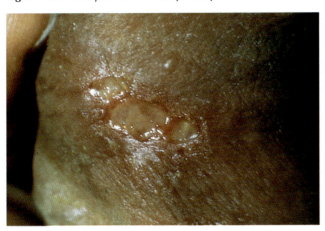

Figure 11.16 Erosions on the penis due to herpes simplex

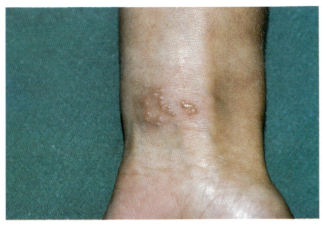

Figure 11.17 Herpes simplex on the wrist, an uncommon site

Genital herpes

This is considered a sexually transmitted disease. In men, any part of the genitalia may be affected, but the penis (Figures 11.15 and 11.16) is most commonly involved. In women, the vulva, vagina and cervix may be the site of lesions. Patients are contagious during the eruption.

The clinical sequence of events in genital herpes simplex is the same as that elsewhere. There is the prodromal symptom of a tingling or burning sensation, then blisters (Figure 11.15) which are followed by pustules and finally erosions (Figure 11.16) rather than scabs. Herpes simplex of the genitalia is often recurrent and the diagnosis can be established by taking swabs from the lesions at the blistering stage for virological examination.

One of the most common reasons for misdiagnosing herpes simplex at sites other than the lips and genitalia is failure to realize that the virus may produce lesions at other sites. Although the face (apart from the lips) is frequently involved, the eruption may appear anywhere on the skin (Figures 11.13 and 11.17). The clinical presentation is that of grouped blisters often in a discoid pattern. The blisters often have an erythematous base which may become pustular and subsequently form a crust before healing.

Herpes simplex very occasionally affects the fingers and is often misdiagnosed as a bacterial infection, as the condition is painful and may give rise to redness and swelling before the blisters are apparent. Herpes simplex affecting the fingers is termed 'the herpetic whitlow' and is common in nurses who have been caring for patients with a tracheostomy; the virus is thought to inhabit the respiratory tract without causing lesions.

Complications

The most common complication is secondary bacterial infection. Repeated herpes simplex infection at one particular site may cause scarring, especially if there is superadded bacterial infection. Herpes simplex infection in the periocular region may spread to the eye where it may give rise to corneal ulcers.

Primary gingivostomatitis and vulvovaginitis
This type of clinical response to primary infection is rare. Why it occurs in some and not in others is not understood. At the onset of the infection, there are no antibodies to the virus, but these appear in high titer as the disease progresses. When the mouth is involved, as occurs most frequently in young children, painful oral lesions develop in association with fever, malaise and

lymphadenopathy. White patches appear in the mouth with surrounding erythema. Ulcers may eventually form. Redness and swelling of the gingiva are characteristic of the infection. In women, vulvovaginitis may occur with white plaques on the vaginal wall and cervix. Subsequently, these areas may ulcerate. In both gingivostomatitis and vulvovaginitis, the characteristic blisters may occur on the surrounding skin.

Eczema herpeticum (Kaposi's varicelliform eruption)
This is a widespread vesicular eruption characterized by lesions predominantly on the face (Figure 11.18) in persons who have atopic eczema.

Systemic herpes simplex infection
When such infection occurs, the central nervous system is the most common and serious site of involvement.

Diagnosis

This can usually be made on clinical grounds alone. In the more difficult cases, virological studies can be helpful in establishing a diagnosis. The virus can be found in the blister fluid and cultured. A rising antibody titer can be demonstrated during the infection.

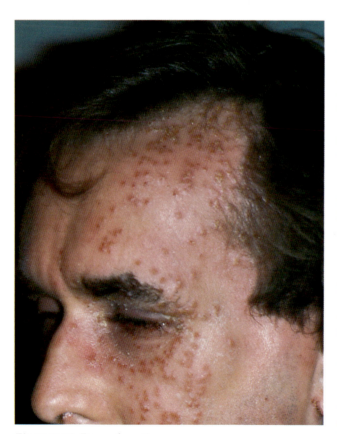

Figure 11.18 *Eczema herpeticum*

Treatment and management
Once the subject has been infected, the virus will lie dormant in the nerves and, under certain circumstances, will advance along the nerve endings into the skin or mucous membranes. In the dormant phase while in the nerve endings, the virus is undetectable and not affected by current antiviral drugs. However, when the virus enters the skin, it becomes susceptible to appropriate antiviral agents.

As an attack of herpes simplex infection is self-limiting, no treatment is required in the majority of cases. However, patients often ask for some form of treatment, and astringent lotions, e.g. spirit, can be given for topical use in the blistering stages of the eruption. If secondary bacterial infection occurs, then topical antibiotics may be given. The organisms most likely to cause secondary infection are the staphylococci, and sodium fusidate ointment is likely to be the most effective treatment.

Recurrent herpes simplex infection is a considerable problem for the patient, particularly if the attacks are frequent. The antiviral drug acyclovir is currently the most effective preparation for treating herpes simplex infections. It may be used topically, taken by mouth or used parenterally in severely ill patients. To be effective in shortening the duration and severity of an episode, it should be used within 24 h of the symptoms developing. Topically, acyclovir should be applied every 4 h for 5 days. If taken by mouth, the dose should be 200 mg five times a day for 5 days. If patients have recurrent infections, it is reasonable for them to have a supply of treatment at home so that they may start treatment as soon as possible. Unfortunately, acyclovir cannot prevent further attacks in patients prone to recurrent outbreaks.

In severe infections, as may be encountered in primary infections or in eczema herpeticum, oral or parenteral acyclovir should be used.

HERPES ZOSTER (SHINGLES)

Skin lesions due to herpes zoster virus occur in the area of skin supplied by one particular sensory root ganglion. Prior to the appearance of the skin lesions, there may be severe pain for 2–3 days in the area supplied by the particular nerve root, which may in some cases give rise to diagnostic problems.

The skin lesions are small blisters with some surrounding erythema (Figure 11.19). They may occur in one or two small groups or throughout the area of skin innervated by the particular sensory root ganglion involved (Figures 11.19 and 11.20). New groups of lesions may appear over a period of a few days after the first lesions have appeared. The blisters tend to be larger (up to 1.0 cm in diameter) than in herpes simplex and not infrequently are hemorrhagic (Figure 11.20).

Herpes zoster usually affects the thoracic nerves. The appearance is characteristic with lesions extending from the spine on the back to the midline on the anterior chest (Figure 11.19) or on the abdominal wall in front (Figure 11.20). The lesions do not usually cross the midline.

Herpes zoster may affect the root ganglia of the sensory cranial nerves. The fifth cranial nerve is the most commonly affected and usually only one division, i.e. ophthalmic, maxillary or mandibular, is involved (Figures 11.21 and 11.22). If the ophthalmic division is affected, keratitis and conjunctivitis may occur in addition to the skin lesions. In the otic type of zoster, in which the geniculate ganglion is involved, there may be an accompanying Bell's palsy and skin lesions in the external auditory canal, and on the pinna and tongue.

Complications

Generalized herpes zoster may occur as a very widespread eruption. In these cases, there is usually a severe underlying disturbance of the patient's immune mechanisms, such as in lymphoma. Generalized herpes zoster is sometimes the presenting manifestation of Hodgkin's disease or leukemia and patients must be investigated for these conditions.

Chickenpox and herpes zoster are caused by the same virus and, in some patients, the two diseases occur together. Secondary infection of the blisters does occur, but is not as common as in herpes simplex lesions, perhaps because herpes simplex more commonly affects the lips.

Postherpetic neuralgia is one of the most distressing symptoms that occurs after the skin lesions have subsided. The complication is seen more frequently in elderly patients and may last for years. Paralysis of the skeletal muscles, not usually permanent, can occur due to the herpes zoster virus. The muscles involved are usually those supplied by the same sensory root involved in the disease.

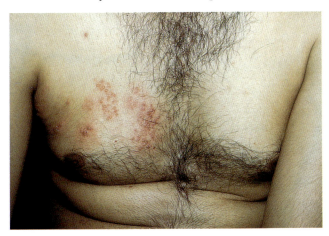

Figure 11.19 *Herpes zoster on the chest. The lesions remain in the area supplied by the intercostal nerve and do not cross the midline*

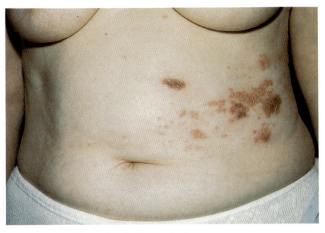

Figure 11.20 *Hemorrhagic blisters in herpes zoster*

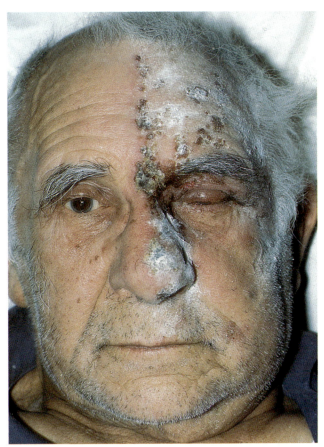

Figure 11.21 *Herpes zoster of the ophthalmic division of the fifth cranial nerve*

Diagnosis

The disease is usually easy to diagnose on clinical grounds once the blisters have appeared. However, if there is difficulty, the virus can be isolated and grown from the blister fluid and identified by virological tests.

Treatment

In the majority of patients, only palliative treatment is required, e.g. mild analgesics. If secondary infection of the blisters occurs, then topical antibiotics may be required. Pain during and after the active stage of the disease may be severe and stronger analgesics may be needed. Drugs of addiction, e.g. pethidine and the opiates, should be avoided because of the possible lengthy duration of postherpetic neuralgia.

Acyclovir reportedly can shorten the duration of lesions. However, it has to be taken orally in high doses, i.e. 800 mg five times a day for 1 week. It must also be started within 48 h and preferably within 24 h of the lesions developing. Unfortunately, treatment with acy-

clovir has no effect on the incidence or severity of postherpetic neuralgia. It is therefore questionable as to whether acyclovir can be recommended for routine use in herpes zoster, although it should certainly be used in immunocompromised patients and in those who have other disorders in whom an attack of herpes zoster may have a deleterious effect.

Systemic corticosteroids and vitamin B_{12} injections have been advocated for herpes zoster to shorten the course of the disorder and prevent postherpetic neuralgia. However, neither of these preparations has proved conclusively to prevent postherpetic neuralgia.

Herpes zoster involving the eye should be managed by an ophthalmologist.

ORF

This virus infection of the skin is acquired by contact with sheep. The lesions, which are nearly always on the hands (Figure 11.23), consist of inflammatory papules which subsequently become hemorrhagic and pustular; they are usually less than 1 cm in diameter, although there may be a surrounding area of erythema.

The differential diagnosis includes anthrax and erysipeloid. The lesions undergo spontaneous resolution within a few weeks; there is no specific treatment.

Figure 11.22 Herpes zoster affecting predominantly the mandibular division, but there is also some involvement of the maxillary division of the fifth cranial nerve

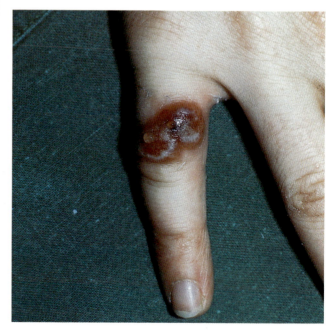

Figure 11.23 Hemorrhagic papules with surrounding erythema in orf

MILKER'S NODULES

This is similar in appearance to orf, but is acquired from cows. The initial lesions usually occur on the fingers and may be multiple or single. They attain their maximum size within 2 weeks in the form of firm brownish nodules which are usually 1 cm in diameter, but may be larger. The lesions are painless and not pustular. No treatment is required unless there is bacterial infection.

HAND, FOOT AND MOUTH DISEASE

This is a viral disease due to Coxsackie A16. Characteristically, there are painful erosions in the oral cavity and small blisters on the hands and feet. The blisters usually occur on the palms and soles, and tend to be small (approximately 0.5 cm) and gray with a surrounding erythematous halo (Figure 11.24). The disorder is self-limiting and lasts about 1 week.

AIDS

AIDS is caused by the human immunodeficiency virus (HIV) which was first isolated in 1982. As its name implies, it depletes the defense mechanisms of the body by interfering with the functions of CD4 T lymphocytes. Thus, there is impaired cell immunity, and subjects are prone to certain other infections and disorders which may be triggered by infectious agents. Patients with AIDS may present to a dermatologist because of severe and persistent infections of the skin or other conditions which, although not considered to be primarily an infection, are manifestations of impaired cell-mediated immunity possibly related to an infective cause.

Infections

These are all common skin infections as seen in current practice, but tend to be more severe, fail to undergo spontaneous resolution and are more resistant to treatment. Dermatophytes, *Candida albicans*, human papillomavirus (warts), molluscum contagiosum, herpes simplex virus (Figure 11.25), herpes zoster virus and staphylococci may be involved. The possibility of underlying HIV infection should be considered if the above infections tend to be severe and persistent.

Kaposi's sarcoma

Prior to AIDS, Kaposi's sarcoma was considered a rare disease predominantly seen in elderly Ashkenazi Jews. The lesions presented as large purplish plaques on the

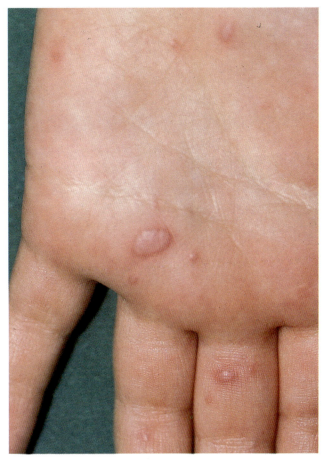

Figure 11.24 Small grayish blisters with surrounding erythema on the palm in hand, foot and mouth disease

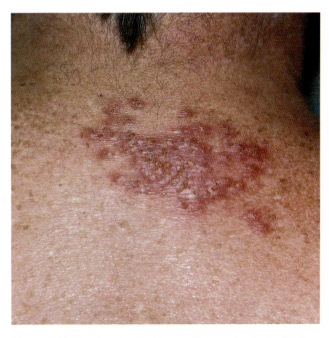

Figure 11.25 Persistent and widespread herpes simplex in AIDS

lower legs and feet (*see* Chapter 15). In AIDS, Kaposi's sarcoma may present as red or purplish macules, papules, nodules or plaques (Figure 11.26). The lesions may present on any part of the body and may also involve the mucous membranes.

Kaposi's sarcoma is a malignant condition affecting either the capillaries or pericapillary tissues. A viral etiology has been suggested.

Other malignancies

There is an increased incidence of lymphoma in AIDS and this may present as skin nodules. There is also an increase of oral squamous cell carcinomas, cervical intraepithelial neoplasia and intraepithelial neoplasia of the anogenital region.

Oral hairy leukoplakia

This is another condition suggestive of AIDS. It consists of white, vertically ribbed, keratinized plaques usually situated on the lateral borders of the tongue (Figure 11.27). It is thought that the condition is due to

proliferation of the Epstein–Barr virus in the oral epithelium. The lesion is often asymptomatic and may coexist or be confused with oral candidoses. Treatment with the antiviral drugs acyclovir and ganciclovir have been reported to clear the condition in some cases.

Seborrheic eczema

A common dermatological feature of AIDS is severe seborrheic eczema which, for many years, has been thought to be associated with an infective cause and was even referred to as 'microbial eczema' 100 years ago. An overgrowth of *Pityrosporum* yeasts are found in seborrheic eczema, but the role of these organisms, if any, in causing eczema is not known. In AIDS, it has been suggested that, because of impaired immunity, there is further overgrowth of the *Pityrosporum* organisms which will aggravate the eczema. Clinically, the seborrheic eczema may be widespread and difficult to control. It must be remembered, however, that seborrheic eczema is a very common disorder and may be severe in many individuals who are not HIV-positive.

Psoriasis

In patients with psoriasis who develop AIDS, the psoriasis may be considerably worse and difficult to control. The immunosuppressive drugs methotrexate and cyclosporine, and PUVA, which is also immunosuppressive, are not advised. Topical treatments and oral retinoids are the treatments of choice. Patients with AIDS may also develop psoriasis and it has been suggested that the virus may act as a trigger of the disease.

Drug eruptions

Patients with AIDS receive many drugs, particularly antibiotics, and there is a higher incidence and severity of drug rashes in these patients. There are no specific drug rashes in AIDS, but all the recognized clinical patterns (*see* Chapter 13) may occur.

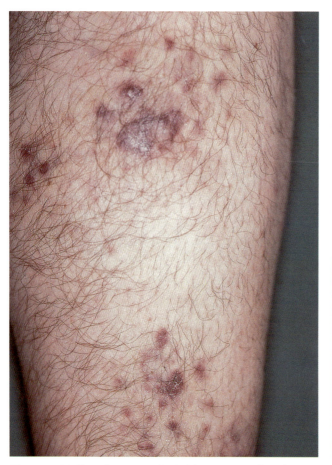

Figure 11.26 *Kaposi's sarcoma in AIDS presents with widespread numerous small purplish papules*

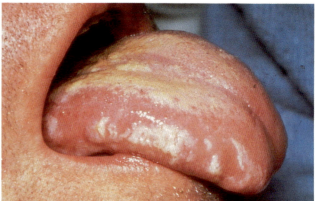

Figure 11.27 *White hairy leukoplakia on the side of the tongue in AIDS*

12

Bacterial infections

Although bacterial infections of the skin still result in an appreciable number of attendances in a dermatological clinic, their incidence has fallen because of the advent of antibiotics and the general improvement in hygiene and standard of living.

IMPETIGO

This is one of the most common bacterial infections seen today and is unfortunately often misdiagnosed before attending the skin clinic.

Impetigo is usually caused by *Staphylococcus aureus*, but it is not uncommon to find a mixed infection with staphylococcus and ß-hemolytic streptococcus. It is important to know that streptococcal infections of the skin may give rise to renal and cardiac complications in the same way that streptococcal infections of the upper respiratory tract may give rise to pathological manifestations that are not respiratory in nature.

Morphological appearances

Impetigo is an infection of the epidermis. In the early stages, a purulent blister (Figures 12.1 and 12.2) may be the first sign of the disorder. However, because the roof of the blister is so thin, it soon ruptures to present as superficial erosions (Figures 12.3 and 12.4). Another form of presentation is the golden crusted lesion caused by seropurulent weeping, which clots and combines with keratin to form crusts (Figures 12.3, 12.5 and 12.6). Satellite lesions are common in impetigo and appear around the older and larger lesions (Figures 12.3 and 12.7).

The original lesions may also coalesce to form large eroded or crusted areas. The hands and face are the most common sites for impetigo probably because of the easy spread from one to the other. The diagnosis of impetigo should be considered when there is asymmetry of the lesions (Figure 12.7), unlike the endogenous eczemas.

Frequently, the diagnosis may be made more difficult because of the previous use of topical steroids, which alter the classical appearances of the lesions by diminishing the crusts and the golden color of the lesions.

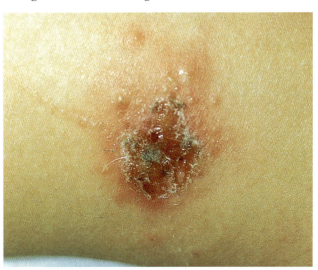

Figure 12.1 Impetigo. Small superficial pustules, the initial lesion surrounding the more typical crusted lesion

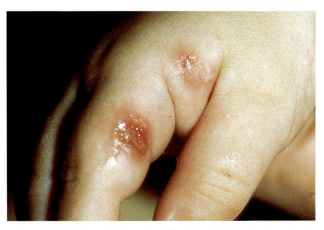

Figure 12.2 Blisters in impetigo. The edge of the lesion is vesicular with a central eroded area

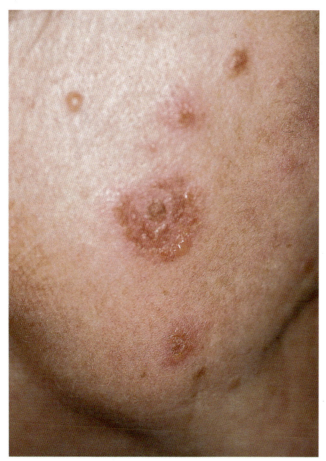

Figure 12.3 *Superficial erosions and crusting in impetigo*

Treatment and management

Impetigo is a contagious disorder and, thus, care over personal hygiene is important. Children should be kept away from school until cured.

Over the last few years, the use of topical antibiotics has declined and systemic antibiotics are now usually recommended for impetigo. Erythromycin and peni-

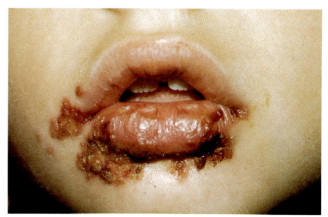

Figure 12.5 *Golden crusts in impetigo*

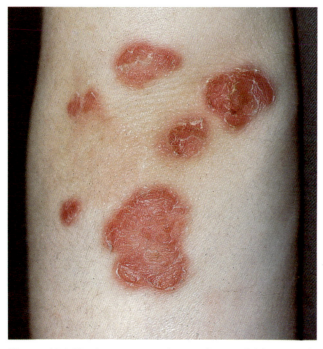

Figure 12.4 *Erythematous erosions and superficial crusts in impetigo*

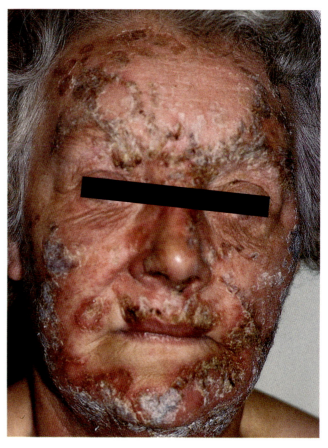

Figure 12.6 *Severe crusting and some erosions in impetigo*

cillin are the drugs of choice. If there is no significant improvement in a few days, swabs must be taken for bacteriological studies and the appropriate antibiotic given. If topical treatment is required, fusidic acid should be used. Any crusts on the lesions should be removed, if possible, with soap and water prior to using the topical preparation. The fusidic acid should be applied four times a day. Treatment for impetigo should be continued until all signs of the disease have cleared.

In patients in whom the impetigo recurs or when it involves the nostrils, it is likely that the organism is harbored in the anterior nares. The topical antibiotic should thus also be applied to this site.

ECTHYMA

This is essentially a deep type of impetigo. It usually begins as a small pustule which erodes through the epidermis and into the upper dermis to produce a shallow ulcer. Oozing occurs with formation of a firm yellow crust.

The most common site is the legs, and lesions occur repeatedly after minor trauma. Because of the involvement of the dermis, healing leaves a superficial scar. Poor hygiene and neglect are predisposing factors.

Treatment

As there is involvement of the dermis, systemic as well as topical antibiotics should be used. The choice of antibiotics is empirical until the results of bacteriological investigations are available.

SECONDARY IMPETIGO

This is where primary skin disease is secondarily infected by staphylococci and streptococci, and clinical lesions, as seen in primary impetigo, are formed. The most common skin disease to become secondarily infected is eczema. The treatment is as for impetigo initially, and the eczema is treated subsequently. In secondary impetigo, the infection may involve the dermis because of preexistent skin disease and, in these instances, systemic antibiotics are also required if the condition is to be quickly controlled.

FOLLICULITIS

Bacterial infection is only one of the causes of this disease. Folliculitis on the back is often seen in association with or as a manifestation of seborrheic eczema. Folliculitis today is most commonly seen in the beard area (Figure 12.8). It is more common in blacks than in whites and is thought to be caused by short curling hairs which grow back into the skin, leading to irritation with secondary infection. People who use cutting oils are liable to develop a folliculitis if the area is continually soaked with the oil.

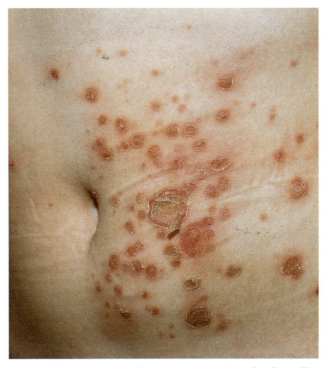

Figure 12.7 *Asymmetrical eruption in impetigo. Small satellite lesions develop around the original affected areas*

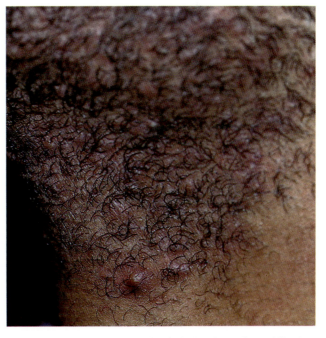

Figure 12.8 *Papules and pustules in the beard area due to folliculitis*

Treatment

If the folliculitis is associated with seborrheic eczema, treatment as for eczema is often all that is necessary to cure the disorder. In some instances, further improvement is obtained with weak keratolytic preparations such as 2% salicylic acid in a spirit or cream base. Folliculitis of the beard area is often difficult to clear other than by not shaving. If the patient does not wish to grow a beard, systemic antibiotics should be given. It is usually necessary to give these drugs for a number of weeks but, even then, there is usually a high incidence of recurrence. Swabs should be taken from the anterior nares, and if the organisms are harbored at these sites, then topical antibiotics, usually fusidic acid, should be applied to the nares twice daily for at least 6 weeks.

ACNE KELOID

This term denotes a chronic folliculitis on the nape of the neck (Figure 12.9). The condition only occurs in males after puberty and is more common in blacks compared with whites and Asians.

Acne keloid presents as pustules, and firm papules and plaques (Figure 12.9), and is a keloidal reaction to inflammatory changes in the hair follicles. Why keloids form is not known. The condition tends to be very persistent. Treatment is not always successful, but tends to consist of topical antibiotics (fusidic acid) and antiseptics. In acute stages, systemic antibiotics are helpful. Intralesional triamcinolone is helpful in inducing resolution of the lesions. Excision of the area and grafting is sometimes necessary.

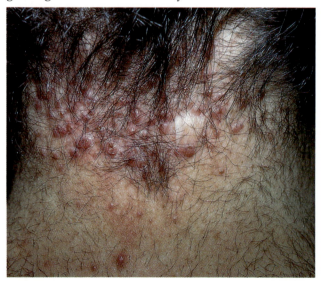

Figure 12.9 *Acne keloid. Firm red papules on the back of the lower scalp*

FURUNCLES (BOILS)

This is essentially a folliculitis, but the infection spreads well away from the follicle into the surrounding dermis. Clinically, the lesion begins as a small red nodule which increases in size and becomes fluctuant within 2–3 days. During this time the lesion becomes 'walled off' in the dermis. The apex of the lesion ultimately becomes yellow (pus) and breaks down to discharge pus and necrotic tissue. When the lesion heals, a small scar is left behind.

A carbuncle is a coalescent aggregation of a number of furuncles that ultimately gives rise to a deep pus-filled ulcer. In terms of pathology, the abscesses around the hair follicles are not walled off from each other.

The most common site for furuncles and carbuncles is the back of the neck, although they may occur wherever there are hair follicles.

Treatment

For a single isolated boil, no treatment other than hot compresses is required. If the lesion is fluctuant, pain can be relieved by a small incision through the center of the lesion. Topical antibiotics are of no therapeutic value in the treatment of the lesion.

Multiple and recurrent boils

The most common cause of recurrent boils is the harboring of the infecting organism in the anterior nares, axillae or perineum. Swabs should be taken from these sites. The appropriate topical antibiotics should be applied twice daily for at least a month to the area where the organism has been found. Bathing with 30 ml of 10% hexachlorophane added to the bath water has been claimed to be of value in decreasing the number of lesions when multiple boils are present. Systemic antibiotics are helpful in the early phase of the lesions and will prevent new lesions from forming. However, unless the underlying source of the organisms is found, systemic antibiotics will not prevent the development of new lesions when the antibiotics are stopped. In all cases of recurrent skin infections, it is wise to think of underlying systemic disease. The most common systemic diseases to present with skin infections are diabetes mellitus and lymphomas. Rarer disorders, such as the dysgammaglobulinemias, should be considered as a last resort.

ERYSIPELAS

This streptococcal infection has become relatively uncommon. It begins as a red indurated plaque of cellulitis with a distinct border. As in other forms of cellulitis, the skin feels hot. There is usually constitutional upset and fever. The most common sites to be affected are the face and scalp, the port of entry being a small crack in the skin of the nostril or external auditory canal. However, if the patient has had any previous wounds or other dermatoses (Figure 12.10), these are obvious points of entry for the organism. Occasionally, erysipelas is recurrent at one particular site, e.g. on the face, and may eventually leave brawny permanent edema. The cause of this recurrent infection may be a chronic otitis externa.

Treatment

Systemic antibiotics, usually penicillin, are required. The affected part, particularly if it is a limb, should be rested. If the disorder is recurrent, it is worth looking for a persistent port of entry in the form of a chronic dermatosis which requires treatment.

TUBERCULOUS SKIN INFECTIONS

As with tuberculosis at other sites of the body, infections of the skin have become increasingly rare. A number of clinical varieties of skin tuberculosis have been described in the past and these clinically descriptive terms are used here.

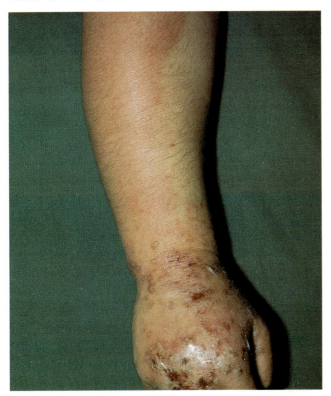

Figure 12.10 *Erysipelas on the forearm. An erythematous indurated area with a well-demarcated edge. The streptococci gained entry into the tissue from eczema on the hand*

Lupus vulgaris

This was probably the most common form of skin tuberculosis seen in the past. The lesion may occur at any site, although it is most frequently seen on the hands and neck. It presents as a reddish-brown nodular plaque (Figure 12.11) and, when pressed with a glass spatula, small brownish nodules ('apple-jelly' nodules) can be seen. The surface of the lesion may be scaly but, usually, it presents as an infiltrated plaque, as the primary changes are in the dermis. If untreated, the disease is progressive and leads to destruction of the tissues and subsequent scarring. In the past, it has led to severe disfigurement.

Tuberculosis verrucosa cutis

This clinical form of tuberculosis is the result of direct inoculation of the skin with tubercle bacilli. It may be granulomatous with superficial pustules and may be misdiagnosed as a chronic boil. Another appearance is that of granuloma with a warty surface (Figure 12.12).

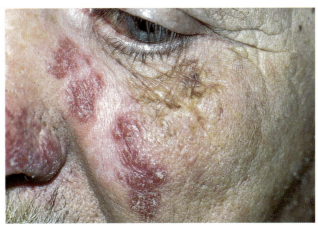

Figure 12.11 *Lupus vulgaris. Reddish nodular lesions on the face*

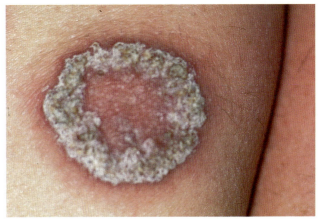

Figure 12.12 *Warty tuberculosis on the buttock*

Scrofuloderma

This is an extension of tuberculous infection to the skin from an underlying focus in the bones or lymph nodes.

Treatment
The therapy for tuberculous infections of the skin is the same as that for tuberculous infections at other sites of the body.

SYPHILIS: PRIMARY LESION OR CHANCRE

The typical lesion is a painless ulcer, with an indurated border, usually less than 1 cm in diameter (Figure 12.13). There is accompanying regional lymphadenopathy. The most common sites for a chancre are naturally on the penis and vulva. However, for a high proportion of women, it is present on the cervix and, therefore, may well escape detection. The chancre may appear anywhere on the skin, the most frequent extragenital sites being the lips, mouth, fingers, breasts and anus.

Secondary syphilis

Lesions of secondary syphilis may appear within 6 weeks and up to 1 year after initial infection. The most common form of skin lesion is a reddish papular eruption on the trunk and limbs (Figure 12.14). The lesions may be widespread or few in number. A not infrequent site of involvement is the palms of the hands which can sometimes help in the clinical diagnosis (Figure 12.15).

At first, the lesions may be discrete papules but, on occasions, they may merge, leading to a confluent scaly dermatosis similar to psoriasis or eczema of the palms. On the genitalia or around the anus, small eroded exudative papules (condylomata lata) (Figures 12.16

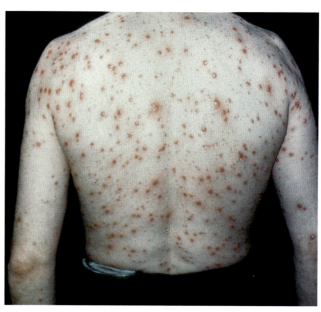

Figure 12.14 Extensive papular eruption in secondary syphilis

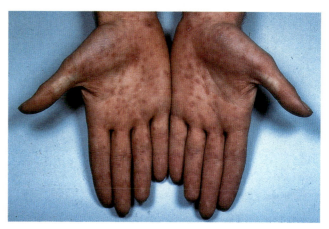

Figure 12.15 Papular eruption on the palms in secondary syphilis. This can be a helpful feature in the diagnosis

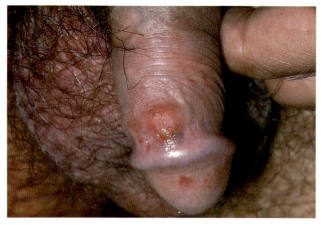

Figure 12.13 Primary chancre on the penis

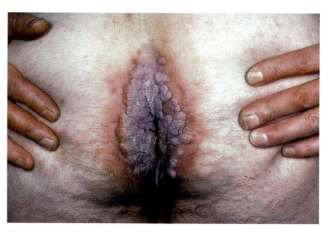

Figure 12.16 Secondary syphilis. Condylomata lata on the perianal skin

and 12.17) may be seen and may have to be distinguished from viral warts – particularly if they are the only manifestation of secondary syphilis. Secondary syphilitic eruption of the skin has always been considered the great mimicker of other dermatoses. Most frequently, it resembles psoriasis or pityriasis rosea but, in any atypical dermatosis of recent onset, secondary syphilis should be remembered.

Hair loss may occur in secondary syphilis. This is usually patchy and the areas affected are not completely bald, as occurs in alopecia areata.

The mucous membranes may also be involved in secondary syphilis. In the mouth and pharynx, there are oval, round (Figure 12.18) or arcuate grayish patches which tend to ulcerate and may give rise to the classical 'snail-track' ulcer.

Accompanying the cutaneous lesions of secondary syphilis may be constitutional upset and lymphadenopathy. Serological tests are always positive in the secondary stage of syphilis.

Tertiary syphilis

Only the skin manifestations of tertiary syphilis are mentioned here and all are very rare today. Nodular

lesions of varying size (2–5 mm) of a reddish-brown color usually appear in groups and spread out in various directions to produce lesions of irregular pattern (Figure 12.19).

Gumma

This is a mass of syphilitic granulation tissue. It begins below the skin, but extends into the skin. The lesions are painless and slow-growing, but frequently break down and ulcerate.

Chronic interstitial glossitis

This presents as extensive and irregular fissuring of the tongue with accompanying leukoplakic changes.

Treatment
Penicillin is still the drug of choice for the treatment of syphilis. It is best for patients with primary and secondary syphilis to be treated in venereology departments so that their contacts can be traced. Patients should also be investigated for the possibility of other venereal diseases.

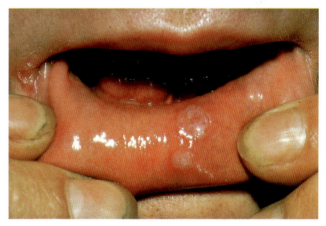

Figure 12.18 *Grayish-white patches on the oral mucous membrane in secondary syphilis*

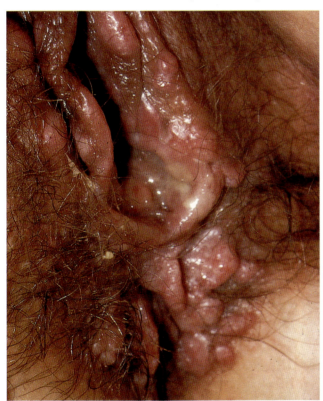

Figure 12.17 *Condylomata lata on the vulva and perineum*

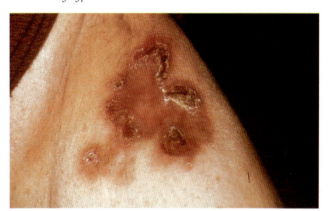

Figure 12.19 *Tertiary syphilis. Infiltrated scaly lesion*

13

Drug eruptions

In this chapter, the skin lesions produced by drugs taken or given systemically will be considered rather than the skin lesions produced by topically applied therapeutic agents.

Almost any drug can produce a skin eruption which may mimic most dermatological entities, or produce bizarre patterns of reaction in the skin. In dealing with a patient who presents with a rash, it is most important to determine, as part of the history-taking, whether the patient has received in the immediate past, or is receiving at present, any drugs.

It also is very important to appreciate that what the patient means by a drug compared with what the doctor means is often very different, and specific questions may have to be asked. The patient usually considers a drug to be those substances prescribed by a doctor for a serious or acute illness. However, it must be remembered that many drugs such as mild analgesics (salicylates and paracetamol), laxatives and tonics can be bought by patients over the pharmacy counter with no prescription from a doctor. These substances may also cause drug eruptions, but are not considered to be drugs by the patient. In addition, any drug which may have been taken for any length of time, e.g. regular hypnotics, tranquillizers or contraceptive pills, are not considered to be drugs by the patient nor thought likely to be responsible for the complaint as the drug has not caused any previous trouble.

Thus, in practice, it is better to ask the patient whether any pills, tablets or medicines of any description have been taken for any complaint, rather than asking "Have you taken any drugs recently?" Both the patient and the doctor must appreciate that, even if the drug has been taken for a long time without previous trouble, it should not be exempt from suspicion of causing the present complaint.

Despite the wide variation in pattern of reaction that may be produced in the skin, there are a number of features that suggest that a drug may be the cause.

(1) The eruption is frequently widespread because it is produced by a circulating agent rather than a topically applied substance;

(2) It commonly appears as an inflammatory response with widespread pruritus;

(3) It is usually of sudden onset; and

(4) It may be associated with constitutional upset such as malaise or fever, and there may be signs of disorder in other organs frequently affected by drugs, such as the bone marrow, liver or kidneys.

It is not possible to be definitive about which drugs cause a specific pattern of skin reaction, but certain drugs are more likely than others to cause recognized dermatological entities. The following examples of significant eruptions should be considered as being possibly due to drugs if a positive history is obtained. However, when considering the possibility that a rash is drug-induced, a good rule to follow is that any drug may cause any type of rash.

TYPES OF DRUG ERUPTIONS

Urticaria and angioneurotic edema

The two drugs that most frequently cause angioneurotic edema (Figure 13.1) and urticaria (Figure 13.2) are penicillins and salicylates. The urticaria due to penicillin usually appears 1–2 weeks after starting the drug, but may occur as long as 6 weeks after commencement. Urticaria following penicillin may be persistent and last for many weeks. Other drugs which may cause urticaria are thiouracil, isoniazid, serum, quinine, acetyl-cholinesterase inhibitors and radiographic contrast media.

Exanthem or morbilliform eruption

This is a widespread macular erythematous eruption (Figure 13.3). Latterly, there may be some scaling or peeling and, occasionally, the lesions are raised with an urticarial appearance (Figure 13.4). At present, the most common cause of this type of eruption is ampicillin. Other drugs which also cause this pattern are gold, phenothiazines, barbiturates, sulfonamides, phenytoin and carbamazepine.

Erythema multiforme

This is a well-recognized dermatological entity with annular erythematous and vesicular lesions occurring predominantly on the hands (Figure 13.5), forearms and feet. There may also be oral lesions (Figure 13.6) usually presenting as ulcers or erosions on the mucous membrane. This type of eruption is most commonly caused by sulfonamides and penicillin.

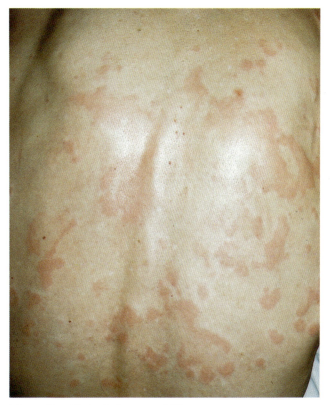

Figure 13.2 Urticaria due to penicillin

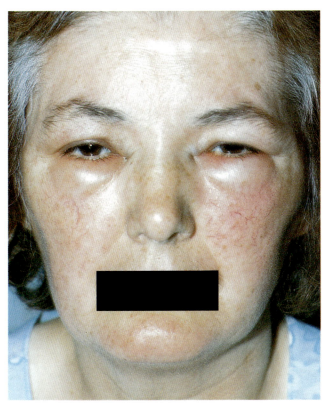

Figure 13.1 Angioneurotic edema around the eyes due to penicillin

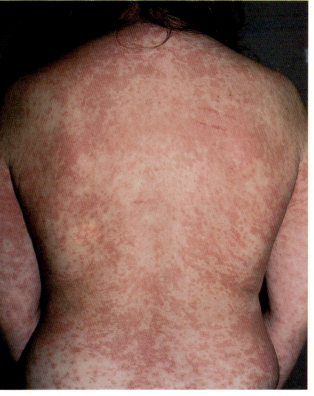

Figure 13.3 Widespread erythematous macular eruptions due to ampicillin

Photosensitivity

This is usually an acute erythematous eruption on light-exposed areas (Figure 13.7) and, in some instances, the inflammation may be so intense as to produce blistering of the skin. The drugs most likely to be responsible are the phenothiazines, particularly chlorpromazine, and the tetracyclines. It is also well recognized as a reaction to the sulfonamides, quinidine, thiazides, nalidixic acid and non-steroidal anti-inflammatory drugs.

Blistering eruptions

The most usual drugs to produce large discrete blisters in the skin (Figure 13.8) are the sulfonamides, but they have also been described after penicillin and in comatosed patients, who are often overdosed with a variety of psychotropic drugs.

Purpura

Purpura (Figure 13.9) is most commonly seen on the legs whatever the cause, and drug-induced purpura is no exception. It may occur following quinidine, chlo-

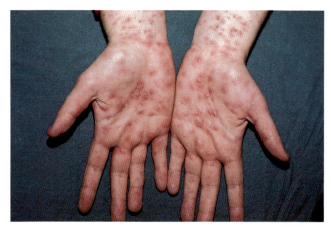

Figure 13.5 Erythema multiforme on the hands due to a sulfonamide

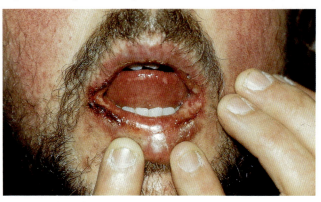

Figure 13.6 Ulceration on the lips and oral mucosa in erythema multiforme

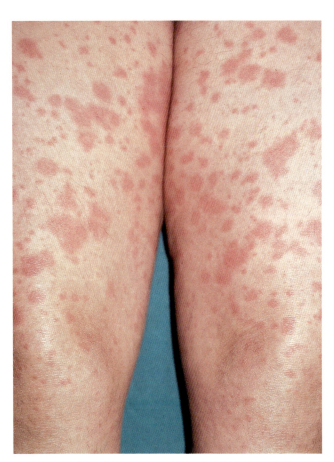

Figure 13.4 Maculopapular eruption, in which some lesions resemble urticaria, due to a sulfonamide

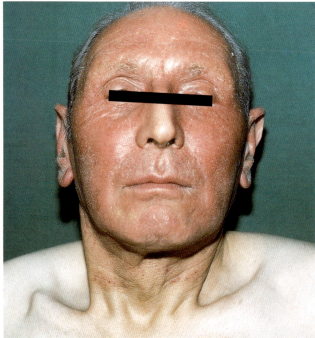

Figure 13.7 Acute photosensitive eruption due to tetracycline

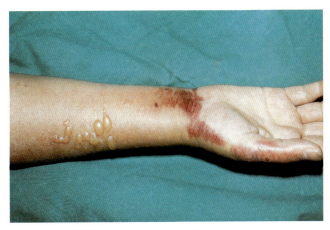

Figure 13.8 Bullous eruption due to sulfonamide

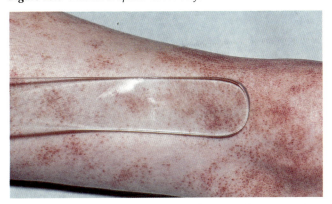

Figure 13.9 Purpura due to a non steroidal anti-inflammatory drug

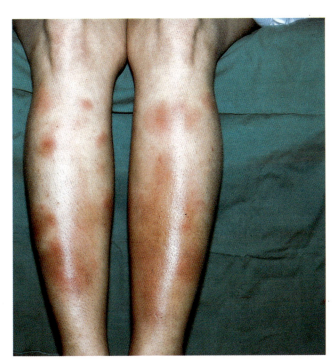

Figure 13.10 Erythema multiforme due to a sulfonamide

ramphenicol, sulfonamides, barbiturates, bleomycin, meprobamate and carbamazepine.

Erythema nodosum

This presents as painful reddish indurated plaques, usually on the front of the legs (Figure 13.10). It can be drug-induced, and the sulfonamides seem to be the most frequent cause of this type of eruption.

Generalized or exfoliative dermatitis

This is essentially an eczematous response of the skin (Figure 13.11). Heavy metals are the most common cause and gold is probably the only heavy metal still used in clinical practice. This eruption has also been noted after barbiturates, quinine and sulfonamides.

Lichen planus-like eruptions

These are sometimes very similar to lichen planus, but are usually more confluent and slightly scaly. The eruption in these instances is referred to as lichenoid. The drugs which have been implicated are chloroquine, mepacrine, thiazides, gold and chlorpropamide.

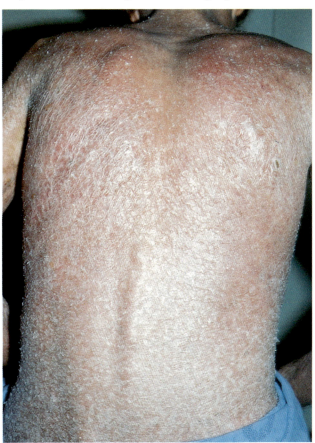

Figure 13.11 Erythroderma due to gold

Acne

This well-recognized complication of systemic corticosteroids is also induced by iodides, lithium, danazol and some oral contraceptives. In the latter, the acne appears to be due to the relatively dominant effect of the progesterone component on the sebaceous glands.

Cutaneous vasculitis

When this is due to drugs, as with other causes, it mainly affects the lower legs. The lesions may be purpuric or purplish papules, nodules and blisters. Drugs usually associated with vasculitis are thiazides, sulfonamides and penicillin.

Lupus erythematosus

A lupus erythematosus (LE)-like syndrome can be induced by drugs. Apart from the classical cutaneous lesions (Figure 13.12), internal organs may also be involved and antinuclear antibodies present. The first drug known to cause this reaction was the hypotensive agent hydralazine. Procainamide and penicillin are now also known to precipitate lupus erythematosus.

Pigmentation

Various types of pigmentation may be seen with drugs. Oral contraceptives may induce chloasma (increased

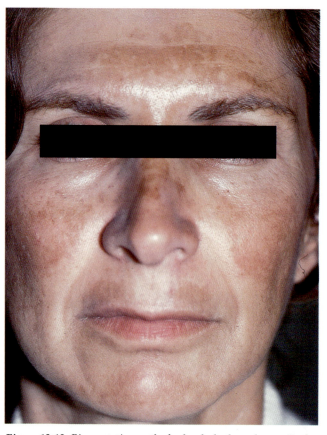

Figure 13.13 Pigmentation on the forehead, cheeks and upper lip due to an oral contraceptive

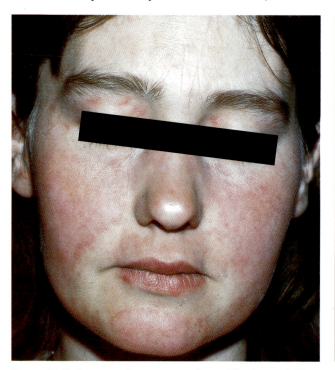

Figure 13.12 Lupus erythematosus syndrome following penicillin

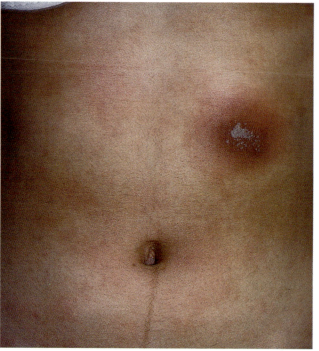

Figure 13.14 Fixed drug eruption. Pigmentation and blisters surrounded by erythema

melanin deposition) on the upper cheeks and forehead (Figure 13.13). Minocycline may cause a bluish-black pigmentation on the cheeks; chloroquine may cause a diffuse bluish-black color on the face; mepacrine produces a yellow discoloration of all the skin areas; and chlorpromazine produces a slate-gray color in the exposed areas.

Pruritus ani and pruritus vulva

This is a complication of broad-spectrum antibiotics. *Candida albicans* is often present in the skin in these cases and it is thought to be due to altered bacterial flora.

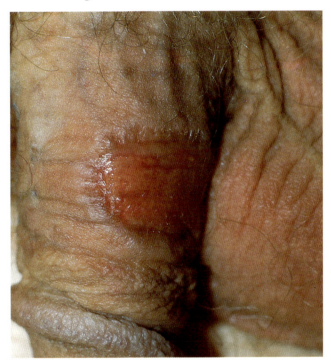

Figure 13.15 Fixed drug eruption on the penis. Genitalia are a common site for a fixed drug eruption

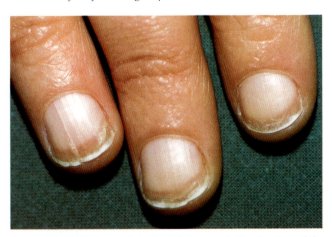

Figure 13.16 Photo-onycholysis with brownish discoloration of the nail due to tetracycline

Fixed drug eruptions

These follow highly distinctive clinical patterns. They consist of circumscribed lesions which reappear at exactly the same site each time the drug is taken. The clinical lesions are variable, but usually consist of an erythematous patch with possible urticarial or bullous formation (Figure 13.14); an erosion may follow (Figure 13.15). This usually subsides within a few days, but residual pigmentation may persist for a considerable length of time. Fixed drug eruptions by nature usually occur only with drugs which are taken infrequently, because if the patient is taking continuous medication, the eruption would be present continuously in the active stages. The drugs most frequently involved are barbiturates and phenolphthalein, which is found in a number of proprietary laxative preparations.

Photo-onycholysis

Separation of the distal part of the nail from the nail bed and brownish discoloration of the nail (Figure 13.16) is a rare side effect of tetracyclines in patients who have been exposed to sunlight. The prognosis is good with recovery of the nails.

MECHANISMS OF DRUG ERUPTIONS

Allergy

It is usually assumed by doctors and patients alike that if a patient develops a rash after taking a drug, then he is 'allergic' to it. However, the varied pattern of drug eruptions and their subsequent behavior, and the fact that antibodies cannot be detected to these drugs, suggest that not all drug reactions are allergic in nature.

Toxic

It would appear from the behavior of many of these reactions that they exert a direct damaging effect on the skin, but the exact biochemical processes involved are not known.

Idiosyncrasy

This is a term used when a patient develops a severe reaction even when only a small dose of the drug is given. This may be due to abnormal enzyme systems in the body that are not present in the majority of people.

Intolerance

Most drugs are either metabolized by the tissues, usually of the liver, or excreted unchanged by the kidney. Thus, if these organs have impaired function and the particular drug is not excreted or metabolized by them, it may accumulate in the body to toxic levels and cause a reaction, which it would not do in a healthy individual. If it is known that a patient has liver or kidney disease, care must be taken before prescribing any drug until it is known that there is no risk from the drug or its metabolic products.

DIAGNOSIS

The diagnosis of drug reactions may prove difficult. Often the only basis for the diagnosis is circumstantial evidence. The clinical picture is still the most useful guide; the time relationship between taking the drug and the development of the rash is very important, as is the pattern of reaction produced.

Unfortunately, there are no safe or reliable tests for substantiating a diagnosis. Intradermal or patch tests are useful only if there is a true allergy and, even then, there is a high incidence of false-negatives. In addition, if a patient has an allergy to a drug such as a penicillin, then even a small dose given intradermally may prove fatal.

An oral test dose of the drug is sometimes suggested after the rash has cleared, but this carries the possibility of inducing an even more severe reaction. Laboratory tests *in vitro* with the patient's serum and drug have been tried, but the number of false-negative results is so high that, at present, the tests are of little practical value.

MANAGEMENT AND TREATMENT

Once a drug is suspected of causing an eruption, it should be stopped. The treatment is dependent on the type of eruption but is largely symptomatic. If there is severe pruritus, then systemic antihistamines should be given in adequate dosages. If there is an inflammatory response in the epidermis with erythema and scaling, topical steroids may prove helpful. Systemic steroids may also be valuable in appropriate cases.

In certain instances when it is considered necessary to use the drug again, desensitization has been attempted. Initially, the drug is given in very small quantities so that no reaction is produced and the dose is then gradually increased. The procedure does not always work and is not without risk.

The questions always raised are whether or not the drug is the cause of the eruption and must it always be avoided in the future? If there is a *definite* history of a reaction following a particular drug and other drugs can be used as alternatives, it is probably advisable to avoid the incriminated drug unless it is a question of life or death. There have been cases in the past when a drug which apparently definitely caused an eruption induced no reaction when given again. It is now known that the disease for which the drug is given can combine with the drug to produce the reaction, so when the drug is given on a second occasion for a different disease, no reaction occurs. This has been recorded with ampicillin, e.g. when administered for glandular fever.

14
Bullous disorders

Although many disease processes affecting the skin (e.g. bacterial infections, viral infections, vasculitis) may cause blisters, there is a group of rare diseases in which the predominant sign is blisters. These diseases are usually known as the bullous disorders and include pemphigus, pemphigoid, dermatitis herpetiformis, epidermolysis bullosa and herpes gestationis. Although all the conditions are rare, they are well-recognized dermatological entities and no comprehensive discussion of dermatological conditions would be complete without mention of them.

PEMPHIGUS

The word 'pemphigus' comes from the Greek *pemphix* meaning 'pustule'. Pemphigus occurs in middle-aged and elderly patients, appearing more commonly in members of the Jewish race. It is most important to appreciate that pemphigus affects not only the skin but also the mucous membranes of the mouth, pharnyx and vagina. One-third of patients with pemphigus may present with lesions at these sites before developing lesions on the skin. Pemphigus has no predilection for any specific site of involvement and may present anywhere on the skin. The lesions tend to become widespread in a short space of time.

Pemphigus is an epidermal disease, and the disorder is one of failure of the epidermal cells (keratinocytes) to adhere together and maintain cell contact. The cells drift apart and the space between the cells fills with fluid, which eventually gives rise to a blister. Because the blister forms *in* the epidermis, the roof of the blister is very thin and ruptures easily. There are a number of clinical presentations of pemphigus, depending on whether the disease process is high up or deep down in the epidermis. When blisters are present in pemphigus, they tend to be flaccid (Figure 14.1) because of their thin easily easily-ruptured roof, giving rise to erosions (Figures 14.2 and 14.3). Crusting of the eroded surface of the skin soon occurs (Figure 14.3) and, thus, patients

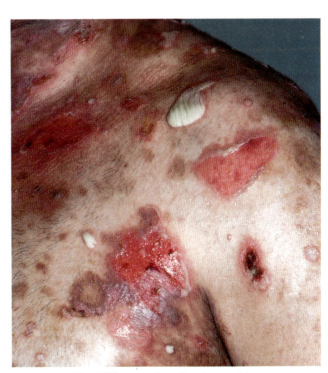

Figure 14.1 Flaccid blisters and erosions in pemphigus

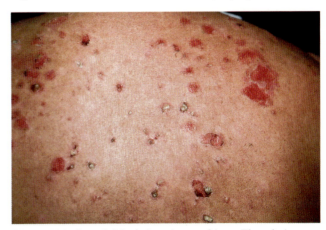

Figure 14.2 Superficial erosions in pemphigus. These lesions are more common than blisters

may present with one of three types of skin lesion – blisters, erosions or crusted scabby lesions, or a combination of any of these.

Occasionally, pemphigus presents with widespread erosions only, and this form of the disease may be misdiagnosed unless it is appreciated that pemphigus may present without blisters. When pemphigus affects the mucous membranes of the mouth, the pharynx or the genital tract in females, it presents as red denuded areas or as superficial ulcers (Figures 14.4 and 14.5), and no blisters are seen. In patients who have persistent erosions in the mouth, pemphigus should be considered in the differential diagnosis.

Etiology

Pemphigus is now considered to be one of the so-called autoimmune diseases. The antibody found in pemphigus is formed against the cell membrane of the epidermal cells and affects cell adhesion. Thus, the epidermal cells do not adhere to each other but drift apart, with blister formation and destruction of the epidermis. The detection of the antibody is now one of the diagnostic tests in pemphigus. The antibody is found in the skin adjacent to the lesions and also circulating in the blood. The antibody can therefore be detected by direct (in the skin) or indirect (in the serum) studies. Usually, a fluorescent technique is used (Figure 14.6). As in all autoimmune disorders, it is not known whether the antibody is primary or secondary.

Treatment

Prior to the advent of corticosteroids, pemphigus was invariably a fatal disease and the mortality still approaches 10% in many published series, although death is usually due to a side effect of treatment. The basis of treatment is oral corticosteroids but, unfortunately, a high initial dose is required. The serious nature of the disorder and high incidence of side effects of treatment make it imperative that the diagnosis is confirmed by histological and immunological investigations.

The initial dose of prednisone should be 60–120 mg daily, depending on the severity of the disease. Once the active process has been stopped and no new lesions are seen, the dose of steroid can be reduced. The speed of reduction depends on the severity of the disease and appearance of new lesions. If it is possible to reduce the dose to 15 mg daily, it is probably advisable to maintain this dose for 6–8 weeks; if no new lesions then appear, a gradual reduction of dose can be attempted. If the

disease is severe at the outset, or new lesions appear with a dose of prednisone above 30 mg daily, other immunosuppressive drugs can be used in addition to steroids to reduce the steroid requirements. The immunosuppressive drugs that have been tried in pemphigus include azathioprine, cyclosporine, methotrexate, cyclophosphamide, gold and dapsone. Which of these drugs is chosen is arbitrary as claims have been made for all of them by different workers. All immunosuppressive drugs have a high incidence of side effects, some of which are serious and, thus, the morbidity from

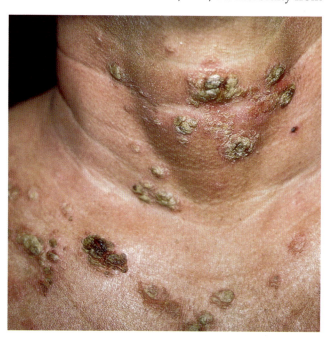

Figure 14.3 Thick crusted lesions in pemphigus

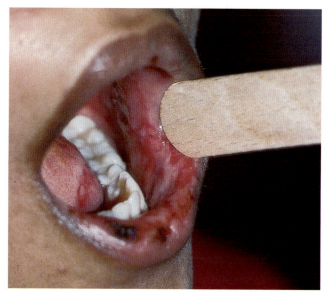

Figure 14.4 Erosions on the buccal mucosa, tongue and lips in pemphigus

treatment in pemphigus, particularly when the disease is severe, is high. Plasmapheresis has also been used to treat pemphigus and there have been favorable results.

Eventually, the disease process in pemphigus may burn itself out and all drugs may be stopped. However, the time taken for this to happen varies considerably between patients, depending on the severity of the disease. Some patients may be able to discontinue treatment after 1 or 2 years whereas others may have to continue for several years.

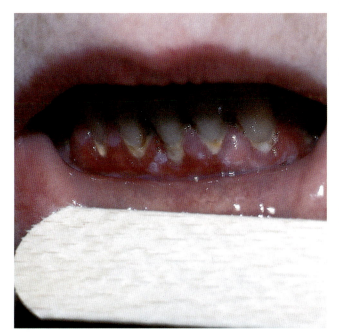

Figure 14.5 *Erosions on the gums in pemphigus*

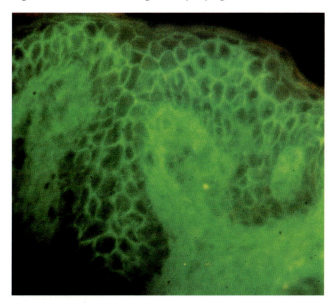

Figure 14.6 *Localization of the pemphigus antibody (bright-green) to the cell membrane of the epidermal cells*

BENIGN FAMILIAL PEMPHIGUS (HAILEY–HAILEY DISEASE)

This disease is considered under the heading of pemphigus because, as with true pemphigus, it is characterized by *intra*epidermal blisters. In benign familial pemphigus, the cause is genetically determined and the cohesion between epidermal cells appears to be at fault so that minor trauma produces splits in the epidermis. The genetic defect is dominant, yet only 70% of patients give a positive family history.

Characteristically, the neck and intertriginous areas (Figure 14.7) are affected. The initial lesion is a small blister which soon breaks to form crusted lesions. The affected area becomes inflamed so that the advanced stage of the disease presents as a red, thickened, moist area with linear clefts where the epidermis has split.

Unlike pemphigus, there is no established auto-immune basis for the disease. It is not a serious condition as is pemphigus, and it only affects relatively small areas of the skin surface. There may be long periods when the patient has no skin lesions. As there is no increased mortality associated with the disorder, it has been considered benign.

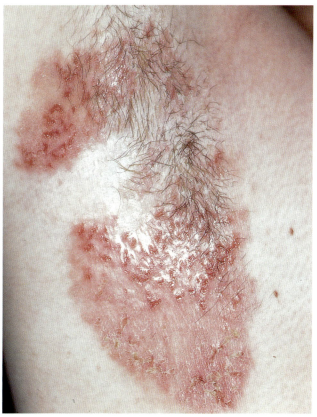

Figure 14.7 *A red moist plaque with characteristic clefts in benign familial pemphigus in the axilla*

Treatment

The role of bacteria in precipitating this disorder is unknown. However, the condition often improves with topical antibiotics or antiseptics. Magenta paint is helpful if the patient is prepared to use it. Systemic antibiotics may also be helpful in acute exacerbations. Anything which causes excessive sweating will aggravate or precipitate the condition. Potent (Group III or IV) topical steroids also help acute exacerbations, but long-term use is not advisable in intertriginous areas.

When the disease is severe and persistent, surgical excision of the affected areas and grafting may have to be considered.

PEMPHIGOID

Pemphigoid is the adjectival form of the word 'pemphigus' and originally meant 'pemphigus-like'. Pemphigoid has now been separated from pemphigus on clinical, histological and immunological grounds.

Pemphigoid is most commonly seen in elderly patients. Unlike pemphigus, the site of blister formation is at the basement membrane between the epidermis and dermis. Thus, the roof of the blister is thicker and is less likely to rupture than in pemphigus. The patient therefore presents with fairly tense blisters, varying in size from a few millimeters to a few centimeters in diameter (Figure 14.8). These may be widespread and involve any part of the skin, although the most common sites are the limbs (Figure 14.9).

Another clinical feature of pemphigoid is the presence of large confluent areas of skin which are erythematous and raised, giving plaque-like lesions. If these are present, it is usual to find the blisters in these red areas and not on the normal-looking skin (Figure 14.9). Mucosal lesions may occur, but are usually confined to the mouth and are less frequent than in pemphigus. If untreated, the disease will run a chronic course over a period of years and does not carry the high mortality seen in pemphigus.

Etiology

Pemphigoid, like pemphigus, is now considered to be one of the so-called autoimmune disorders. The antibody found in pemphigoid is different from that present in pemphigus and is active against the basement membrane. The antibody can be detected in the skin at the edge of the blisters and in the blood. Thus, the antibody can be detected by immunofluorescent studies on the skin (direct; Figure 14.10) or in the blood (indirect). The point to be stressed is that, at present, it is not certain whether the antibody is primary or secondary, but its detection has helped in the differential diagnosis of blistering eruptions.

Treatment

Oral steroids form the basis of treatment in pemphigoid. The initial dose should be 40–60 mg daily and, once new lesions cease to appear, the dose should be gradually

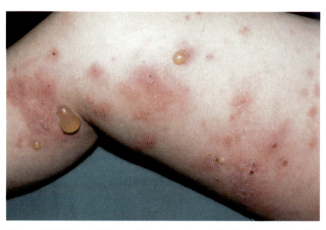

Figure 14.8 Tense blisters of varying size on the leg in pemphigoid

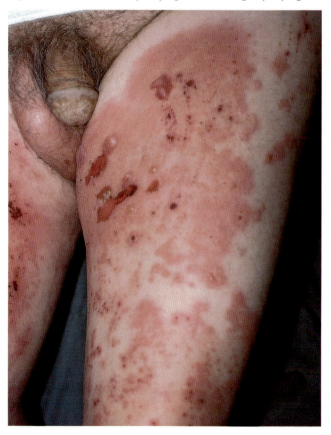

Figure 14.9 Blisters situated on extensive erythematous urticarial plaques in pemphigoid

reduced. A maintenance dose of 10–15 mg prednisone may be required for some time until a spontaneous remission occurs. The average duration of pemphigoid is approximately 2 years, but a small proportion may have a recurrence.

In addition to steroids, other immunosuppressive drugs are used in pemphigoid. The most commonly used is azathioprine, but cyclosporine and cyclophosphamide have also been used. The benefit from these drugs is not usually apparent for 6 weeks after beginning the drug. These drugs do not replace prednisone but are given with it in an attempt to reduce the steroid requirements needed to control the disease.

MUCOUS MEMBRANE (CICATRICIAL) PEMPHIGOID

This disease is so called because, clinically, it mainly affects the mucous membranes but, when skin lesions are present, they tend to be tense blisters and histologically are subepidermal as seen in pemphigoid. The other name for this disorder is cicatricial pemphigoid because it causes scarring at sites of involvement. Immunologically, the disease is also similar to pemphigoid in that a linear band of IgG is found at the dermoepidermal junction in the perilesional tissue of both the skin and mucous membrane lesions.

Mucous membrane pemphigoid is usually a disease of individuals in late middle-age and in the elderly. It may affect the mucous membranes of the eyes, mouth, nose, larynx, esophagus, anus and genitalia. The conjunctivae are most frequently involved and changes are often present even when the patient is asymptomatic. At a later stage, there is redness, soreness and eventual scarring of the conjunctivae (Figure 14.11) which, if severe, may lead to blindness.

In the mouth, the presentation is that of recurrent mouth ulcers and soreness. Involvement of the esophagus may lead to dysphagia. When the skin is involved, unlike pemphigoid, the blisters often heal with scarring.

Treatment

When the disease is mild, only symptomatic treatment is necessary. Unfortunately, no treatment has been shown conclusively to stop scarring of the conjunctiva. There have been claims that dapsone or sulfapyridine may halt the process, but it is too early to say whether this is so.

Dapsone and sulfapyridine appear to heal the mouth ulcers and have beneficial effects on the skin lesions. Systemic steroids are also helpful for the oral and skin lesions but, because the disease tends to be chronic, they may have to be taken for a considerable time. The dose required to control the oral and skin lesions is variable but it may be as little as 5–10 mg prednisone daily, although higher doses are often required. Azathioprine and cyclophosphamide have also been claimed to be helpful in this disease.

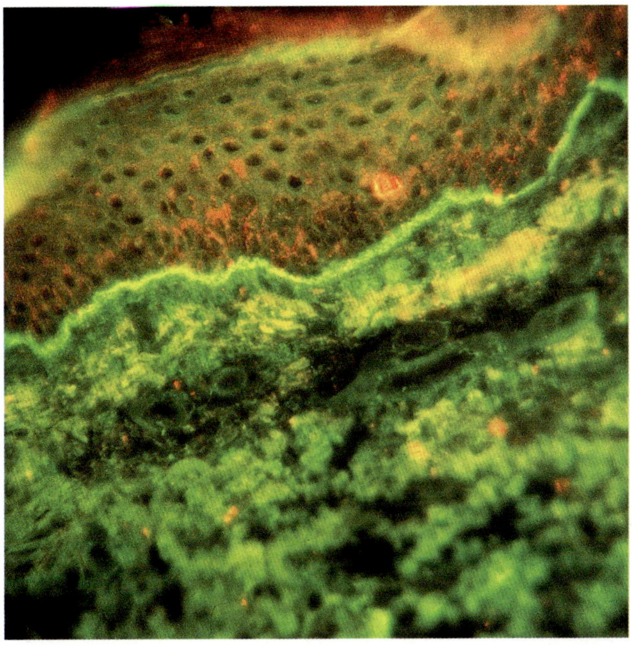

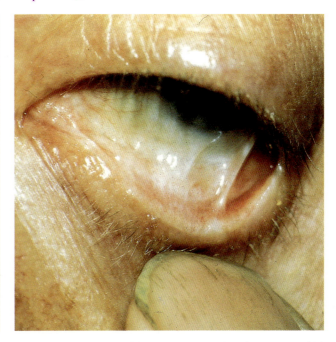

Figure 14.10 *Pemphigoid antibody (bright-green) seen along the line of the basement membrane*

Figure 14.11 *Scarring of the conjunctiva with a characteristic fold, as seen in mucous membrane pemphigoid*

DERMATITIS HERPETIFORMIS

Dermatitis herpetiformis may begin at any age, but onset is rare in childhood and in the elderly. The most common age of onset is in young adulthood. The lesions occur most frequently on the elbows and extensor surfaces of the forearms (Figures 14.12–14.14), knees (Figure 14.15), buttocks (Figure 14.16) and areas of pres-

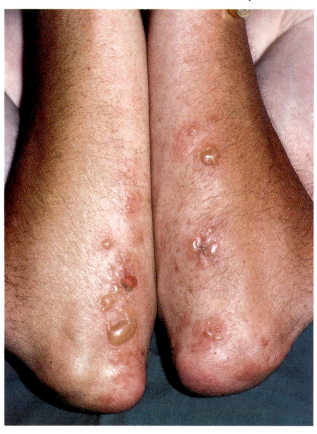

Figure 14.12 *Blisters on the elbows and extensor forearms, the most common site in dermatitis herpetiformis*

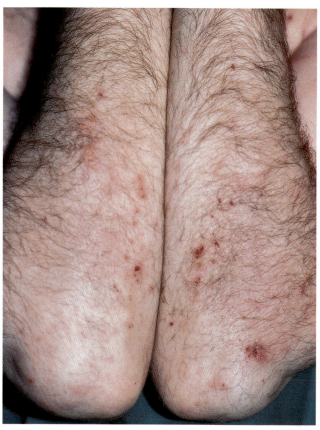

Figure 14.14 *Excoriated papules on the extensor forearms in dermatitis herpetiformis. The blisters are ruptured because of the excoriation due to the intense irritation*

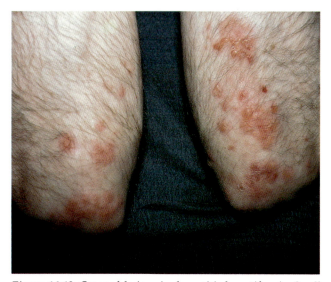

Figure 14.13 *Grouped lesions in dermatitis herpetiformis. Small blisters on an urticarial base*

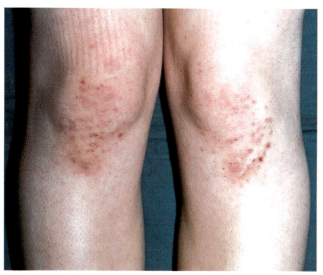

Figure 14.15 *Excoriated papules on the knees in dermatitis herpetiformis*

sure from clothing. However, the lesions may occur on any part of the skin, and the skin over the scapulae is another common site. The typical lesion is a small blister (Figure 14.12), and the lesions may be grouped (Figure

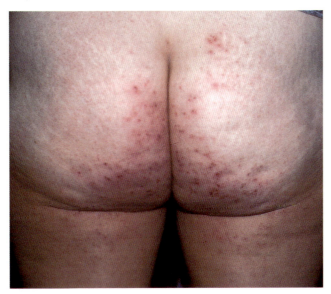

Figure 14.16 *Excoriated papules on the buttocks. This is the second most common site for lesions in dermatitis herpetiformis*

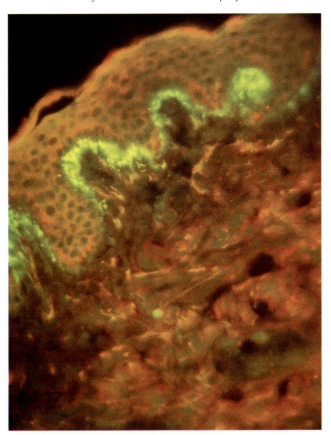

Figure 14.17 *Deposits of IgA in the dermal papillae of the uninvolved skin in dermatitis herpetiformis is diagnostic*

14.13), hence the term 'herpetiform'. The blisters are often found on an urticarial base and, not infrequently, the urticarial lesions show no clinical blister formation. The lesions are intensely irritating and, because of this, the patient frequently presents with an excoriated papular eruption rather than blisters, which have been destroyed by continual scratching (Figures 14.14–14.16).

Dermatitis herpetiformis is a chronic and persistent disorder, but approximately 15% of patients may have a remission of skin lesions after a number of years. The severity of the eruption varies considerably from patient to patient; in some the rash is generalized whereas, in others, it is confined to the elbows.

Etiology

The rash of dermatitis herpetiformis has now been shown to be due to gluten. A gluten-free diet will clear the rash, and reintroduction of gluten to the diet causes a recurrence of the rash. The small intestine mucosa is also gluten-sensitive and approximately 90% of patients have a demonstrable enteropathy similar to celiac disease, although the enteropathy is invariably mild. Very few patients have symptoms of malabsorption, although a number are found to be iron- and folate-deficient on investigation. In addition, there is a high incidence of autoantibodies in dermatitis herpetiformis, especially antinuclear, gastric–parietal cell and thyroid antibodies. This is associated with an increased incidence of autoimmune disease, particularly thyroid disease, pernicious anemia and early-onset diabetes.

As in celiac disease, there is a very high incidence of the histocompatibility antigens HLA B8/DR3/DQ2. Also, as has been shown in celiac disease, there is an increased incidence of lymphoma in patients with dermatitis herpetiformis. Whether this is due to gluten acting upon an abnormal immunological system or solely due to abnormality of the immune system predisposing to malignant change is not known.

The blister is subepidermal and the primary pathology in the skin occurs in the dermal papillae just *below* the basement membrane. It has been established that, in the *uninvolved* skin of patients with dermatitis herpetiformis, there are deposits of class A immunoglobulins (IgA) on the reticulin fibers in the dermal papillae. IgA is the principal immunoglobulin produced by the gastrointestinal tract, and it is likely that an immune complex related to gluten is formed and deposited on the reticulin fibers of the skin. Reticulin is involved in the disease process, and antireticulin and antiendomysial antibodies are detected in the blood. The detection of IgA deposits in the uninvolved skin is the simplest and most reliable test for establishing the diagnosis of dermatitis herpetiformis (Figure 14.17).

Management and treatment

All patients with dermatitis herpetiformis should be fully investigated, including a biopsy taken from uninvolved skin for detection of IgA deposits, a full blood count, a small intestinal biopsy, an autoantibody screen, blood glucose and liver function tests.

Initial treatment should commence with dapsone which, in the majority of patients, will control the rash within a few days. Relapse occurs equally quickly when the dapsone is stopped. The average dose of dapsone to control the skin lesions is 100 mg daily, although a smaller dose may be successful in some patients and a higher dose necessary in others.

Dapsone has a relatively high incidence of side effects (*see* Chapter 25) and, if it cannot be tolerated, sulfapyridine or sulfamethoxypyridazine should be tried. None of these drugs heal the intestinal pathology.

A gluten-free diet is the ideal treatment for dermatitis herpetiformis. Such a regimen will correct the enteropathy as well as clear the skin lesions and, eventually, no drugs will be required. However, it should be stressed that it takes, on average, 6 months of following the diet before drug requirements begin to fall andmore than 2 years before patients can do without drugs. The diet must be strict to be effective. A number of patients find the diet too difficult or a social handicap and these patients will have to take drugs. A gluten-free diet has to be considered a lifelong treatment.

Patients with dermatitis herpetiformis should be followed up, particularly if they take dapsone, to be certain they are not anemic due to either the drug or malabsorption. These patients have a high incidence of autoimmune disorders, particularly thyroid disease, pernicious anemia and diabetes mellitus. Thus, autoantibody screens and other necessary investigations should be performed yearly or every 2 years. The increased incidence of lymphoma should also be borne in mind, although there is a suggestion that a gluten-free diet may protect patients from this complication.

LINEAR IgA DISEASE

This disease is so called because it is characterized by a linear band of IgA deposits at the dermoepidermal junc-

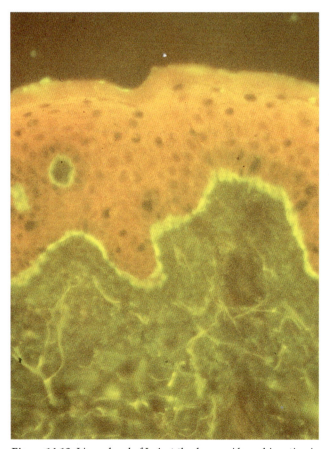

Figure 14.18 *Linear band of IgA at the dermoepidermal junction in linear IgA disease*

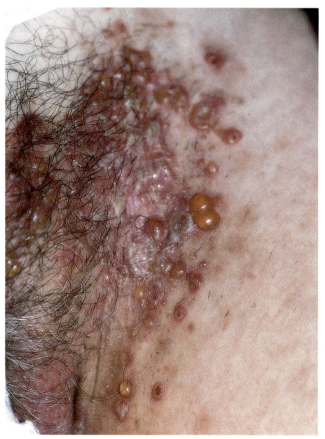

Figure 14.19 *Linear IgA disease. Small grouped blisters in the groin, a common site for this disease*

tion (Figure 14.18). It is usual to distinguish two forms of the disease, one in children and the other in adults. In children, it is sometimes called benign chronic bullous disease of childhood and has a relatively good prognosis. The disease tends to burn itself out by puberty whereas the adult form tends to be persistent, although clinical remissions may occur.

In adults, the clinical picture is variable; it may resemble dermatitis herpetiformis with small grouped blisters (Figure 14.19) or it may be similar to pemphigoid with large blisters on an urticarial base. The eruption may occur on any part of the body, but the groins and axillae are often affected. The rash is usually well controlled by dapsone or sulfapyridine.

In the childhood variety, the eruption has two sites of predilection: the lower trunk, groins and upper thighs, and the central area of the face, especially around the mouth. The rash consists of blisters of varying size on an urticarial base and is usually controlled by dapsone or sulfapyridine.

The cause of linear IgA disease, both in children and adults, is as yet unknown.

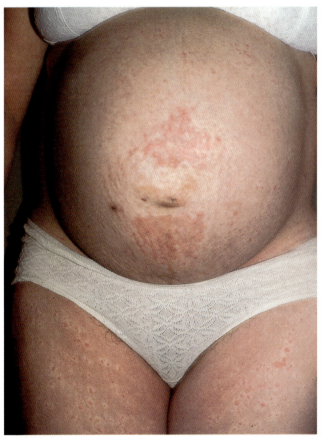

Figure 14.20 *Herpes gestationis. The rash begins on the abdomen around the umbilicus*

PREGNANCY RASHES

As two of the three recognized eruptions associated with pregnancy may have blisters, it is convenient to consider them here. The incidence of rashes directly due to pregnancy is thought to be 1:250 pregnancies. Papular eruption of pregnancy and erythema multiforme of pregnancy occur with equal frequency, but herpes gestationis is rare.

Papular eruption or prurigo of pregnancy

This eruption may occur at any time in the pregnancy and may be widespread, involving the trunk and limbs. The lesions are small firm papules which are invariably excoriated and crusted. The rash runs a variable course and may resolve before the end of the pregnancy or extend into the postpartum period. The cause of this type of rash is unknown, and treatment is symptomatic with Group II topical steroids and oral antihistamines. There are no serious consequences to the mother or fetus, and the rash does not usually recur in subsequent pregnancies.

Toxic erythema or erythema multiforme of pregnancy

This eruption may also begin at any time during pregnancy or in the postpartum period, although the most common time is late in pregnancy. The eruption usually affects the trunk and upper limbs. As the name implies, there may be a variety of different skin lesions, including patchy erythema, urticaria, blisters and so-called target lesions. The duration is variable and the rash may clear before the end of pregnancy. The exact cause is unknown, but there are no serious risks to the mother or fetus. If the eruption is not severe, symptomatic treatment is all that is required. If it is severe, systemic steroids may be necessary. An initial daily dose of 20 mg prednisone is usually sufficient to suppress the eruption. There is a relatively high risk of the rash recurring in subsequent pregnancies.

Herpes gestationis

This is a rare eruption in pregnancy and, unlike the papular or erythema multiforme type of eruptions, herpes gestationis has been shown to be associated with definite immunological findings. Biopsy of perilesional skin shows deposition of C3 complement and occasionally IgG at the dermoepidermal junction. The serum contains a factor which is capable of binding complement to normal skin called the HG (herpes gestationis) factor.

The rash may begin at any time during pregnancy or early in the puerperium. Characteristically, the eruption commences around the umbilicus (Figure 14.20) and then gradually spreads to the trunk and thighs. If it is severe, it may become generalized to involve the face, palms and soles. The eruption is polymorphic and, although it begins as a papular or urticarial rash, blisters usually appear and some may be large. The rash tends to persist until the pregnancy is over and possibly for a few weeks postpartum. There is a high incidence of recurrence in subsequent pregnancies. Fortunately, there is no serious risk to the mother or fetus although, if the rash is severe, labor may be induced prematurely.

Treatment is symptomatic if the eruption is not severe; otherwise, systemic steroids at the dosage recommended for erythema multiforme of pregnancy should be effective in suppressing the rash.

EPIDERMOLYSIS BULLOSA

This rather cumbersome name is used to describe a group of congenital blistering disorders that are all genetically determined. In the simple form, there is spontaneous blister formation on the hands and feet from birth and later in life at sites of even slight trauma to the skin. In this form, the blisters heal and leave no scars. In the more severe forms, there may be scarring and subsequent contractual deformity of the hands and feet. The teeth and nails (Figure 14.21) may also be abnormal in certain forms of epidermolysis bullosa. The more severe forms may involve the mucous membranes of the mouth, pharynx and esophagus, with the most serious complication being esophageal stricture.

Treatment

In the simple form, no treatment is usually required, although topical steroids may shorten the duration of the blisters. In the more severe forms, the disorder can be improved by systemic steroids, but any benefit has to be weighed against the complications of long-term steroid therapy.

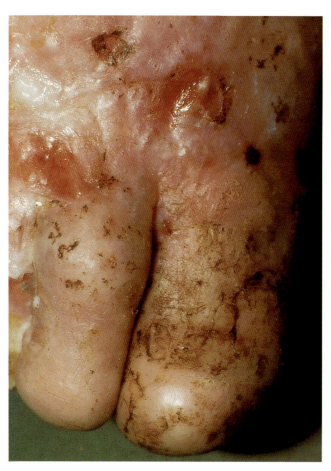

Figure 14.21 Loss of nails and blisters, erosions and scarring in epidermolysis bullosa

15

Malignant conditions of the skin

BASAL CELL EPITHELIOMA

This is sometimes referred to as a basal cell carcinoma or by the common name of rodent ulcer. Basal cell epithelioma is the most common malignant tumor of the skin. It usually occurs on the face, most usually below the eyes or on the sides of the nose (Figure 15.1). Basal cell epithelioma appears to be induced by ultraviolet light as the condition is much more common in countries like South Africa and Australia. The degree of pigmentation of the skin is also an important factor, the tumor being more frequent in fair-skinned people and rarely developing in blacks. Basal cell epithelioma is sometimes also seen in the skin many years after radiotherapy for non-malignant conditions, e.g. tinea capitis, but fortunately the use of radiotherapy for non-malignant skin conditions is now, or should be, a thing of the past. Multiple basal cell epitheliomata, usually on the trunk, are seen many years after prolonged arsenic therapy (Figure 15.2) but, again fortunately, this is becoming rare. It may take 30 or 40 years for basal cell epitheliomata to appear after radiotherapy or arsenic.

Basal cell epithelioma is usually a condition of middle-aged and elderly persons, but very rarely may be seen in younger people, usually in those of European descent who have lived in countries which have a great deal of strong sunshine. It may occur in children or teenagers as part of a genetically determined disorder associated with skeletal abnormalities.

Clinical presentations

Ulcer
The most common morphology is for the lesion to begin as a small papule which then spreads outwards, leaving a central ulcer (Figure 15.1). Telangiectasia may be seen in the raised and pearl-colored edges which are characteristic of basal cell epithelioma (Figure 15.3). Once the lesion ulcerates, it bleeds and patients often present with a persistent scab which fails to heal (Figures 15.1 and 15.4). If this is the case, the edges should be care-

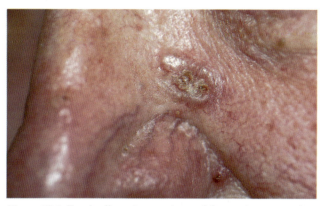

Figure 15.1 *Basal cell carcinoma at one of the most common sites. There is a raised pearly edge and central ulcer*

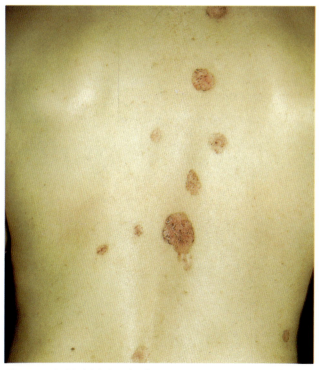

Figure 15.2 *Multiple basal cell carcinomata on the trunk following previous arsenic treatment for psoriasis*

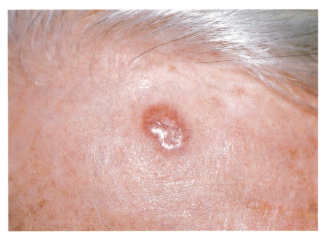

Figure 15.3 *Basal cell carcinoma. Pearly plaque with central depression and telangiectasia*

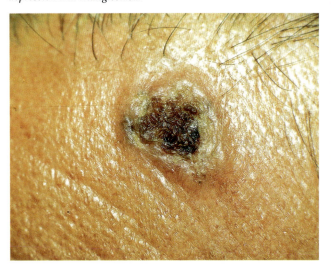

Figure 15.4 *Basal cell carcinoma. Persistent scab on the forehead with a raised pearly edge*

fully examined to see if they are raised and pearly (Figures 15.1 and 15.4). If in doubt, the scab should be removed with a pair of forceps. If left untreated, the lesion will spread over the skin in an annular fashion and inwards to involve the underlying structures.

Cystic type
Occasionally, there is no ulceration but a continual enlargement, and the presenting feature is then a cystic pearl-colored lesion (Figure 15.5) with an irregular surface and no ulcer. Telangiectasia can usually be seen on the surface.

Morpheic type
This is a relatively rare form, but can present diagnostic difficulties if it is not known. The presenting feature is a firm whitish plaque usually on the face (Figure 15.6). There may or may not be ulceration. This type of lesion is due to a fibrotic reaction to the carcinoma with an attempt to heal. It is very slow-growing and persistent. Occasional scarring in a basal cell epithelioma may be seen. If features of the original lesion are still visible, the diagnosis should be easier to establish.

Pigmented type
Occasionally, the cystic or classical ulcer becomes pigmented (Figure 15.7), when it may be difficult to distinguish the lesion from a malignant melanoma, particularly if the whole structure is pigmented.

Superficial type
This is a form of basal carcinoma usually seen on the trunk (Figure 15.2). The lesion tends not to be invasive (hence its name) but to spread on the surface in all directions. The patient usually presents with a discoid erythematous lesion, which may have small ulcers in it and a raised pearly edge (Figure 15.8).

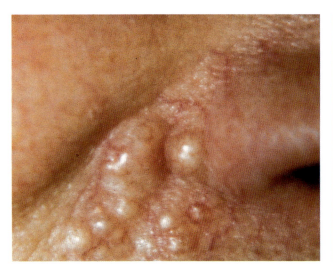

Figure 15.5 *Cystic basal cell carcinoma. A group of pearly colored papules with no ulceration*

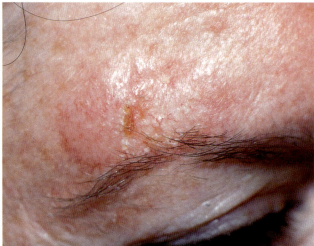

Figure 15.6 *Morpheic basal cell carcinoma. Firm whitish plaque above the eyebrow*

Prognosis

The prognosis of a basal cell carcinoma is usually excellent because it does not metastasize and is very slow-growing. Thus, if the patient seeks advice early, there should be a complete cure. If the lesions are left untreated, they may prove fatal after many years as they will erode deeper structures and will then often prove to be untreatable.

Treatment

Radiotherapy

Before radiotherapy, the lesion should be biopsied to confirm the clinical diagnosis. If radiotherapy is carried out at a reputable center, then the cure rate is of the order of 95%. This treatment is simple and is probably the treatment of choice for elderly patients. However, when dealing with younger persons, it should be remembered that radiotherapy given in a therapeutic dose for carcinoma will probably produce scarring and telangiectasia in the site 5–10 years later.

Surgery

Excision is the treatment of choice in younger persons and offers a cure rate of 95% in competent hands.

Curettage and cautery

For lesions less than 1 cm in diameter, it has been shown that a 90% cure rate can be produced using this type of treatment. Although the recurrence rate is higher than with surgery or radiotherapy, the cosmetic result with small lesions may be better.

Topical cytotoxic drugs

5-Fluorouracil has been used in the treatment of the superficial type of lesion. However, the cure rate is low and the agent certainly has no part in the treatment of the other types of basal cell carcinomata.

SQUAMOUS CELL EPITHELIOMA

The common sites for squamous cell epitheliomata are the exposed areas of skin (Figure 15.9) and lips. The backs of the hands (Figure 15.10), pinnae and lips (Figure 15.11) appear to be particularly prone to develop squamous cell epitheliomata. Because the lesions are more common on exposed rather than unexposed skin, sunlight has been incriminated as the cause of these lesions as seen with basal cell epitheliomas. However, squamous cell lesions are common on the lips and backs of the hands, and these are extremely rare sites for basal cell lesions. Squamous cell epitheliomata also occur at sites of chronic trauma and in some chronic skin disorders, e.g. discoid lupus erythematosus.

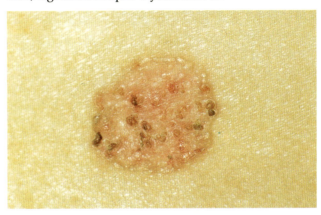

Figure 15.8 *Superficial basal cell carcinoma. Usually found on the trunk and shoulders, the lesion spreads laterally rather then inwardly. The edge is pearly, but the center tends to be red and scaly with small scabs or superficial ulcers*

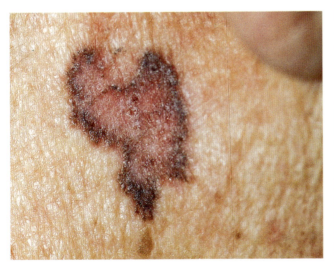

Figure 15.7 *Pigmented basal cell carcinoma. The edge of the lesion is raised and pigmented*

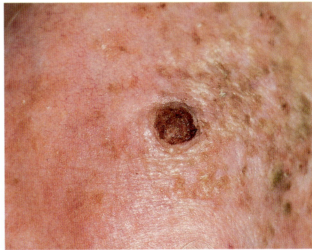

Figure 15.9 *Squamous cell carcinoma presenting as a persistent ulcer on the forehead*

Clinical features

The epithelioma begins as a small nodule which grows to form an oval or circular tumor (Figure 15.10). The lesion may break down and present as an ulcer (Figure 15.9) usually, but not always, with rolled edges. It may alternatively present as a scabbed nodule (Figure 15.10). On the lip, it may present as a small *persistent* fissure or ulcer (Figure 15.11) and such lesions should be biopsied.

Prognosis

Although this type of carcinoma has an excellent prognosis compared with carcinomata involving internal organs, it does not have as good a prognosis as do basal cell epitheliomata. The squamous cell lesion has the ability to metastasize. However, if it is treated early, the prognosis is good.

Treatment

The diagnosis should be established by biopsy and treatment is then by surgery or radiotherapy, or both.

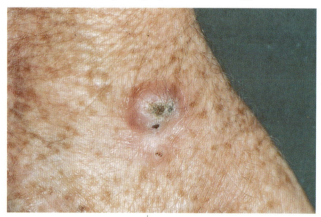

Figure 15.10 *Squamous cell carcinoma on the back of the hand presenting as a nodular lesion with a superficial ulcer*

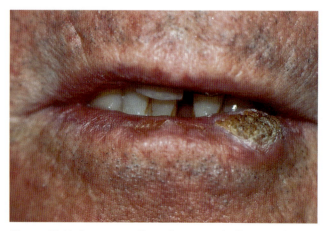

Figure 15.11 *Squamous cell carcinoma on the lip, an infiltrated ulcerated lesion*

KERATOACANTHOMA

Although this lesion is not malignant, it is convenient to discuss it here because it is often the differential diagnosis when considering basal and squamous cell carcinomata.

Keratoacanthoma is not uncommon. It presents as a small papule which rapidly grows in size over a period of 3 months. The lesion is often raised 0.5 cm above the surrounding skin surface and is usually 1–2 cm in diameter. The edges are rolled and there is a central depression with a thickened keratin plug (Figure 15.12). If this becomes detached, the lesion may well be similar to an ulcerating epithelioma. If left untreated, the keratoacanthoma will maintain the size achieved during its 3-month growing period for a further 3 months and then involute after another 3 months.

Treatment

Because of the differential diagnosis, it is important that keratoacanthomata are biopsied to establish the correct diagnosis. Once this has been done, it would be acceptable to leave the lesion alone and await its spontaneous resolution. However, because the most common site is the face, the patient will often ask for treatment. If the lesion is 1 cm or less in diameter, then curettage and cautery are the simplest treatment. With larger lesions, radiotherapy will be necessary. The cause of keratoacanthomata is as yet unknown.

MALIGNANT MELANOMA

This is a relatively rare tumor compared with basal cell carcinomata, although there has been an increase in the incidence of malignant melanoma over the last 20 years. Although not proven, this is thought to be due to increased exposure to sunlight. The malignant

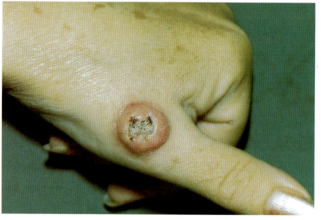

Figure 15.12 *Keratoacanthoma. Raised reddish nodule with a central keratin plug*

melanoma may occur anywhere on the skin surface, but there is a higher incidence on the legs in females and on the back in males compared to other parts of the body.

Malignant melanomata do *not* always arise in pre-existing moles or pigmented nevi, but the percentage arising from moles and that arising at sites with no preceding lesion are not known.

Clinical features

The lesion is usually, but *not always,* pigmented (Figure 15.13). If any of the following features are reported, then malignant melanoma should be suspected:

(1) An increase in size of a pigmented lesion. There may also be satellite pigmented lesions (Figure 15.14);

(2) An alteration in pigmentation of the lesion. The skin surrounding the lesion may also show alteration of pigmentation, either an increase (Figure 15.15) or decrease; and

(3) Ulceration or bleeding of a pigmented or non-pigmented lesion.

Prognosis

There is now reasonable evidence to show that the deeper the lesion, both histologically and in actual measurement, the worse the prognosis. Thus, clinically, those lesions which are not, or only just, palpable have a good prognosis while those which are nodular have a poorer prognosis.

Some melanomata tend to spread laterally and give rise to macular areas of pigmentation; this type of lesion is referred to as a superficial spreading melanoma (Figure 15.16). Lesions invading the deeper tissues are referred to as nodular melanomas (Figure 15.15).

However, what determines whether melanomata spread laterally or become invasive is not known. In addition, there is variation in the prognosis among patients with tumors of similar depths of invasion.

Hormonal and immunological factors play some part in the prognosis, and appear to influence the spread and growth of metastases.

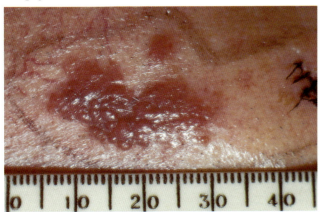

Figure 15.13 *Amelanotic melanoma with satellite lesions*

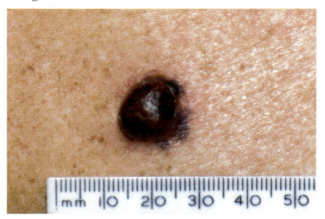

Figure 15.15 *Nodular malignant melanoma. Irregular areas of macular pigmentation extend from the base of the nodule*

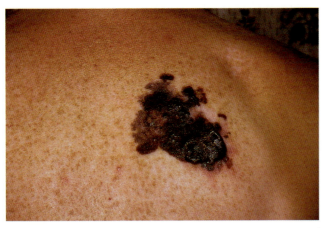

Figure 15.14 *Malignant melanoma with satellite lesions and variable pigmentation*

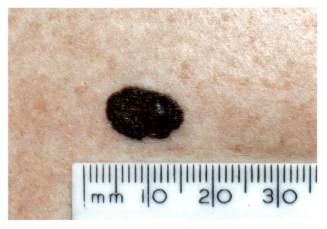

Figure 15.16 *Superficial spreading malignant melanoma*

Treatment

Surgical excision is the treatment for malignant melanoma. It now appears that very wide and deep excisions do not influence the prognosis as much as other factors and therefore are not necessary. Removal of regional lymph nodes is carried out only if there is clinical evidence of involvement. If possible, regional perfusion of the affected part of the body, e.g. leg, with cytotoxic drugs is sometimes performed.

Lentigo maligna

This variant of malignant melanoma presents as a macular pigmented area usually on the face (Figure 15.17). There is a very gradual increase in size. The lesion may be present for 20–30 years before it becomes nodular and develops into a malignant melanoma. Surgical excision is necessary when the lesion becomes nodular, and is usually recommended in young persons in the macular stage. However, in the elderly, cryotherapy is often employed in the macular stage.

INTRAEPIDERMAL EPITHELIOMA

Bowen's disease

This carcinoma *in situ* is more common in women than in men. The lesion is confined to the epidermis and may not become invasive for many years. It is, however,

potentially malignant and may change to a squamous cell epithelioma. The lesion may involve any part of the skin, although the lower leg is the most common site. It usually presents as a solitary reddish-brown scaly plaque (Figure 15.18). The edges may be slightly raised

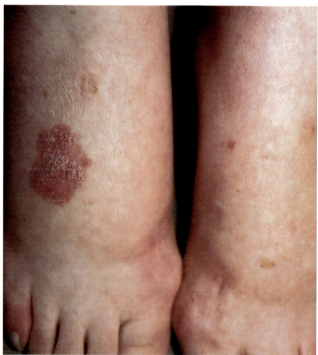

Figure 15.18 Bowen's disease. A unilateral persistent red scaly patch on the foot

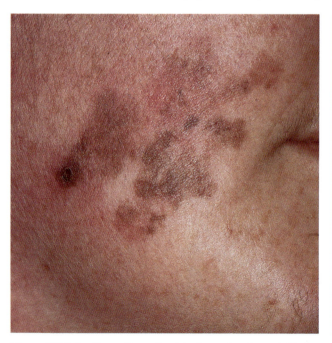

Figure 15.17 Lentigo maligna. Persistent macular pigmented lesion on the face. The lesion gradually enlarges over the years

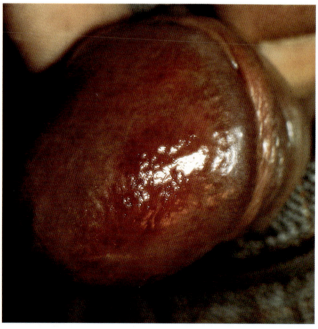

Figure 15.19 Erythroplasia of Queyrat. Persistent red moist area on the glans penis

with papillomatous growth. It is very slow-growing but persistent.

Treatment
The diagnosis should be established by biopsy. If the lesion is small, it can be removed by curettage and cautery or excision; if it is over 2 cm in diameter, a graft will probably be necessary after surgery. Radiotherapy, cryotherapy or topical 5-fluorouracil may also be used.

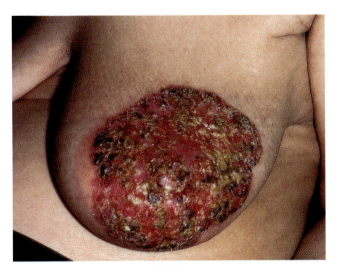

Figure 15.20 Paget's disease of the breast

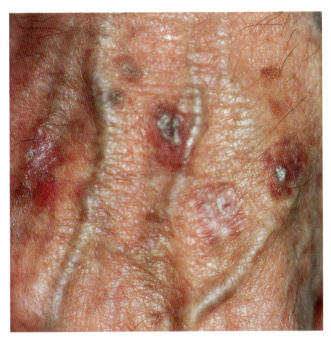

Figure 15.21 Actinic keratoses on the back of the hand presents as a persistent grayish scaly lesion

Erythroplasia of Queyrat

This is the name given to intraepidermal carcinoma of the glans penis (Figure 15.19). The lesion presents as a persistent red moist area with a velvety appearance.

Treatment
The treatment of choice is topical 5-fluorouracil. This is usually successful, and radiotherapy and surgery are not necessary.

Paget's disease

This is also an intraepidermal carcinoma. The most common site is the nipple and areola of the female breast in the middle-aged. It usually presents as unilateral erythema and scaling, and looks eczematous (Figure 15.20). In the later stages, there may be destruction of the nipple. Unfortunately, the condition is usually part of an intraductal carcinoma and treatment is therefore mastectomy.

ACTINIC KERATOSES

These lesions are not in themselves malignant, but may eventually turn into squamous cell epitheliomata. As the name implies, they are found on the areas of skin exposed to light, and are more common in fair-skinnned people and in those living in climates which have a great deal of sunshine.

The lesions are discrete and raised with a thick scaly surface (Figure 15.21). They are grayish-brown and usually numerous. There are usually other signs of excessive exposure to ultraviolet light, such as pigmented patches and thinning of the skin. The top of the lesion may be knocked off by trauma to leave a small superficial ulcer.

Treatment

The lesions are purely epidermal and may be treated with cryotherapy or electrocautery. If the lesions are numerous, the best treatment is with 5-fluorouracil.

SKIN LYMPHOMA

Cutaneous T-cell lymphoma

Previously termed 'mycosis fungoides', this lymphoma is confined to the skin in the early stages and continues predominantly as a skin disorder, but may eventually involve the internal organs. It is rare in childhood, but may begin in early adult life or subsequently at any age. In the early stages, the disease presents as persistent erythematous scaly patches (Figure 15.22) on any part of the skin and may resemble eczema or psoriasis. The lesions may persist in this form for many years before becoming infiltrated nodules and plaques (Figure 15.23) which may eventually ulcerate. Although the disease is invariably fatal, the course of the disease may occur over many years, and elderly patients frequently die due to other causes.

Treatment

In the early stages, the lesions can be clinically cleared and irritation suppressed by Group III and IV topical steroids. However, these drugs do not affect the malignant cells in the skin, but only suppress the accompanying inflammatory reaction. PUVA (*see* Chapter 25) and topical nitrogen mustards are both used to treat cutaneous T-cell lymphoma in the early stages. However, whether these treatments affect the ultimate prognosis is not known, but both treatments certainly clear the lesions. In more severe stages with tumor development, radiotherapy is effective in clearing the tumors. Total body electron-beam treatment has been used to induce remissions when the disease is extensive and unresponsive to PUVA.

KAPOSI'S SARCOMA

There are two distinct patterns of Kaposi's sarcoma. The first was described in elderly subjects and usually began on the lower leg and foot. It was most commonly seen in Ashkenazi Jews. The second pattern is seen in AIDS (*see* Chapter 11).

In the elderly non-AIDS patient, Kaposi's sarcoma presents as purple nodules and plaques on the lower leg and foot (Figure 15.24). The disease usually runs a protracted course over many years with new lesions gradually appearing, but some may also involute spontaneously. The lymph nodes, mucosal surfaces and internal organs, particularly the small intestine, may all be affected.

In the past, Kaposi's sarcoma was thought to be a multifocal neoplastic lesion arising from the capillary cells. More recently, it has been suggested that the process begins in the perivascular tissues. Viruses, genetic factors and altered immunity have all been implicated as being of etiological significance.

If the lesions are only confined to one limb and are not causing significant pain or discomfort, no treatment is necessary. If there are symptoms, the lesions may respond to radiotherapy, and surgical excision of individual lesions is sometimes necessary. Cytotoxic drugs have been used in extensive disease.

OTHER LYMPHOMAS

Sarcomata, leukemia and Hodgkin's disease all may appear as infiltrated papules or plaques in the skin which occasionally are the presenting feature of these disorders. The diagnosis is established by biopsy.

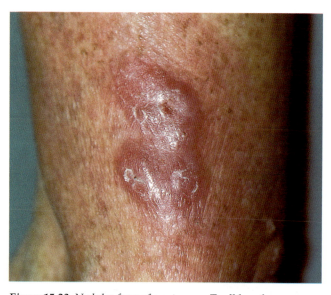

Figure 15.23 Nodular form of a cutaneous T-cell lymphoma

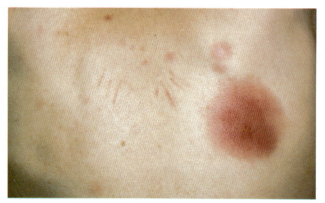

Figure 15.22 Asymmetrical reddish-brown patch on the back, one of the forms of a cutaneous T-cell lymphona

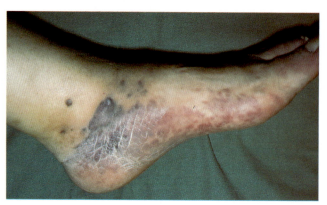

Figure 15.24 Infiltrated purplish plaques and nodules in Kaposi's sarcoma

16

Acne and rosacea

ACNE

Acne is now used synonymously, with and has virtually replaced, the term 'acne vulgaris'. Acne is essentially a disorder of adolescence. It has been estimated that up to 80% of all adolescents will have some degree of acne, varying from a few comedones to severe cystic lesions. The most common age of onset is at puberty, but acne may appear 1–2 years before. However, it should also be appreciated that acne may begin after puberty and even in the third and fourth decades (particularly in women). The natural history is variable. The disorder may last only a few months in the mildest forms but, usually, it will persist from puberty to the late teens or early twenties. In some patients the acne will persist into adult life even until middle age, although the severity of the disease will probably be less. It is not possible to predict at what age it will resolve, and caution should be exercised in telling patients they will grow out of it!

Pathology

Acne is a disease which affects the pilosebaceous unit. The primary defect appears to be excess keratin production at the opening of the pilosebaceous unit which prevents the escape of sebum. A comedo (blackhead) subsequently forms; this is a mass of keratin and sebum. The upper portion of the blackhead is darkened by melanin from melanocytes in the adjacent epidermis; the lower part of the comedo remains a yellowish-white color. Comedones are sometimes referred to as 'open' or 'closed', i.e. not reaching the surface of the skin to be extruded. In the latter instances, the sebaceous gland continues to produce sebum, and the gland begins to swell and eventually ruptures intradermally. The sebum which escapes into the dermis is an irritant which then leads to a foreign-body reaction. Thus, there is erythema and pus formation, and the area tends to be 'walled off' by connective tissue cells, and healing occurs with subsequent fibrosis. The degree of inflammation and subsequent scarring varies greatly between patients even if the sebaceous glands rupture, and may well depend on the composition of sebum and on how irritating the sebum is to the surrounding tissues. In some cases of severe inflammation, cyst formation occurs, the so-called acne cyst. It should be stressed that the pathology of acne does not appear to be initiated or continued by bacteria.

Etiology

The basic causes of acne are not yet known, but it is undoubtedly in some way related to hormones because of the onset at or around the time of puberty and the fact that acne is often worse premenstrually. However, it appears that an end-organ effect rather than the circulating levels of hormones are the cause of acne.

Clinical features

Site
Acne lesions occur on the face, upper chest, on the back above the waistline, shoulders and occasionally neck (Figures 16.1–16.3). These tend to be the areas which have more sebaceous glands per unit surface area than other parts of the skin. The lesion may occur only on the face or on parts of the face, i.e. forehead, cheeks or along the chin, with sparing of the trunk. Conversely, the lesions may occur only on the trunk with no involvement of the face. The back is more commonly affected than the chest and usually more severely.

Types of lesion
The initial lesion is the comedo or blackhead (Figure 16.4). If the comedones are closed, then the gland ruptures and, depending on the degree of inflammation, the clinical appearance varies. If the inflammatory reaction is not severe, a red papule forms (Figure 16.5); in more severe inflammatory reactions, clinically visible pustules appear (Figure 16.6). Finally, cyst formation may occur (Figure 16.7), with cysts up to 2 cm in diameter. Because of the inflammation, the skin surrounding the lesions is red compared with the unin-

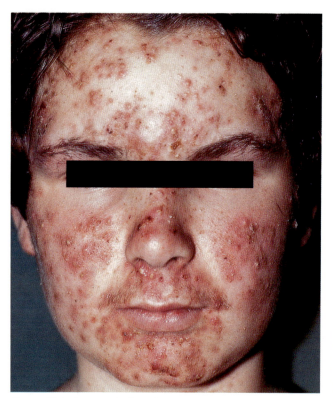

Figure 16.1 Acne on the face, the most common site

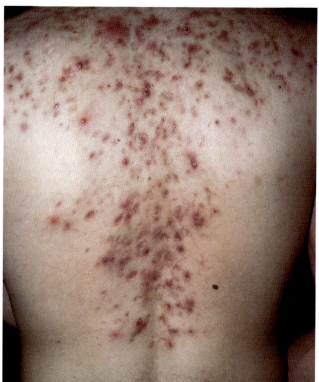

Figure 16.3 Acne on the back may occur lower than on the chest, but usually remains above the waist

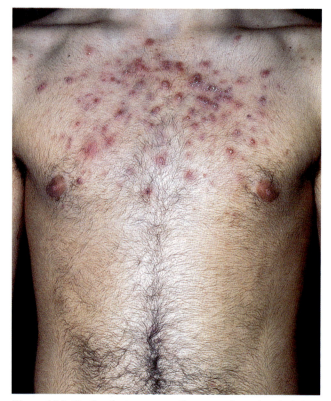

Figure 16.2 On the chest, acne usually occurs above the nipple line

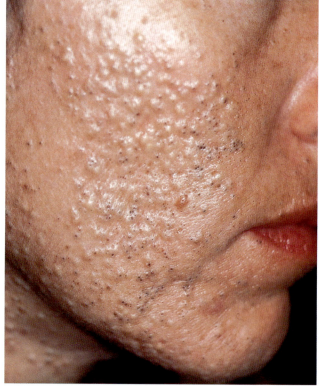

Figure 16.4 Comedones or blackheads in acne

volved skin. If the inflammatory response has been severe, there is fibrosis and scarring with scars often appearing as small depressed pits (Figure 16.8). Occasionally, as with other scars, keloid formation may occur (Figure 16.9). It should be stressed that just as the sites of involvement vary between patients, so may the types of lesion, i.e. some patients have only comedones while others have only papules and pustules, and some have only cysts. Alternatively, there may be patients with all types of lesions. The reasons for such variation are not known.

Management and treatment

A large number of people do not seek treatment for their acne and are aware that the disorder has no internal consequences. However, because the lesions are unsightly and most frequently occur during adolescence, many do ask for help. It appears that the patient's personality is important in deciding whether to seek medical advice. If a patient does ask for treatment, the worst possible approach is to tell them they will grow

out of their troubles by the time they are 21 years old and therefore do nothing for them.

General measures

Diet
In the past, great emphasis has been placed on diet, and patients have been advised to cut out chocolates, sweets and fatty meats and to reduce their fat and/or carbohydrate intake, depending on what is fashionable at the time. However, there is no worthwhile evidence as yet

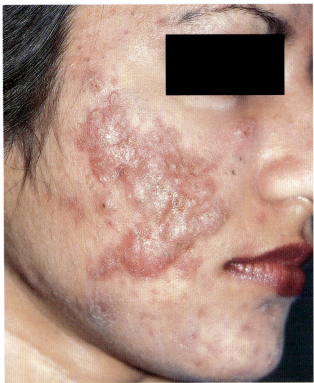

Figure 16.7 Cystic lesions on the cheek in acne

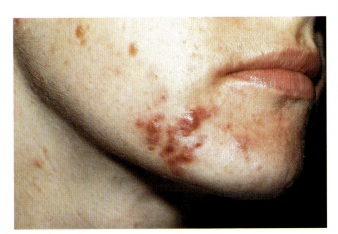

Figure 16.5 Erythematous papules on the chin in acne

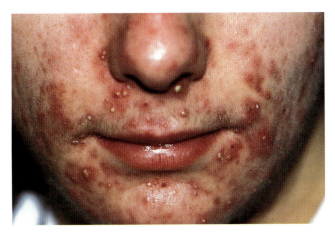

Figure 16.6 Pustules and papules in acne

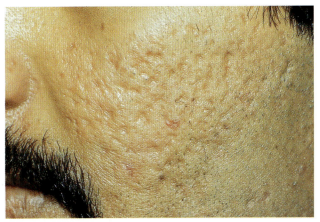

Figure 16.8 Scarring due to acne. The scars are characteristically pitted

to show that manipulation of the diet has a part to play in the management of acne.

Cleansing

It is often implied that patients with acne do not wash frequently enough. Although frequent washing with soap and water may help slightly by removing excess keratin and sebum, thereby decreasing comedo formation, the lack of washing with soap and water does not cause acne. Because acne is not primarily an infective condition, antiseptic soaps and lotions are not indicated.

Debridement

Removal of large comedones produces definite cosmetic improvement and is sometimes helpful in preventing superficial pustulation, but has no effect on deeper inflammatory lesions. Comedones should be removed after soaking the area with a hot towel for a few minutes, using a comedo extractor.

Sunlight

Ultraviolet light is often beneficial in acne probably due to the peeling effect it has on the skin, which prevents blockage of the pilosebaceous units. In summer, patients should be instructed to get some sun whenever possible.

Artificial ultraviolet light may be given in some cases if benefit is derived. Occasionally, some patients appear to be made worse by ultraviolet light, but this is more often due to heat and humidity, which causes swelling of the keratin and further blockage of the pilosebaceous units.

Topical treatment

Keratolytics

Any substance which breaks up keratin may unblock the pilosebaceous unit and allow drainage of the sebum.

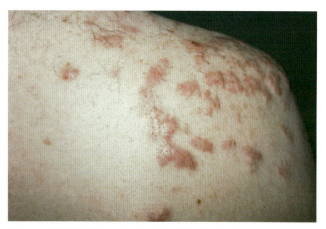

Figure 16.9 *Keloids on the shoulder following inflammatory lesions of acne*

Sulfur 1–5%, salicylic acid or resorcinol, in either a spirit or cream base, have all been used in the past and may have a beneficial effect on acne. These preparations should be applied at night. It is advisable to start with a 1% preparation and increase the strength if the patient can tolerate the resultant skin soreness.

Benzoyl peroxide is another keratolytic used in many proprietary preparations at strengths varying from 2.5–10%, usually in a cream or gel base. The point of using keratolytics is to achieve a satisfactory clinical response without causing excessive dryness and peeling of the skin. Most topical preparations are useful only for comedones, and superficial papules and pustules.

Retinoids

Two topical preparations, one of isotretinoin and the other of tretinoin, are available for the treatment of acne. They act by increasing exfoliation of corneocytes of the stratum corneum. The result is similar therefore to keratolytics. Topical retinoids tend to be irritants and therefore tend to cause redness, peeling and soreness, which some patients are unable to tolerate.

Antibiotics

The role of topical antibiotics in the treatment of acne is debatable. Some studies have claimed that they are as effective as systemic antibiotics while others have shown that they are no more effective than keratolytics. The antibiotics most commonly used are clindamycin, erythromycin and tetracycline. Many microbiologists do not support the widespread use of antibiotics because of the risk of developing resistant organisms.

Systemic treatment

Antibiotics

Antibiotics are usually the first line of systemic treatment. Tetracyclines and erythromycin are most commonly used for acne. All have to be taken for weeks before any significant improvement is apparent. Thus, patients are usually only reviewed after 6–8 weeks. If there is no improvement after 3 months, then a change of treatment either to different antibiotics or non-antibiotic oral treatment should be considered.

The initial dose of tetracycline or erythromycin ranges from 250–500 mg twice daily. If significant improvement is obtained, it may be possible to reduce the dose and maintain the improvement. Antibiotic treatment may have to be continued for many months or even years while the disease is active.

Antibiotics do not alter the natural history of the condition, but appear to be only suppressive. The tetracyclines minocycline and doxycycline are currently in vogue as they can be taken as a once-daily dose, but they are considerably more expensive than tetracyline.

Hormones and antihormones

Androgens and progesterone stimulate sebaceous glands and therefore make acne worse whereas estrogens tend to suppress their activity and thus improve acne.

Cyproterone acetate is an antiandrogen that suppresses sebaceous gland activity and improves acne, but can only be used in women. Cyproterone acetate should be combined with an estrogen to prevent conception, and the patient should be told that the two drugs combined act as a contraceptive. The regimen consists of cyproterone acetate 50–100 mg daily for 10 days and ethinylestradiol 35 μg daily for 21 days, both drugs commencing on the fifth day of the menstrual cycle. When the ethinylestradiol is finished, there should be a break for 7 days before beginning another course.

This regimen can be given for a number of months. It is not effective in all patients, but over 70% show significant improvement, usually during the second month of treatment. However, if the acne is still active, there will be a recurrence usually a few months after the drugs are stopped; further courses may be necessary.

The current contraceptive pills have either no effect on acne, or may aggravate or improve it. The response depends on the particular progesterone and the amount of estrogen in the pill. Contraceptives containing the progesterone norgesterol tend to aggravate and sometimes precipitate acne. The estrogen in the pill improves acne and, thus, the greater the amount of estrogen, the better the effect on acne. Clearly, the balance between the estrogen and progesterone is important and patients vary in their response to progesterones and estrogens. As a general rule, patients with acne or a past history of acne should be given pills with at least 30 μg of ethinylestradiol (or an equivalent estrogen content) and the progesterone norgesterol should be avoided. Oral contraceptive pills containing only progesterone tend to aggravate acne and should also be avoided.

There is now a contraceptive containing ethinylestradiol 35 μg and cyproterone acetate 2 mg, and is taken for 21 days of the menstrual cycle. It is possible to use the cyproterone acetate because, as well as being an antiandrogen, it also has progesterone-like properties, although any effect on the sebaceous glands is outweighed by the antiandrogen effect.

Oral corticosteroids are occasionally used in acne in cases of severe and widespread cystic acne of sudden onset, usually around puberty. The severe reaction in the skin is accompanied by fever and leukocytosis.

Retinoids

The retinoid isotretinoin is probably the most effective currently available treatment for acne. In a significant proportion of patients, it appears to actually cure acne, i.e. no recurrence when treatment is discontinued.

Isotretinoin is usually reserved for patients with severe or persistent acne that has failed to respond adequately to antibiotics. It may also be considered for patients whose acne relapses quickly when antibiotics are discontinued. The isotretinoin dosage ranges from 0.5–1.0 mg/kg/day. The higher the dose, the greater the chances of cure. The course lasts 16 weeks and treatment should not be stopped sooner even if the acne has cleared. If treatment is discontinued after shorter periods, there is likely to be a recurrence of the acne.

Isotretinoin treatment has side effects. The most important is that it is teratogenic, therefore female patients must be instructed on this point before commencing treatment. The most common side effect is cheilitis (Figure 16.10), which may occur to some extent in all patients. Dry skin predisposing to eczema is common particularly on the face and upper limbs.

Other side effects include mild hair loss (which is reversible), dry eyes and nose bleeds. Cheilitis and dry skin are treated with ample moisturizers and emollients. Occasionally, weak (Group I) topical steroids are necessary for the eczema.

A non-medical problem associated with isotretinoin therapy is that it is expensive, and this unfortunately will limit its use.

Isotretinoin appears to be effective in acne as it reduces the size of the sebacous gland and, as a consequence, sebum production. How isotretinoin produces these effects on the sebaceous glands is not known.

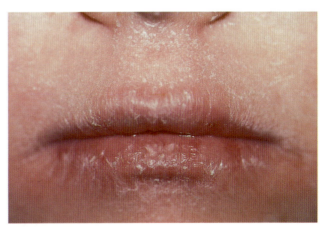

Figure 16.10 *Cheilitis due to isotretinoin, the most common side effect*

Intralesional therapy
The most effective way to treat acne cysts is with intralesional triamcinolone. This appears to counteract the inflammation and prevent scarring.

INFANTILE ACNE

Very occasionally, typical acne lesions may appear on the cheeks of infants during the first few months of life and then subside. This is probably the effect of maternal hormones.

ROSACEA

This is a disorder of young and middle-aged adults. Although the cause is unknown, it appears to be a disorder of the blood vessels in the skin on the face. Rosacea only affects the face. It may affect all of, or only parts of, the face.

The characteristic lesions are ery-thema, papules, pustules and telangiectasia (Figures 16.11 and 16.12). The erythema and telangiectasia may affect only the cheeks and nose, and the papules and pustules may occur only on the cheeks, forehead or chin. All or some of these areas may be involved.

In the early stages, there may be an exaggerated flushing of the skin in response to heat, certain types of food or emotional stress. Subsequently, this erythema persists and telangiectasia begins to appear. The next stage is the development of papules and pustules.

A variation of rosacea is rhinophyma (Figure 16.13). This is thickening of the skin of the nose with associated gross hypertrophy of the sebaceous glands. It is usually the lower third of the nose which enlarges as a hyperemic lobulated mass of tissue pitted by the orifices of the sebaceous glands.

Ocular involvement may occur in rosacea (Figure 16.14). This usually takes the form of rosacea keratitis. The patient may initially complain of sore eyes but, subsequently, pain and photophobia develop.

In addition to the keratitis, there may be blepharitis, conjunctivitis, iritis and even episcleritis. If these are left untreated, the keratitis may lead to ulceration and corneal opacities.

The natural history of rosacea is variable, but it tends to be a chronic disorder persisting for a number of years.

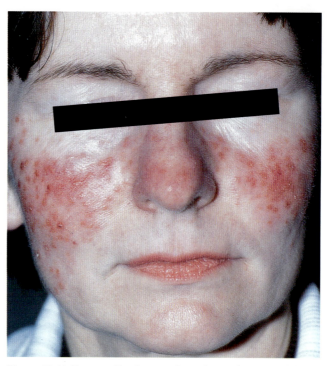

Figure 16.11 Rosacea. Erythema and papules on the nose and cheeks

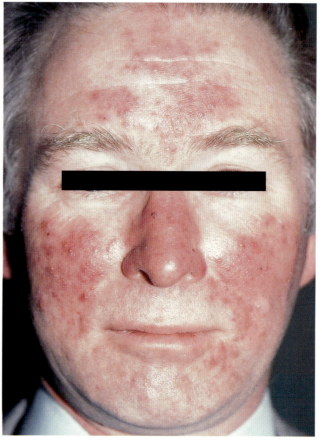

Figure 16.12 Erythema, papules and pustules in rosacea

Treatment

General advice

In the past, it was often assumed that patients with rosacea also had chronic gastritis and, for this reason, they were told to omit alcohol, spicy food, and strong tea and coffee. The benefit obtained from cutting down on these substances probably occurs because they tend to cause reflex vasodilatation of the blood vessels of the skin of the face. There is no evidence that patients with rosacea do in fact have gastritis.

Topical measures

The only drug (when used topically) which has a significant effect on rosacea is metronidazole. This is usually used as a cream or gel. Proprietary preparations are now available. They should be applied twice daily for at least 2 months. Relapse rates are high when treatment is discontinued.

It is important not to prescribe topical steroids for rosacea, particularly Groups II, III or IV. Although these preparations may initially have a beneficial effect, there may well be a rebound flare-up of the rosacea when the preparation is stopped.

Systemic therapy

The most effective treatment at present for rosacea is with tetracyclines. As with acne, the mechanism of action is not understood.

The regimen is similar to that for acne, usually 250 mg twice daily for at least 6 weeks, and the dose is then titrated against the activity of the disease process. Many patients can be controlled with a tetracycline dose as low as 250 mg twice weekly, but may relapse when the drug is stopped.

A small proportion of patients will not respond to tetracyclines; in these cases, a course of metronidazole should be given. The dose is 200 mg daily for 6 weeks, which is then titrated against the severity of the condition as with tetracyclines.

The eye complications of rosacea are best cared for by an ophthalmologist because of their potentially serious sequelae, but these are also often helped by systemic tetracyclines.

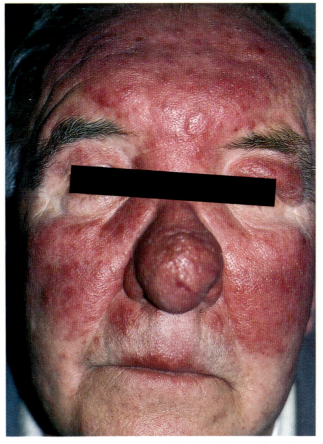

Figure 16.13 Rhinophyma associated with erythema and papules on the cheeks and forehead

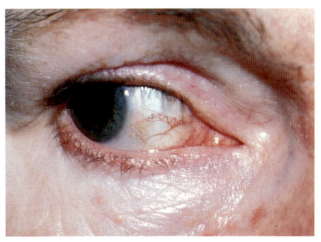

Figure 16.14 Eye involvement in rosacea

17

Lupus erythematosus, scleroderma and dermatomyositis

These three diseases are among the *collagen disorders* and have specific manifestations; there may also be systemic involvement.

LUPUS ERYTHEMATOSUS

Two diseases carry this name, the so-called chronic discoid form and the acute systemic variety. It is still uncertain whether there is any direct relationship between them (other than in name). Some authorities consider that, on occasions, the chronic form may pass into the systemic form while others maintain they are two entirely separate entities.

Chronic discoid lupus erythematosus

This disorder affects men and women equally, and usually commences in early or middle adult life. It tends to be a chronic disease lasting many years, but the natural history has been altered as it is now readily controlled by potent topical corticosteroids.

Sites of involvement
The most common site of involvement is the face (Figure 17.1), and the disorder frequently appears for the first time after exposure to sunlight. Lesions may also appear on the scalp, ears, neck, hands (Figure 17.2) and very occasionally on the arms and upper trunk. The lesions may be solitary, few in number or numerous and, even in the last instance, they tend not to be symmetrical. Discoid lupus erythematosus may affect the fingers and toes and is sometimes referred to as chilblain lupus erythematosus.

Morphology
In the early stages, the lesion is a well-defined red plaque (Figure 17.3). The surface is scaly (Figure 17.2) and there is follicular dilatation. The scale extends into

the follicles and, if the scale from a lesion is removed in one piece, the follicular scales then appear as small prominent spines on the undersurface. However, if the superficial scale has been shed but the keratin remains in the hair follicles, the dilated follicles appear to be plugged with keratin (Figures 17.3 and 17.4). The size of the plaque is variable; it may be as small as 0.5 cm, but

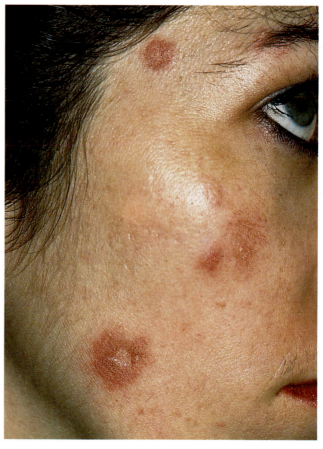

Figure 17.1 *Discoid lupus erythematosus on the face. Red infiltrated patches and the lowermost lesion shows scarring*

is frequently 2–3 cm in diameter. Occasionally, the lesions merge to form a large confluent plaque involving the entire forehead or cheek. As the disease progresses, there is scarring (Figures 17.1, 17.5 and 17.6) and atrophic change in the skin; telangiectasia and pigmentary changes may occur. Occasionally, the lesions break down and ulcerate and, very rarely, after many years may progress to a squamous cell carcinoma.

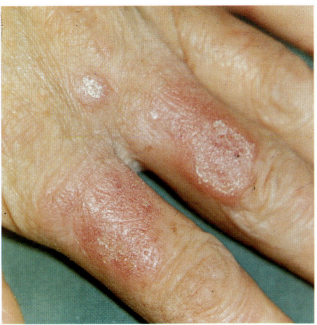

Figure 17.2 *Discoid lupus erythematosus on the fingers. Well demarcated lesions with a scaly surface*

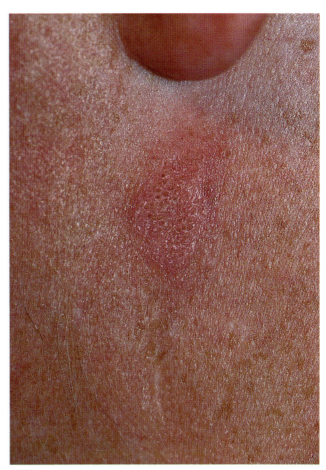

Figure 17.4 *Follicular plugging in discoid lupus erythematosus*

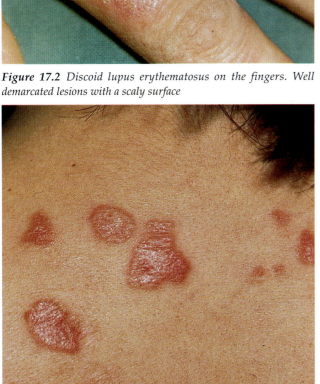

Figure 17.3 *Red plaques with follicular plugging on the upper back in discoid lupus erythematosus*

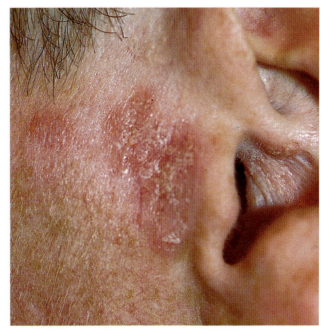

Figure 17.5 *Scarring in the center of a lesion of discoid lupus erythematosus*

The mouth or vagina are sometimes involved. At these sites, the lesions appear as persistent erosions.

If the scalp is involved, there will eventually be hair loss as there is destruction of the hair follicles (Figure 17.7). Chilblain lupus erythematosus presents as purplish patches on the fingers and toes (Figure 17.8).

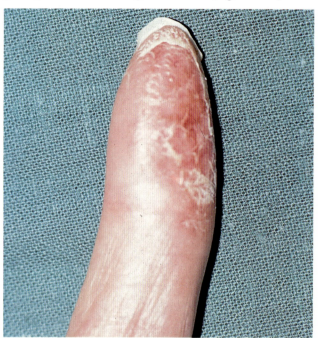

Figure 17.6 *Red scaly atrophic lesion on the finger in discoid lupus erythematosus*

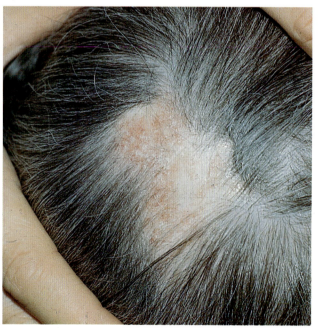

Figure 17.7 *Discoid lupus erythematosus. Red scaly scarred area in the scalp with hair loss. There is destruction of the hair follicles due to the scarring*

In the end stages of the disorder when the disease process has run its course, the site of involvement appears as white thickened scar tissue. It is not uncommon to see the disease still active at the periphery of a lesion while the center is inactive, thus giving rise to a red annular scaly lesion with a white atrophic center.

Treatment

As has already been mentioned, discoid lupus erythematosus is adversely affected by sunlight and, thus, patients should avoid sun exposure as much as possible. Sun-barrier preparations should be used for lesions on the head and neck prior to patients going outdoors during the summer months (*see* Chapter 23).

Topical steroids

The powerful topical corticosteroids (Group IV) have improved the treatment and management of chronic discoid lupus erythematosus. Many lesions will respond to twice-daily applications of these steroid preparations. The use of these drugs has to be continued until the disease process is completely suppressed. Topical steroids should be used in short courses and not indefinitely once the lesion has resolved. If there is relapse, then the steroid should be used again.

Systemic steroids

In patients with plaques resistant to topical corticosteroids, systemic steroids such as prednisone at a dose of 30 mg / day are usually effective within a few weeks. A maintenance dose of approximately 10 mg / day is sometimes necessary until the disease burns itself out.

Antimalarial drugs

Mepacrine at a dose of 100–200 mg daily is often effective at suppressing discoid lupus erythematosus. However, the drug causes yellow staining of the skin which patients may find unpleasant. Chloroquine sulfate 100 mg twice daily and hydroxychloroquine 400 mg

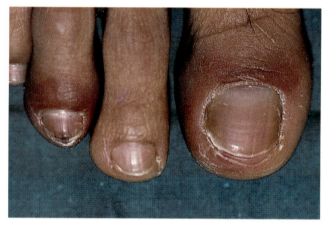

Figure 17.8 *Purplish patches on the toes in chilblain lupus erythematosus*

daily are also effective but, if used for any length of time, may cause retinal damage. Thus, these patients should be seen regularly by an ophthalmologist.

Thalidomide

In widespread disease particularly with mucous membrane involvement, thalidomide 400 mg daily is often effective.

Systemic lupus erythematosus

As the name implies, this is a systemic disorder which may or may not have cutaneous manifestations. It is essentially a vasculitis and organs may be involved either singly or together. The presenting symptoms of systemic lupus erythematosus (SLE) are numerous, but the more common are skin lesions, fever, fatigue, arthropathy, renal involvement and pleural or pericardial effusions.

Approximately half the patients with SLE have skin lesions. Although the cutaneous manifestations are not constant or regular, they may in some cases present with clinical patterns which are distinct enough to suggest the diagnosis. The face is the most common site to be involved and the 'classical' eruption is the 'butterfly' pattern across the nose and malar prominences (Figure 17.9). Initially, this is simply an erythema but, with more severe involvement, the erythema increases and approaches the appearances of a cellulitis with exudation and crusting. Frequently, the eruption is more extensive, involving all exposed areas with a diffuse erythema (Figure 17.10); it may finally become generalized, involving unexposed areas . Hair loss of a diffuse type occurs in a small percentage of patients and has been known to be the presenting symptom. The skin lesions, when they resolve, do not scar as in the chronic discoid type of LE, but often leave residual hyperpigmentation.

There is often telangiectasia on the posterior nail-folds and splinter hemorrhages on the nail bed (Figure 17.11). The knees and elbows may show erythema, telangiectasia and scaling, which may break down and

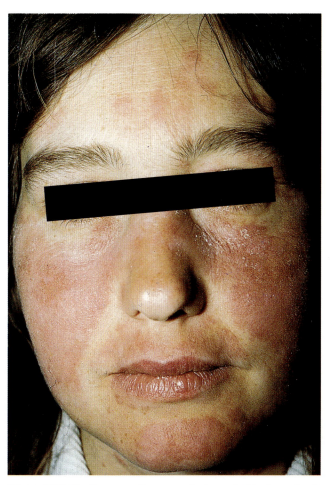

Figure 17.9 *Erythema on the nose, cheeks and chin in systemic lupus erythematosus*

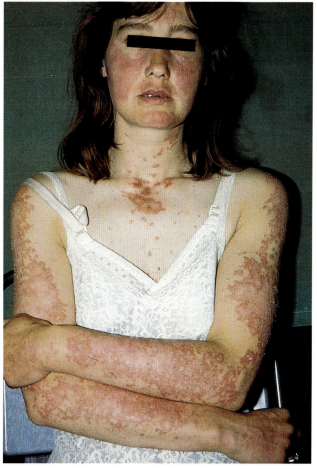

Figure 17.10 *Photosensitive eruption in systemic lupus erythematosus*

ulcerate. Occasionally, these lesions may be seen at other parts of the body. Very rarely, the presenting sign is purpura due to thrombocytopenia.

Diagnosis

Skin biopsy for routine histological studies may show only non-specific inflammatory changes. Direct immunofluorescent studies show deposition of IgG and/or IgM and C3 complement in the region of the basement membrane. This finding is also present in the uninvolved skin in sun-exposed skin. The band of immunoglobulins is much wider and more irregular than that found in pemphigoid.

Serological studies show the presence of antinuclear antibodies. These are present in all patients, but they may not appear for some time after the clinical onset of symptoms. Lupus erythematosus cells are present in approximately half the patients, but it should be remembered that they are not specific to SLE.

Treatment and prognosis

The management of SLE will vary according to the clinical extent of the disease, which organs are involved and the severity of the involvement. Systemic steroids are the most useful drugs in the acute stages of the disease, and the initial dose depends on the severity.

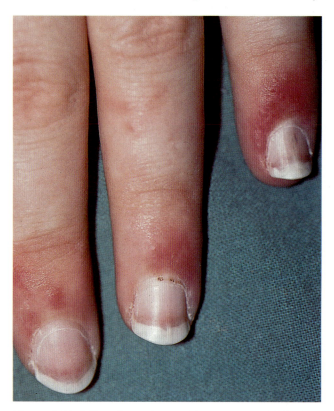

Figure 17.11 *Splinter hemorrhages of the posterior nail fold. These are thrombosed dilated capillaries. Erythema of the posterior nail fold is also a common feature in systemic lupus erythematosus*

The immunosuppressive drugs azathioprine and cyclophosphamide have been used in combination with systemic steroids, but there are conflicting reports as to their value. The antimalarial drugs chloroquine and hydroxychloroquine may be helpful in controlling the disease, but long-term use is associated with the risk of retinal damage.

Plasmapheresis has been used in severely ill patients in addition to drug therapy. Not infrequently, the disease will go into remission, when the dosages of steroids and immunosuppressive drugs can be reduced and, in some cases, stopped.

Although the cause of SLE is unknown, sunlight is best avoided as it can produce an acute exacerbation in some patients. Some drugs, such as penicillin and procainamide, have been known to produce a lupus erythematosus-like illness that is completely reversible when the drug is stopped; this induced type usually has an excellent prognosis. The prognosis for non-drug-induced SLE is variable. It may prove fatal within a short space of time whereas, in others, the disease will smolder on and result in death usually due to renal involvement. However, the disease is not invariably fatal, although the morbidity is high. In some instances, there may be acute exacerbations from time to time with general good health in between.

SCLERODERMA

As with lupus erythematosus, there are two types of scleroderma, a localized cutaneous form and a systemic form which has cutaneous manifestations.

Localized scleroderma

This is sometimes referred to as 'morphea'. It consists of hardened plaques in the dermis with overlying atrophic epidermis. The lesions may occur at any site and are usually round or oval, but sometimes linear. In the early stages, the lesion presents as a firm white plaque (Figures 17.12 and 17.13), often with a surrounding violaceous border, which subsequently becomes pigmented (Figure 17.13). If the area is particularly hairy, loss of hair will be noted. If the face is involved, there may be underlying atrophy of the muscles. There is usually no systemic involvement associated with morphea.

Prognosis and treatment

In the majority of patients, the lesions tend to improve gradually and there may be complete resolution, although this may take 5–10 years. The cause is unknown and, unfortunately, there is no effective treatment at this time.

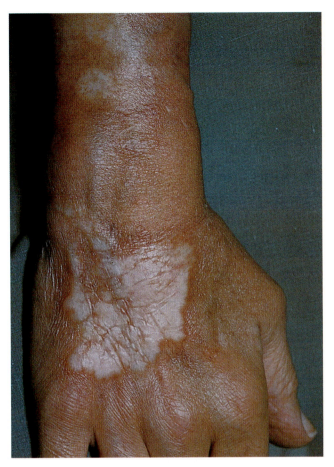

Figure 17.12 *Localized scleroderma (morphea) on the back of the hand*

Systemic scleroderma

This chronic disorder, sometimes referred to as systemic sclerosis, may involve a few or many organs. The pathological changes are more pronounced in the connective tissue due to alteration of the collagen. The skin is usually involved as are the gastrointestinal tract and lungs. When the gastrointestinal tract is affected, there is usually involvement of the esophagus with altered peristalsis and, ultimately, dysphagia. The small intestine may be affected, giving rise to malabsorption, as well as the large bowel, giving rise to constipation. When the lungs are involved, there is a diffusion defect. The kidneys and heart may also be affected.

The skin changes are often preceded by Raynaud's phenomenon, which may be present for a number of years before other skin changes are apparent. Raynaud's phenomenon may become severe and lead to necrosis of the fingertips (Figure 17.14).

The common sites of involvement in patients with sclerodermatous changes in the skin are the face, hands and forearms. The patient may first notice difficulty in moving the fingers; the skin, which has a shiny appearance, becomes immobile and tight, and this may lead to deformity of the hand (Figure 17.15). There may be atrophy of the pulp space on the tips of the fingers, giving the appearance of thin tapering digits (Figure 17.16). The expression on the face may be altered because of the skin tightness; patients are not able to

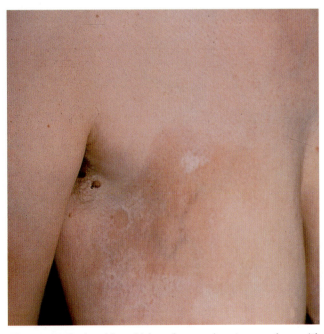

Figure 17.13 *A white thickened area due to morphea with surrounding pigmentation*

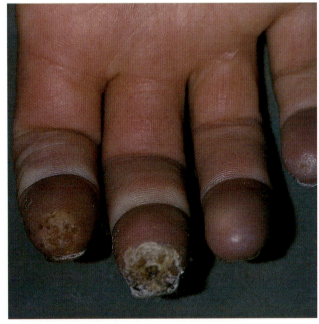

Figure 17.14 *Necrosis of the fingertip associated with severe Raynaud's phenomenon in systemic sclerosis*

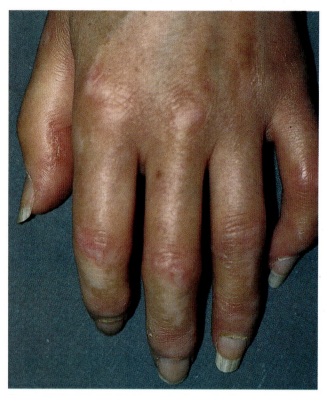

Figure 17.15 *Shiny tight skin on the fingers leading to deformity of the fifth finger in systemic sclerosis*

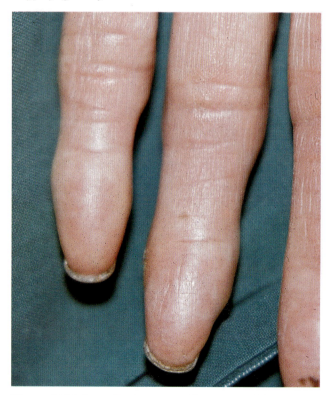

Figure 17.16 *Loss of pulp space with tapering of the digits in systemic sclerosis*

smile and may notice that they cannot open their mouths wide enough to insert a spoon.

In the later stages, there may be macular patches of telangiectasia on the cheeks (Figure 17.17). As in SLE, there may be dilated capillaries and nail-fold hemorrhages. Cutaneous calcinosis is a fairly frequent manifestation of systemic sclerosis. It is common on the hands, particularly the tips of the fingers where it may present as persistent ulcers, whereas elsewhere it presents as hard white nodules.

Prognosis and treatment

There is a variable prognosis in this disorder. Some patients may die from the disease within 1–2 years of the first signs appearing, particularly if the heart or kidneys are involved. On the other hand, patients may show very slow progression of the disorder over 20–30 years and may in fact die due to intercurrent illness.

Treatment is unsatisfactory. At the present time, there is no known measure which can significantly alter

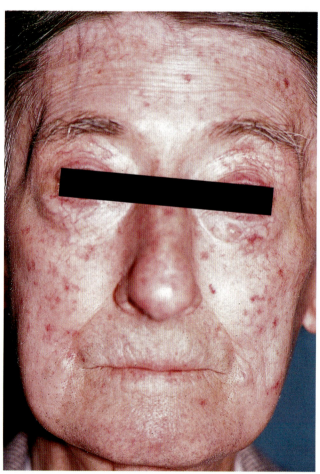

Figure 17.17 *Macular telangiectasia on the face in systemic sclerosis*

the course of the illness. Systemic steroids, other hormones and immunosuppressive agents have all been tried without obvious benefit. If Raynaud's phenomenon is present and severe, patients should be advised to avoid the cold or carrying heavy shopping bags and cases, etc.

The anabolic steroid stanozolol and infusions of prostacyclin have been shown to be helpful in the control of Raynaud's phenomenon. Simple measures, such as physiotherapy to improve the mobility of the hands and arms, are points worth paying attention to.

DERMATOMYOSITIS

Dermatomyositis is a disorder involving skin and skeletal muscle. It may first present in either childhood or adult life. In adults, but not children, the disease is associated with internal malignancy in approximately 50% of cases.

Skin lesions

These usually begin around the eyes as a purplish erythema (Figure 17.18). There may be accompanying edema which, in some instances, may be so severe as to force the eyes to close. The neck, chest, arms and occasionally the whole body may be similarly involved. Subsequently, the skin may become scaly and, occasionally in the severe forms, blisters may appear.

In the later stages when the edema has subsided, there remains a reticulate erythema and patchy pigmentation which may progress to atrophic changes in the skin. Nail-fold capillary dilatation and thrombosis may be seen as in lupus erythematosus. Erythematous patches over the dorsal aspect of the interphalangeal and metacarpophalangeal joints are a characteristic feature of dermatomyositis. The lesions over the metacarpophalangeal joints are often linear (Figure 17.19).

As in scleroderma, the patients may have Raynaud's phenomenon and develop cutaneous calcinosis. However, in dematomyositis, the calcinosis tends to occur around the joints, particularly the knees and elbows (Figure 17.20). Calcinosis is more likely to occur in the juvenile cases.

Muscle

Muscle involvement
The involvement of the muscles is variable as with the skin lesions. In the mild forms, there is weakness of the

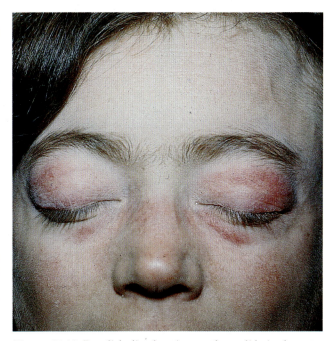

Figure 17.18 Purplish discoloration on the eyelids in dermatomyositis

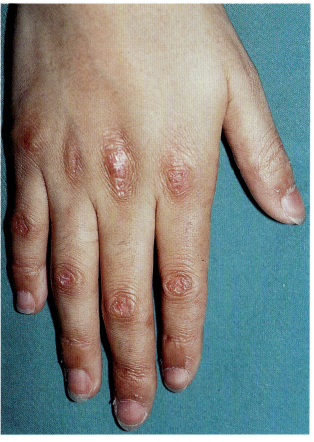

Figure 17.19 Erythematous, scaly, atrophic patches over the metacarpophalangeal and proximal interphalangeal joints in dermatomyositis

muscles usually in the shoulders, upper arms, pelvic girdle and thighs. The weakness may be minimal and scarcely noticed but, in those more severely involved, there will be obvious impairment of muscle activity (e.g. patients often notice this because of difficulty in climbing up or going down stairs).

In the most severe cases, there may be involvement of all muscles and difficulty in swallowing and breathing, which may result in death. In the juvenile form, the disease tends to be chronic with severe wasting of the muscles, particularly those of the shoulders (Figure 17.21) and pelvis.

Occasionally, the skin lesions may be severe but the muscle involvement minimal or *vice versa*.

The diagnosis is usually confirmed by muscle enzyme and electromyographic studies.

Prognosis and treatment

The prognosis is variable. Clearly, in adults, a search must be made for internal malignancy. If the disease is not associated with a carcinoma, dermatomyositis may be in itself fatal. In other instances, the disease will run a protracted course over many years before burning itself out, leaving permanent wasting of the muscles. Finally, in other patients, it may be transient and leave little residual change in either skin or muscle.

In the acute stages, relatively high doses of systemic steroids, e.g. prednisone 60 mg daily, are necessary. Once the acute stage is over, the dose can be reduced to the maintenance level, which must be maintained until the disease burns itself out. Other immunosuppressive drugs, including azathioprine, cyclophosphamide and methotrexate, have been tried when moderate doses of prednisone, e.g. 20 mg daily, failed to control the disease.

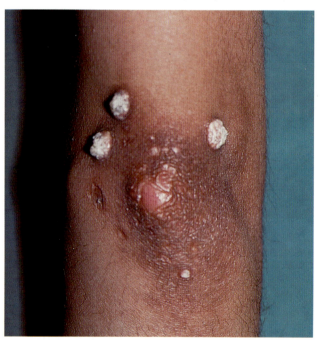

Figure 17.20 Calcinosis around the elbow in dermatomyositis

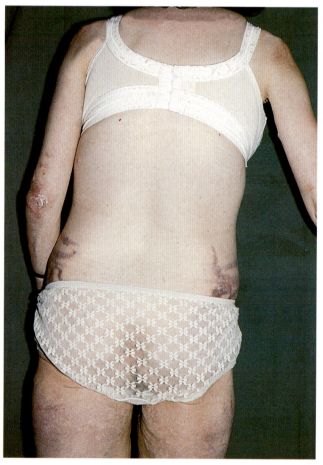

Figure 17.21 Wasting of the muscles around the shoulders, upper arms, pelvis and thighs in dermatomyositis

18

Nevi and benign skin tumors

Nevus is the Latin word for 'mole' and literally means 'blemish' or 'lump' on the skin. There is a certain amount of confusion over its use. Some people use the term to imply congenital lesions, i.e. lesions present at birth, but not all nevi are present at birth; others use the term to imply benign pigmented lesions. It is probably best used in its literal sense as described above and only with an appropriate adjective to describe the lesion.

PIGMENTED NEVI

These are lesions in which melanocytes of the epidermis undergo changes which give rise to specific cells termed 'nevus' cells. These cells may be found in either the epidermis or dermis or both. Thus, although nevus cells are derived from epidermis, they appear to migrate into the dermis.

By implication, a nevus is a defect in the development of the skin. Not all of the melanocytes in a lesion show complete progression to nevus cells. Melanocytes showing only slight changes are often referred to as immature nevus cells while those in which the changes are complete are called mature nevus cells.

When there is focal proliferation of melanocytes in the epidermis only (this occurs in the basal layer of the epidermis where melanocytes are found), the nevus is called a junctional nevus because, histologically, the change is at the junction of dermis and epidermis. This so-called junctional activity is seen when nevi undergo malignant change, but junctional activity in a nevus does *not* in itself imply malignant change.

Nevi in which nevus cells are found in both the epidermis and dermis are referred to as compound nevi whereas those in which the cells are entirely dermal are termed intradermal nevi. It has been assumed in the past that those nevi which are wholly intradermal are unlikely to undergo malignant change. However, this assumption has been challenged. It is argued that even intradermal nevi may have some epidermal component which is not seen on two-dimensional microscopy. However, the implication is that it is only the nevus cells in the epidermis which undergo malignant change.

Pigmented nevi are not all present at birth, and may appear in infancy and childhood. They appear to be hormone-dependent in some instances, appearing for the first time at puberty, during pregnancy and in women taking the contraceptive pill.

Every adult has a few pigmented nevi, the number varying greatly. The average number is around 15 to 20. The clinical importance of pigmented nevi (apart from their cosmetic significance) is whether they may develop into malignant melanomata. Everyone has a number of these lesions and malignancy is uncommon, so the chances of malignancy developing are very small indeed.

Clinical features

Pigmented nevi can be grouped on morphological grounds.

Flat lesions
These are macular pigmented lesions varying in size from a few millimeters to a few centimeters (Figure 18.1). On occasions, they may be extensive and cover large areas of skin, e.g. half a limb. Histologically, these are junctional. The most common sites are the palms and soles. There is no reason to remove these lesions unless they change their clinical features.

Slightly raised lesions
These vary in size, but are usually a few millimeters in diameter. Coarse hairs are frequently present. Histologically, they are often referred to as compound as it is easy to see both intradermal and junctional areas on microscopy.

Sessile and dome-shaped lesions

These frequently bear coarse hairs (Figure 18.2) and histologically are predominantly intradermal. Pigmented nevi, usually the compound or intradermal varieties, may be numerous in some individuals (Figure 18.3) who may well have over 100 such nevi on the skin.

Epidermal or warty nevi

Histologically, these lesions are different from the pigmented nevi described above. They do not appear to arise from melanocytes, but consist of a proliferation of epidermal cells (keratinocytes). However, there is often increased melanocytic activity. Clinically, the lesions present as raised warty (rough surface with clefts) lesions and are often linear. These lesions may be extensive (Figure 18.4).

Treatment and management

There are three main reasons to remove pigmented nevi. First and most important, they should be removed if it is suspected that they are becoming malignant. A lesion should be suspected of malignancy if:

(1) It suddenly enlarges;

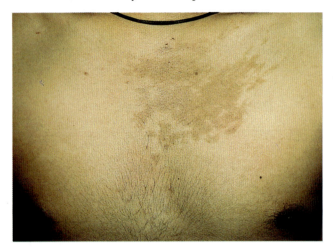

Figure 18.1 *Macular pigmented (melanocytic) nevus*

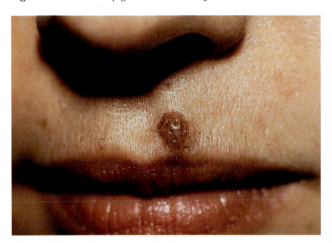

Figure 18.2 *A pigmented papule, the most common presentation of a melanocytic nevus. Coarse hairs are frequently present*

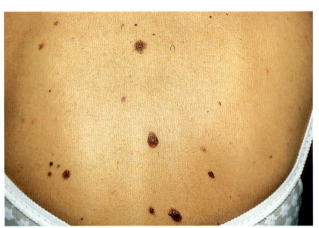

Figure 18.3 *Numerous melanocytic nevi. There is variation in size and shape of the lesions*

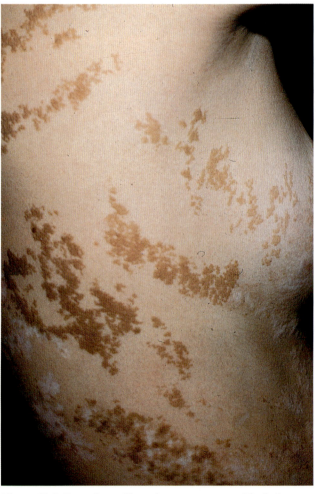

Figure 18.4 *Extensive epidermal or warty nevus. The lesions are usually linear*

(2) There is an alteration in the pigmentation of the lesion itself or of the surrounding skin; and

(3) There is bleeding or ulceration of the lesion.

The second reason for removal is if the lesion is prominent and situated on a part of the skin that is subjected to trauma from clothing, e.g. brassière straps, and is causing discomfort to that part. The third and probably the most common reason for removal is cosmetic.

All pigmented nevi that are to be removed should be surgically excised whatever the indication. No other forms of therapy should be attempted.

JUVENILE MELANOMA

This is a term applied to a nevus which usually appears in childhood and grows rapidly. On microscopy, the features are similar to those seen in a malignant melanoma, but a juvenile melanoma is always benign. As a general rule, pigmented nevi rarely undergo malignant change prior to puberty.

BASAL CELL PAPILLOMA OR SEBORRHEIC WART

These lesions are very common. They are not caused by viruses. Seborrheic warts are disorders of middle-aged and elderly persons. They are usually oval or circular and most frequently occur on the face and trunk. Initially, they grow fairly rapidly and then remain stationary. The lesions are pigmented, and have a cleft surface and greasy appearance, hence the name seborrheic (Figures 18.5 and 18.6). They do not regress as do viral warts and they do not become malignant. If the patient wants them removed, the procedure should be curettage and cautery under local anesthesia.

SKIN TAGS OR FIBROEPITHELIAL POLYPS

These usually occur in middle-aged persons. The most common sites are the neck and axillae (Figure 18.7). They may be few or many in number. They are benign and are easily removed by snipping the base with scissors with cauterization to stop the bleeding.

DERMATOFIBROMA

This is a relatively common lesion particularly on the lower leg in females. It is usually only seen in adults.

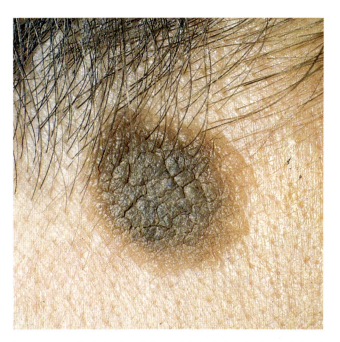

Figure 18.5 Typical seborrheic wart. The lesion is pigmented and raised, with a cleft surface and greasy appearance

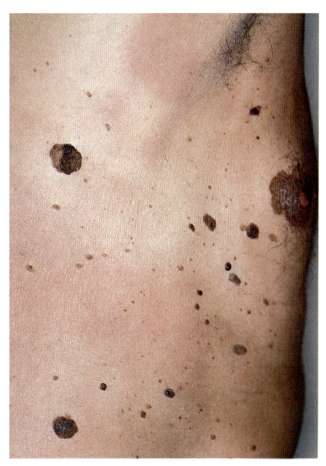

Figure 18.6 Numerous seborrheic warts on the trunk. Lesions are usually multiple

The cause is not known, although trauma or a reaction to insect bites has been suggested.

The lesion is a firm, brownish, dermal nodule usually about 0.5 cm in diameter (Figure 18.8). It is a collection of chronic inflammatory cells with proliferation of collagen and dermal vasculature. The brown color is thought to be due to iron and not melanin.

The lesions are benign and can be left. Their importance is in the differential diagnosis of malignant melanoma. If treatment is required, surgical excision is the most appropriate.

KELOIDS

These are the result of an abnormal response to trauma by the connective tissue of the dermis whereby excess collagen is formed. Undoubtedly, the most common cause of a keloid is surgery (Figure 18.9), but the lesions are also seen following trauma and infection of the dermis, whether viral or bacterial.

In Asians and blacks, spontaneous keloids occur usually on the trunk and upper arms (Figure 18.10). Keloids are more common in blacks than in whites and this should be borne in mind before embarking on removal of benign tumors in blacks.

Clinically, a keloid is a firm raised lesion with a smooth surface (normal epidermis). If it presents at the site of surgery or trauma, there is no difficulty in diagnosis (Figure 18.9), but spontaneous keloids may present diagnostic problems (Figure 18.10).

The treatment of keloids is far from satisfactory. Intralesional steroids (triamcinolone) may flatten the lesions and make them less apparent. Occasionally, keloids are excised, but the wound should be infiltrated with triamcinolone at operation and/or radiotherapy given after surgery. Both these measures are attempts to suppress fibroblast activity leading to further keloid formation.

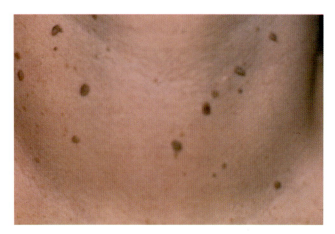

Figure 18.7 Skin tags or fibroepithelial polyps on the neck. The lesions are frequently pigmented

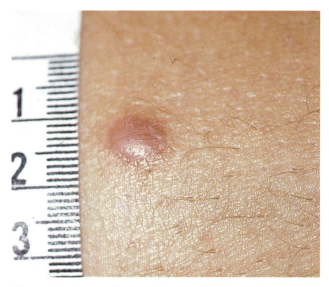

Figure 18.8 Dermatofibroma. A firm, reddish-brown dermal nodule

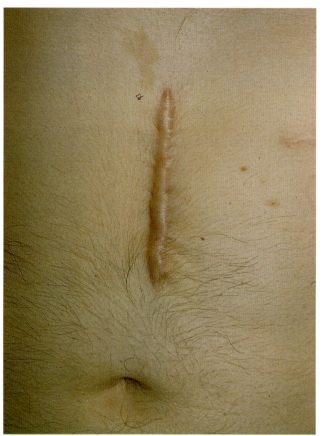

Figure 18.9 Keloid developing in a surgical scar

HEMANGIOMATA

These are divided into congenital and acquired types. The former may be further subdivided into those arising from immature vessels and those arising from mature vessels.

Immature hemangiomata (strawberry nevi)

These are only rarely present at birth. They usually appear within the first week of life as a small red spot and then rapidly enlarge. They are raised above the skin surface and are deep red in color (Figure 18.11).

The hemangiomata may continue to enlarge until the age of 18 months although, frequently, they stop increasing in size before then. The eventual size they attain varies considerably from a few millimeters to as much as 10 cm in diameter. After 18 months, size and appearance usually do not change but, after the age of 3 years, they begin to shrink and become paler, and should disappear completely by the age of 5 or 6 years.

Management and treatment
From the natural history, it can be seen that all lesions will disappear. If there is any residual scarring or puckering of the skin, this can be dealt with after complete resolution. The best cosmetic result will be obtained if the lesions are not treated at all.

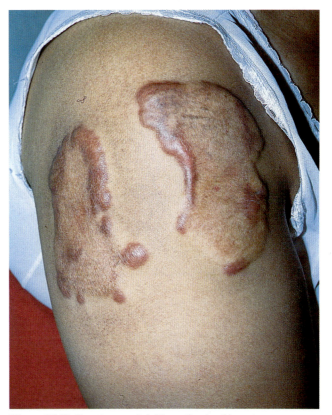

Figure 18.10 Spontaneous keloids on the shoulder

Occasionally, if the hemangioma is near the eye, its growth could cause the eye to close and hence interfere with the development of binocular vision. In these instances, resolution of the lesion can be induced by radiotherapy.

Mature hemangiomata (port-wine stains)

These lesions are present in full extent at birth, which distinguishes them from the immature hemangiomata. They are macular (Figure 18.12). Unfortunately, they persist throughout life and do not undergo resolution.

These hemangiomata may vary from a few to many centimeters in size. The most common sites are the face, neck and upper trunk. They are a severe cosmetic disability, particularly if extensive.

Management and treatment
Until recently, there was no effective treatment for this unsightly lesion. Laser treatment is now giving good results, particularly in adults. If this therapy is not available, the hemangioma should be camouflaged by a suitable cosmetic preparation. There are now many camouflage technicians attached to plastic surgery and dermatology departments, and referral to these centers can be helpful.

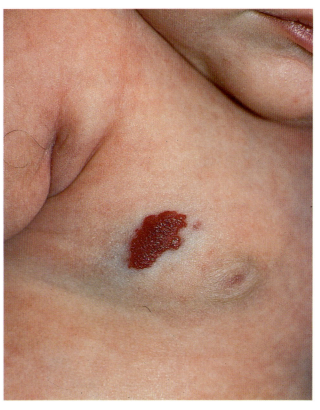

Figure 18.11 Immature capillary hemangioma (strawberry nevus)

Deep hemangiomata

A small percentage of mature hemangiomata are raised and are related to abnormalities of the deeper vessels.

Acquired hemangiomata

Pyogenic granuloma

This lesion is so called because it was thought to be due to infection by a *Staphylococcus*. It is usually a solitary raised red papule (Figure 18.13) that bleeds with the slightest trauma. It may occur anywhere on the body. The cause is unknown but, sometimes, there is a history of previous trauma. The most effective treatment is curettage and cautery under local anesthesia.

Campbell de Morgan spots (cherry angiomata)

These are small raised bright-red angiomata which tend to occur on the trunk in middle-aged and elderly individuals. They are relatively common but they have no special clinical significance. No treatment is indicated, but they can be removed by surgery or cautery.

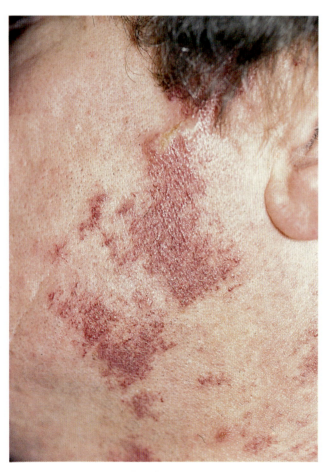

Figure 18.12 *Mature capillary hemangioma (port-wine stain)*

Spider nevi

These are common lesions that may occur at any age. There is a small central red papule from which superficial vessels radiate (Figure 18.14). They usually occur on the face, arms, hands and upper trunk. The lesions are usually solitary and do not imply internal disease. However, occasionally they are multiple and due to

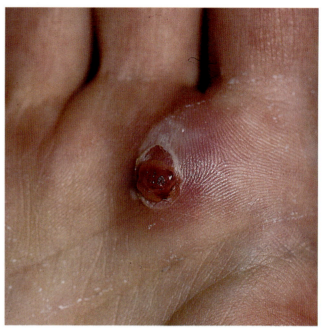

Figure 18.13 *Pyogenic granuloma (acquired hemangioma)*

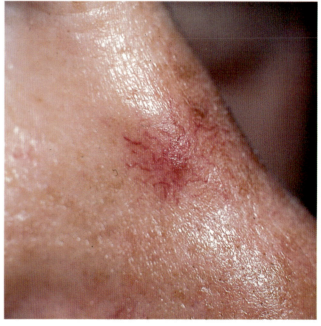

Figure 18.14 *Spider nevus. A central red dot with small vessels radiating from the center*

underlying liver disease. They may also appear in pregnancy and frequently disappear after the confinement.

If treatment is required, the most satisfactory is cautery of the central papule without local anesthesia. If the latter is used, it causes vasoconstriction and the central papule will no longer be visible.

HEREDITARY TELANGIECTASIA

This is a rare but important disease. Small hemangiomata are present on the face, lips (Figure 18.15) and tongue. The importance of the disease lies in the fact that the hemangiomata also occur in the gastrointestinal tract and may bleed, causing a severe hemorrhage. If there is a large bleed, the fall in blood pressure results in the disappearance of the hemangiomata on the face and lips, and thus the diagnosis is missed.

LYMPHANGIOMATA

This is a relatively rare lesion. It presents as grouped blisters (Figure 18.16) on any part of the body. The blisters are deep and the fluid is easily expressed. Frequently, there are hemangiomatous elements associated with a lymphangioma such that the lesion may then have a vascular appearance. The only treatment available is surgery but, unfortunately, the recurrence rate is high.

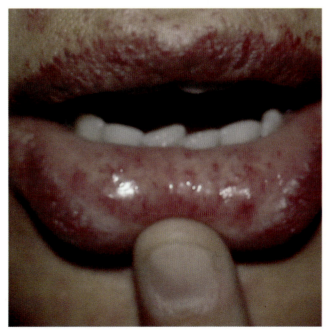

Figure 18.15 *Hereditary telangiectasia. Lesion on the lips involving both skin and mucosal surfaces*

NEVUS SEBACEUS

This lesion is derived from sebaceous gland cells, and usually occurs on the scalp (Figure 18.17) and becomes apparent during infancy. The typical appearance is a yellowish plaque with a slightly irregular surface. There are no hair follicles at the site of the nevus, so the lesion usually presents as a bald patch. The importance of these nevi is that one-third will undergo malignant change in adult life and, therefore, surgical excision is advisable at around puberty. Basal cell carcinoma is the usual malignancy that develops.

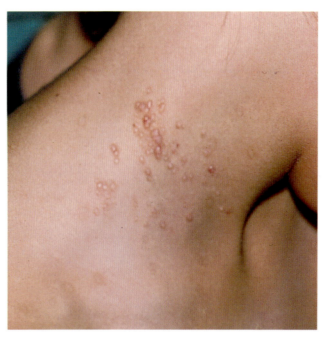

Figure 18.16 *Lymphangioma. Small firm 'blisters' that are easily compressible with a glass spatula and do not rupture*

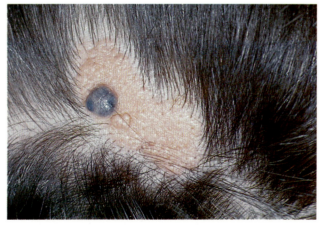

Figure 18.17 *Nevus sebaceus. The typical lesion is a yellowish plaque whereas the pigmented papule indicates neoplastic change (a pigmented basal cell carcinoma)*

19

Urticaria and erythema multiforme

URTICARIA

Urticaria is sometimes referred to as 'hives' or 'nettle rash' by patients. Urticaria is essentially a localized edema of the skin or mucous membranes of the upper respiratory tract. It is due to acute vasodilatation of the blood vessels and increased permeability of the capillary walls causing fluid to pour out into the dermis with resultant swelling of the skin. The vasodilatation and increased permeability is caused by various chemical mediators in the skin which are released under certain conditions. Histamine is one of the substances which can cause an urticarial response and this can be shown by injection of histamine into the skin.

However, it is now thought that, in urticaria, histamine is only one of many substances which can cause the clinical lesion.

Morphology

The initial lesion is an erythematous patch (there is no scaling in urticaria) caused by capillary vasodilatation. The lesion subsequently becomes raised (Figures 19.1–19.3) and may finally have a white center caused by the pressure of intercellular fluid forcing the blood out of the capillaries (Figure 19.3).

An urticarial lesion may vary in size from a few millimeters to many centimeters (Figures 19.1 and 19.2) and, on occasions, may involve large confluent areas of skin. The urticarial lesions often have a 'geographical' pattern rather than a regular configuration.

If the palms or soles are involved, the typical urticarial pattern is not present, the affected area being tense, red and swollen. When the fingers or toes are affected, the swelling may interfere with movement.

Urticaria not infrequently involves the face, producing an alarming picture with swelling around the eyes (Figure 19.4) and/or lips and gross disfiguration. When urticaria takes this pattern, it is sometimes referred to as angioneurotic edema (although this is not a particularly acceptable term to use).

Urticarial skin lesions may be associated with swelling of the tongue, pharnyx and larynx. This is a serious condition as it may cause the patient to asphyxiate. The condition may occur within minutes of the first symptoms appearing.

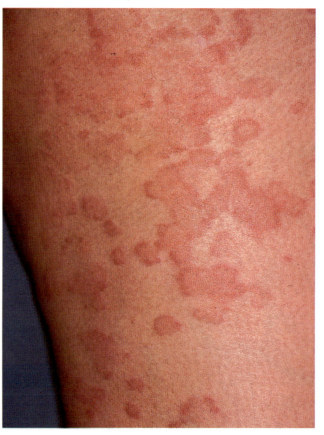

Figure 19.1 *Urticaria on the thigh. Raised red smooth lesions*

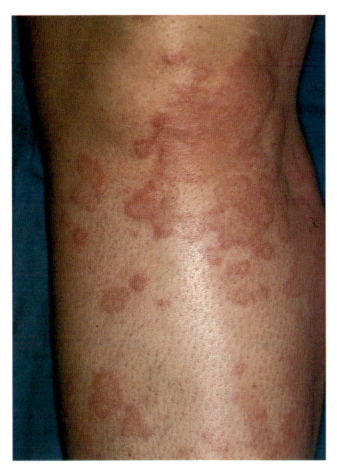

Figure 19.2 Urticaria on the leg. Lesions are of varying size

Organs other than the skin may be affected in association with urticaria (whatever the cause of the latter), e.g. swelling of the joints, bronchospasm, the gut (in the form of colicky abdominal pains); very rarely, there is anaphylactic shock.

Course

An urticarial lesion tends to last for only a few hours, although it may last for as little as a few minutes and, occasionally, for as long as a few days. When the lesion first forms, it is intensely irritating. In patients who give a long history of urticaria, it is important to establish that an individual lesion does, in fact, 'come and go'. In those patients who are never free from the eruption, it is not the original lesions which persist. As stated above, lesions tend to last for a few hours and then clear, but new lesions will then appear at other sites.

The natural history of urticaria is variable. It depends to a certain extent upon whether there are any obvious precipitating factors. In the patients in whom there are no such obvious factors, the disease may last from a few days to many years. In some instances, the patient is never free of lesions whereas, in others, they may be clear for a few days or even weeks before the rash recurs.

Urticaria may also run a variable course in those patients in whom there is an obvious cause (e.g. penicillin). It may last for only a few days or may persist for weeks despite no further penicillin intake.

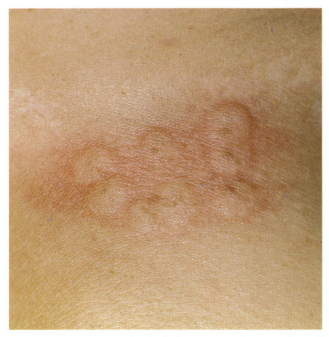

Figure 19.3 Urticaria with raised white center and surrounding red flare

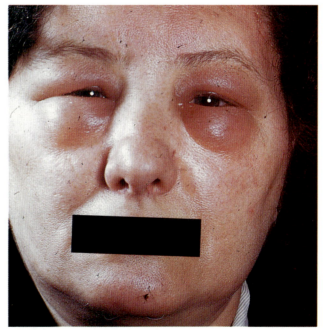

Figure 19.4 Angioedema around the eyes

Causes

In the majority of patients with chronic urticaria seen in a skin clinic, no cause is found for the eruption. In an acute episode, which is often self-limiting, it is much more common to find a cause.

Drugs

These are the most common known cause of urticaria seen today. Penicillin is the most frequent offender, but compounds containing salicylates also produce a relatively high incidence of urticarial eruptions. As mentioned in the chapter on drug eruptions (Chapter 13), any drug can cause any rash, so it is important to ask patients who have urticaria whether they have taken (or been given) any drugs during the last few months.

The number of drugs known to produce urticaria is now so numerous that it would be of no value to name them here but, except for drugs taken orally or given by injection, it is important to remember that inhaled medication or drugs absorbed through a mucous membrane have also to be considered when searching for the offending substance. It is also important to ascertain whether the patient has received any inoculations or blood transfusions.

Foods

In most cases of urticaria, the patient assumes that some particular food is the cause. Certainly in chronic urticaria, this is very rarely the case. Usually, if a patient is sensitive to a particular food, there is a definite history of ingestion of this food just before the eruption. The most common food to cause urticaria is probably shellfish. It is probably unwise to specify other foods here as the patient should be asked whether any particular food was ingested before the rash appeared. Elimination diets and skin testing have not proved to be helpful in establishing whether the patient is sensitive to a particular food. However, these procedures often have a 'negative' therapeutic value for, when carried out and shown to be negative, they help to convince the patient that the causative agent of the skin trouble is not something being ingested.

Apart from the food itself, certain food additives have been implicated as the cause of chronic urticaria. Tartrazine and other azo dyes are used as coloring substances in food and have been reported to cause urticaria. The same dyes are often used to color tablets (including antihistamines given in the treatment of urticaria). Preservatives such as sodium benzoate and benzoic acid have also been mentioned as possible etiological factors. The foods which contain such preservatives are pickles, sauces, instant coffee, preserves, fruit juices and some tinned foods.

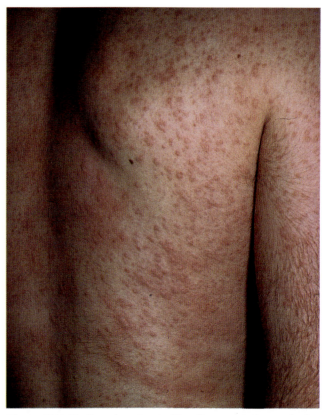

Figure 19.5 Cholinergic urticaria. Usually seen on the trunk after exercise, the lesions tend to be smaller than in other forms of urticaria

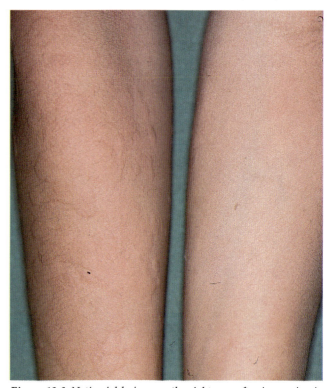

Figure 19.6 Urticarial lesions on the right arm after immersion in cold water

It has been suggested that challenge doses of these dyes and preservatives should be given by mouth to determine whether they are the cause of urticaria and, if there is considered to be a positive response (worsening or induction of urticaria), then a diet free of those substances should be followed. It should be stressed that this approach to the problem is an oversimplification for, in practice, it is difficult to evaluate the provocation test and, even if positive results are obtained, elimination does *not* result in a 100% cure.

Physical factors

Heat

In some subjects, heat from whatever source will produce urticarial lesions. The lesions usually appear within minutes or a few hours of the increase in temperature of the skin. In a number of patients, exercise will produce urticaria. This form of urticaria may have the morphology of the lesions described above or consist of very small (2–3 mm) but numerous wheals. It is thought that the chemical mediator may be acetylcholine, and this type of urticaria has been termed cholinergic (Figure 19.5).

Cold

Cold may also produce urticaria (Figure 19.6). It usually occurs on the exposed areas of the arms or legs. Two types of cold urticaria have been described, one which occurs within minutes of a fall in skin temperature, and another which may appear many hours later. The history of cold urticaria can be substantiated by applying a block of ice to the skin for a few minutes and observing the response.

Trauma

In some individuals, trauma to the skin produces urticarial lesions. These may appear within 2–3 minutes or, like cold urticaria, develop several hours later. This type of urticarial response has been termed 'dermographism' and can easily be substantiated by stroking the skin with a blunt instrument; the urticaria will follow in the line of the trauma (Figure 19.7).

Sunlight

Some persons develop urticaria on areas exposed to the rays of the sun. This is referred to as solar urticaria and is caused by the release of chemicals in the skin caused by ultraviolet irradiation.

Psychogenic factors

There is no doubt that urticaria is aggravated by tension, worry, stress, etc. but so are many other diseases. It cannot be stated with any certainty whether or not urticaria can truly be caused by such factors.

Genetic factors

There is an increased incidence of urticaria in persons with a past or family history of atopy. There is also a rare condition termed 'hereditary angioedema' which is transmitted as an autosomal dominant trait, and a family history is usually, but not always, present.

The disorder is characterized by recurrent swellings of the skin and mucous membranes, and fatalities may occur due to laryngeal obstruction. The disease is characterized by a deficiency of the enzyme called c-1 esterase inhibitor. The deficiency may be in the quantity of this enzyme or due to an inactive form.

Internal diseases

There are recorded instances of urticaria in association with carcinoma, lymphomas, hepatic disorders, renal disorders and collagen diseases. However, whether the underlying systemic disease is directly causing the urticaria or is coincidental has yet to be determined.

Treatment and management

An accurate patient history is important in the management of urticaria. It is imperative to know whether any drugs had been taken before the eruption and whether they can be implicated. If they can, then they must be avoided in the future. If the patient is still taking drugs, they should be stopped or, if possible, substituted.

At present, there is no reliable test either *in vitro* or *in vivo* for confirming whether a particular drug is the

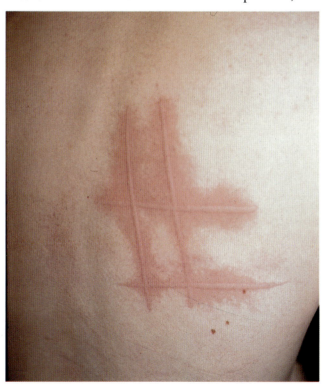

Figure 19.7 *Dermographism. Urticarial lesions with surrounding flare at sites of trauma*

cause of the eruption. If the eruption is of sudden onset, then it may be worth enquiring about any particular food, such as shellfish, which the patient does not usually take. As mentioned above, skin tests which attempt to determine the cause of urticaria have not proved helpful. Oral provocation tests with drugs and food additives may be tried but, as already noted, they are difficult to evaluate, as are the results of elimination diets, in a disease with such a variable course.

If it can be established that urticaria is caused by physical factors, then the appropriate advice should be given to minimize the effects of these factors.

Antihistamines

These drugs are the mainstay in the treatment of urticaria. They are usually given orally but, in severe and acute urticaria, they can be given by intramuscular or intravenous injection to obtain quicker control of the condition. Which antihistamine to use is usually the personal choice of the treating physician. All antihistamines appear to have a similar therapeutic effect, but some tend to cause drowsiness (the main side effect of these drugs) more readily than others. At night, however, it may be helpful to have a drug which has the effect of making patients drowsy, and trimeprazine tartrate and promethazine hydrochloride appear to be the best drugs for this purpose.

A number of antihistamines are now made in slow-release or long-acting formulations and are sometimes helpful in minimizing the soporific effects. Often, urticaria is not controlled because the dose of antihistamine given is too small. The dose should be increased until the urticaria is controlled or until side effects from the antihistamine are intolerable. The H$_2$ blocker cimetidine combined with antihistamines has been reported to be helpful in controlling urticaria that is not controlled by antihistamines alone.

Corticosteroids

These drugs should only be used in emergencies such as angioneurotic edema with involvement of the tongue and larynx. Corticosteroids are also indicated in anaphylactic shock. In both instances, they should be given intravenously. Systemic corticosteroids should not be used to control chronic urticaria. They do not appear to be as effective as antihistamines and, on a long-term basis, are far more hazardous. Topical corticosteroids have no part to play in the treatment of urticaria.

Adrenaline

Subcutaneous adrenaline is still one of the most effective measures for controlling acute urticaria, particularly when there is involvement of the mouth and larynx.

Tracheotomy

This is indicated as an emergency procedure when the patient is asphyxiating because of laryngeal or pharyngeal swelling.

Topical measures

Because the epidermis is intact in urticaria, topical drugs do not penetrate to the site of pathology in therapeutic concentrations. Topical measures are therefore useless in urticaria.

Psychotropic drugs

Drugs to control anxiety and depression should only be used if there are specific indications.

Anabolic steroids

The anabolic steroid danazol is helpful in preventing attacks in hereditary angioedema and has to be taken indefinitely.

URTICARIA PIGMENTOSA (MASTOCYTOSIS)

This is a disorder caused by tumors of mast cells. There are two distinct forms of urticaria pigmentosa, one which occurs in childhood and another which appears in later life.

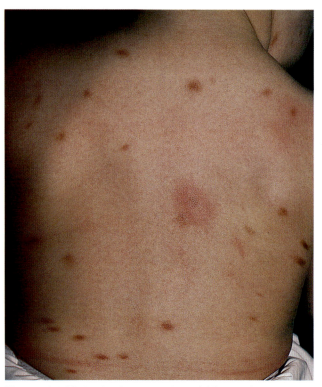

Figure 19.8 Urticaria pigmentosa in a child. Macular pigmented lesions which urticate after trauma

Childhood variety

The lesions may be present at birth or appear within the first few months of life. The most common lesion is a small pigmented macule found predominantly on the trunk (Figure 19.8). The lesions may be few or numerous. Occasionally, they present as small pigmented papules or nodules.

The diagnosis is made by gently scratching the lesions. This slight trauma releases histamine from the mast cells and an acute urticarial lesion develops. Occasionally, there is a more severe response and blistering occurs. The parents of the child will often notice urticarial lesions after slight trauma to the child's skin such as drying after bathing.

The natural history of childhood or congenital mastocytosis is that the lesions usually disappear by adulthood.

Adult variety

This is sometimes referred to as 'acquired' mastocytosis. The lesions may appear at any time and are initially few in number, but slowly become more numerous (Figure 19.9). They are similar to the lesions of congenital or childhood mastocytosis, although the lesions may be redder in appearance. As in childhood mastocytosis, urticaria is produced by slight trauma to the lesions (Figure 19.10).

It is thought that the adult variety is a neoplastic disease of the mast cells, and mast cell tumors develop at other sites, notably the liver, spleen and bones. The disease may progress to an acute form of mast cell 'leukemia' and the patient may die of the disease. The course of the disease is over many years, and may take 20–30 years from the development of the skin lesions to the more serious aspects of the disorder.

A number of treatments have been reported to be helpful in controlling the irritation and whealing that occur in this disorder, but such treatments are only symptomatic. These treatments include oral antihistamines, oral sodium cromoglycate and PUVA (see Chapter 25). If the disease progesses to a malignant phase with bone marrow involvement, appropriate cytotoxic drugs will be necessary.

ERYTHEMA MULTIFORME

This is a distinct symptomatic complex with an appropriate name because the lesions are characterized by a

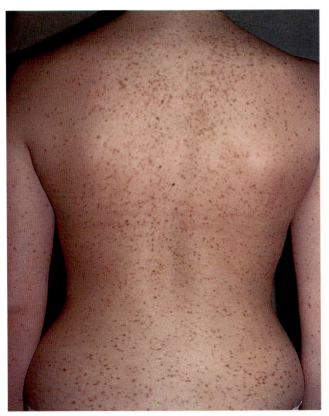

Figure 19.9 *Adult urticaria pigmentosa (mastocytosis). Numerous macular pigmented lesions*

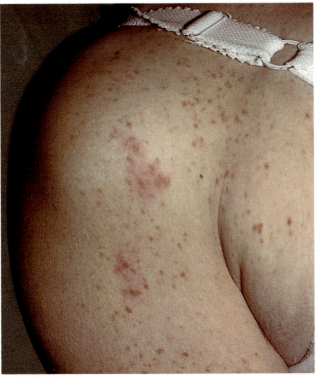

Figure 19.10 *Adult urticaria pigmentosa. Urticated lesions after mild trauma*

variable morphology. The primary pathology of erythema multiforme is that of a vasculitis in the skin.

Morphology and distribution of lesions

In erythema multiforme, the lesions may be erythematous macules or papules, or urticarial, purpuric or blistering. There may be only one (Figure 19.11) or two (Figure 19.12) or all of the various types of lesion present in a given patient.

In the classical form of erythema multiforme, the initial lesion is an erythematous macule which is transformed into a papule (or blisters; Figures 19.13 and 9.14) which extends peripherally with central clearing. As the border extends, a new lesion frequently develops in the center which may be purpuric (Figure 19.15), and as many as three or four rings may be noted. This gives rise to so-called iris or target lesions.

The most common site for erythema multiforme is the extremities of the upper limbs (Figures 19.16 and 19.17). The eruption in erythema multiforme is symmetrical (Figures 19.11, 19.16 and 19.17). Occasionally, the lesions may be widespread, occurring on the trunk and limbs and producing confluent lesions (Figure 19.11).

In a severe form of the disorder known as the Stevens–Johnson syndrome, there is involvement of the

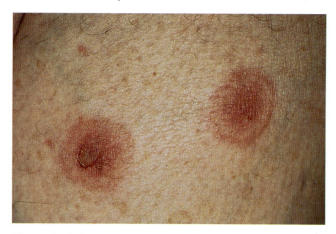

Figure 19.13 Early target lesions in erythema multiforme. A blister is surrounded by an annular erythematous area

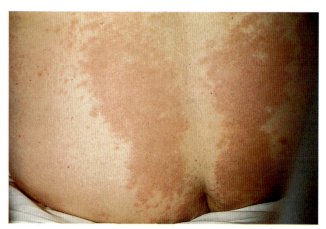

Figure 19.11 Symmetrical urticarial plaques on the back in erythema multiforme

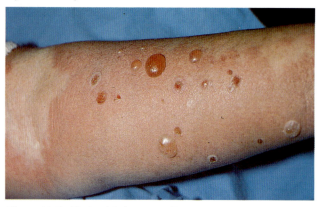

Figure 19.12 Urticarial plaques and blisters in erythema multiforme

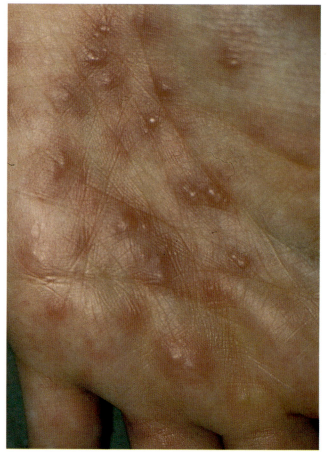

Figure 19.14 Blisters on the palm with surrounding erythema, early lesions in erythema multiforme

mucous membranes of the mouth (Figure 19.18), eyes and genitalia (Figure 19.19). Very occasionally, the eye lesions become severe, progressing to an iritis, uveitis and even panophthalmitis.

Course

In the mild form of erythema multiforme, the lesions are often asymptomatic and clear within 2–3 weeks of onset. Occasionally, there may be slight constitutional upset with the onset of the lesions. In the more severe forms, the patient may be extremely ill with fever and headache. In some patients with the Stevens–Johnson syndrome, the disease may prove fatal.

It is not uncommon for patients to develop recurrent attacks of erythema multiforme. The interval between epidoses may vary from a few weeks to a few years.

Etiology

The exact cause of erythema multiforme is unknown, but it is probably an immunological disorder with the

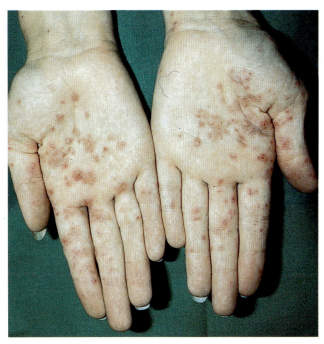

Figure 19.16 *Symmetrical eruption in erythema multiforme*

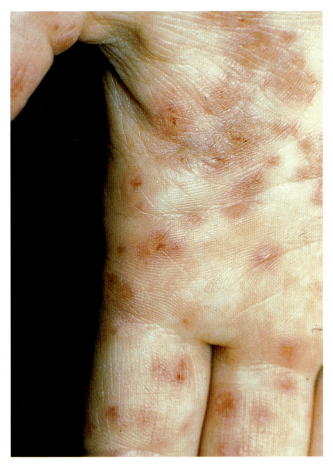

Figure 19.15 *Target lesions on the palms. Central purpura with surrounding annular erythema multiforme*

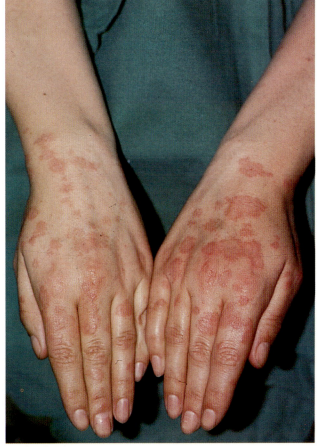

Figure 19.17 *Symmetrical eruption on the backs of the hands in erythema multiforme*

cutaneous blood vessels being the target for the end result of the disease process. In the majority of patients, there is no obvious precipitating factor, but the following have been reported to precipitate attacks.

Viral infections

This refers particularly to herpes simplex (Figure 19.20), but measles has also been found to trigger the condition.

Bacterial infections

This refers particularly to streptococcal infections, but also includes meningococcal infections.

Mycoplasma

This organism has been implicated in the causation of erythema multiforme and is also known to cause so-called primary atypical pneumonia.

Drugs

Any drug may cause erythema multiforme. In the past, sulfonamides and barbiturates were frequent offenders. More recently, erythema multiforme has been associated with terbinafine.

Radiotherapy

Radiotherapy in the treatment of malignancy has been implicated as precipitating erythema multiforme.

Treatment and management

In the mild forms of the disease, no treatment is required as the disease is self-limiting. If there is irritation, systemic antihistamines should be given. In the more severe forms, particularly Stevens–Johnson syndrome, systemic corticosteroids are required and hospitalization is necessary.

In all instances, a careful history should be taken to determine whether there is a possible precipitating factor (e.g. a particular drug) which can be avoided in the future.

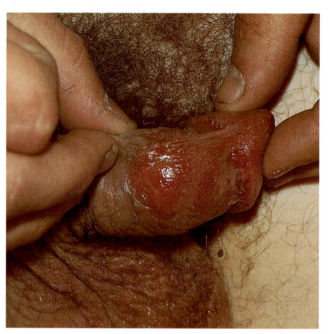

Figure 19.19 *Ulceration on the genitalia in the Stevens–Johnson variant of erythema multiforme*

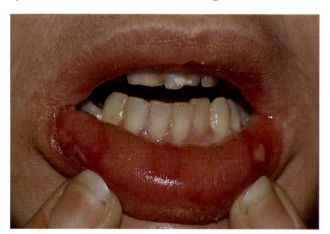

Figure 19.18 *Stevens–Johnson syndrome. Ulcers on the lips*

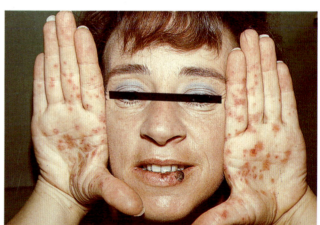

Figure 19.20 *Erythema multiforme triggered by herpes simplex. The end stage of the herpetic lesion on the lip is seen with the early lesions of erythema multiforme on the palms*

20

Cutaneous manifestations of systemic disorders

The title of this chapter is neither satisfactory nor precise, but it is difficult to create a better one. It implies that the skin lesions to be discussed here are either due to a primary pathology in another organ or are possibly part of a generalized disease affecting many tissues. Strictly speaking, it could be argued that the majority of skin lesions (e.g. psoriasis, eczema) are the end result of a generalized process regardless of whether the primary fault is immunological, genetic or infective. In this chapter, those diseases in which the end result of the disease process affects organs other than and in addition to the skin are discussed.

METABOLIC DISEASES

Diabetes mellitus

Necrobiosis lipoidica
This is the characteristic skin lesion associated with diabetes mellitus. Approximately half the patients with necrobiosis lipoidica have glycosuria. The other half are usually considered to be latent diabetics and may develop diabetes later in life. The disorder appears to be more common in women than in men.

The lesions characteristically develop on the anterior aspect of the lower leg (Figure 20.1). The initial lesion is usually an erythematous papule or plaque which gradually extends in an annular fashion. Thus, eventually, the lesion has a raised erythematous edge and, in the center of the lesion (where the disease first began), there is thinning of the epidermis and degeneration of the dermal collagen. The skin in the center of the lesion has a brownish-yellow color and the underlying small veins in the dermis are visible (Figure 20.1). Occasionally, the atrophic epidermis breaks down and ulcerates.

The lesions tend to be persistent and, unfortunately, there is no successful treatment. Control of the diabetes, if present, does not appear to influence the lesions.

Topically applied and intralesional injections of corticosteroids have been tried, but the results have not been impressive.

Granuloma annulare
It is probably incorrect to attribute this disorder to diabetes mellitus, but some studies have suggested that the basic pathological process is similar to that seen in other tissues in patients with diabetes.

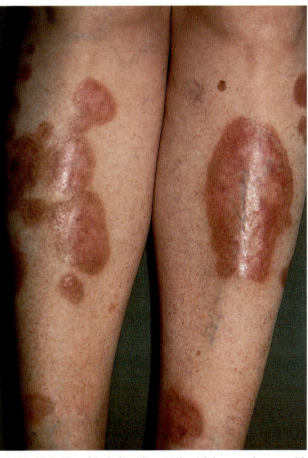

Figure 20.1 *Necrobiosis lipoidica. Yellowish-brown plaques with atrophy in the center of the lesion*

The lesions characteristically occur on the posterior aspects of the hand, fingers, extensor surfaces of the elbows and knees, and around the ankle joints (Figure 20.2). They commence as firm papules and nodules in the dermis of the skin. The lesions usually then extend in an annular pattern with healing of the lesion in the center, thus giving rise to an annular non-scaling lesion (Figure 20.2). The lesion may be of the normal skin color or, not infrequently, it may be violaceous in color.

The lesions may occur in patients of any age, including young children. As diabetes mellitus appears to be no more common in these patients than in the general population, no particular search for diabetes should be undertaken.

Approximately half the lesions will clear spontaneously within 2 years of onset. If treatment is required, intralesional injections of triamcinolone appear to offer the best chance of cure.

Xanthomatosis

A xanthoma is a deposit of excess lipids in the skin. Clinically, the lesion may appear as a papule, nodule or plaque with a whitish-yellow color. The classification may be based on purely clinical morphology, biochemical criteria or in relation to specific underlying disease. There is, in any case, a considerable overlap and, thus, the lesions are best considered according to their clinical appearances.

The diseases that are most commonly associated with xanthomata are the primary disorders of lipid metabolism (some of which are hereditary), diabetes mellitus, hypothyroidism, nephrotic syndrome and liver disease (usually biliary cirrhosis).

Xanthelasma

This is the most common form of xanthoma and presents as a yellowish-white plaque (Figure 20.3) on the upper eyelid or just below the lower eyelid. It usually commences on the medial side of the lid and progresses laterally. It may occur as a single lesion or affect all four eyelids. Xanthelasmata may occur in subjects who do not have a generalized biochemical disorder, but they may be a manifestation of a hyper-lipoproteinemia.

Nodular xanthomata

These lesions usually occur on the extensor surfaces of the limbs, particularly over the joint surfaces (Figure 20.4). They present as painless yellowish nodules and vary in size from a few millimeters to 1–2 cm across.

Papular xanthomata

Occasionally, multiple xanthomata appear as numerous small papules over a matter of a few weeks in so-called eruptive xanthomata. They usually appear on the trunk, buttocks and upper limbs (Figure 20.5).

Plaques

Lipid deposits in the skin and along the tendon sheaths may often present as plaques. They may also be nodular, particularly over large tendons.

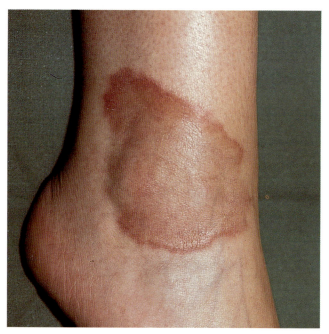

Figure 20.2 *Granuloma annulare. Annular infiltrated edge*

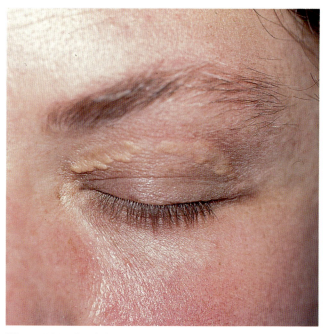

Figure 20.3 *Xanthelasma. Yellowish-white linear plaque on the upper eyelid*

Treatment and management

The treatment of xanthomata depends on which underlying metabolic disorder has produced the lipid deposits in the skin. Thus, the patient must be investigated to determine whether the lesions are secondary to one of the above-mentioned diseases, e.g. diabetes mellitus, or whether they are due to a primary metabolic defect. If the lesions are secondary, then the treatment is that of the primary disorder. If the xanthomata are due to a primary metabolic abnormality, then further investigation is required to determine the biochemical profile, as treatment by dietary restriction and/or drugs will depend on those results.

In patients with xanthelasmata in whom no biochemical disorders are found, the lesions may be removed by either surgery or electrocautery under local anesthesia.

GOUT AND RHEUMATOID NODULES

Gouty tophi usually present as nodules on the ears (Figure 20.6), hands or, occasionally, on the extensor surface of the joints of the limbs. The tophus is formed by the deposition of urates in the dermis and subcutis and, thus, the lesion is frequently attached to the skin. Occasionally, the lesion may be present without the classical history of gouty arthritis.

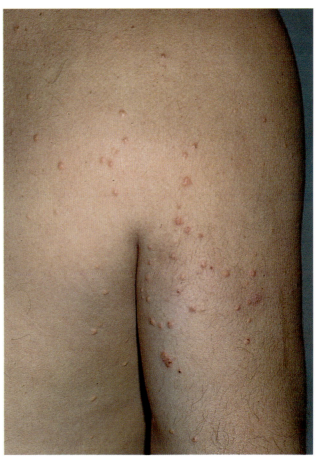

Figure 20.5 Eruptive xanthomata. Small yellowish-red papules on the upper arm and trunk

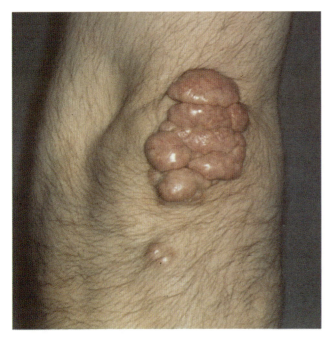

Figure 20.4 Xanthomata. Reddish-yellow nodules on the elbow

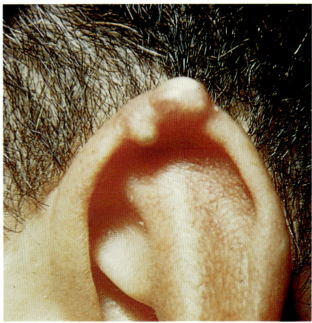

Figure 20.6 Gouty tophi on the pinna

Rheumatoid nodules do not usually present to a dermatologist as these patients are usually under the care of a rheumatologist for their 'rheumatic' condition. Occasionally, however, rheumatoid nodules develop in patients who have no joint problems. The most common sites are the hands, but the nodules may also occur in the feet and elbows (Figure 20.7), and are painless.

ERYTHEMA NODOSUM

This distinct clinical entity is a reaction in the skin and

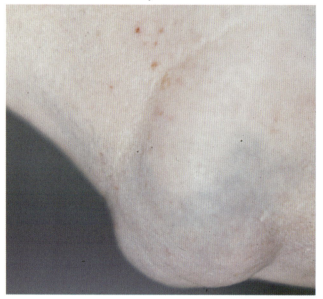

Figure 20.7 Rheumatic nodule on the elbow

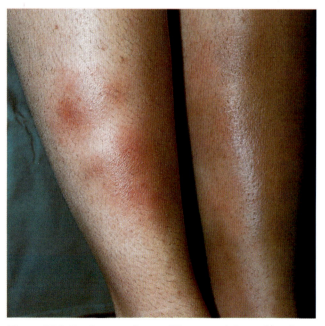

Figure 20.8 Erythema nodosum. Discrete nodules and confluent plaques on the front of the legs

subcutaneous tissues (the primary site of pathology being the blood vessels) to various stimuli, many of which signify internal disease. The lesions occur characteristically on the anterior surface of the legs below the knees (Figure 20.8). Occasionally, they may occur on the backs of the legs, extensor surfaces of the arms and, rarely, on the back of the neck. The lesions are red tender nodules that vary in size from 1–10 cm in diameter. Occasionally, the nodules join to form a confluent plaque (Figure 20.8). The lesions are painful in the initial stages. They may remain red and tender for 2–3 weeks, after which they become less painful, turn purple and involute. Not all of the lesions appear simultaneously and, thus, new ones may appear while older ones are beginning to resolve. The pathological process in the skin in erythema nodosum is usually self-limiting and the skin lesions should have cleared within a month of onset.

Etiology

The most common known causes are streptococcal infections, primary tuberculous infection, sarcoidosis and drugs. Less frequent causes include meningococcal septicemia and lymphogranuloma venereum. In some patients, no cause can be found.

Management and treatment

Clearly, the most important part of management is to investigate the patient to determine the presence of any of the above-mentioned disorders and, if so, to give the appropriate treatment. The treatment of the erythema nodosum lesions will depend on their severity. In the mild forms, rest and simple analgesics are all that is required. In the more severe forms, the patient will be more comfortable in bed and, if the lesions are severe, systemic corticosteroids will control the inflammatory response. However, it must be stressed that systemic corticosteroids can only be given *after* the patient has been investigated to establish the cause of the condition.

SARCOIDOSIS

This is a well-recognized clinical entity with a specific histology, although the etiology remains unknown. Sarcoidosis was, in fact, first noted as a skin disorder, but has subsequently been found to involve any or all organs. Sarcoidosis in the skin may, therefore, be part of the general involvement of the body by the process or it may be the only organ affected.

The skin lesions are due to dermal or subcutaneous granulomatous infiltrates. They appear as smooth papules, nodules or plaques (Figure 20.9). The lesions may be skin-colored, pink or purplish in whites, but hypo- or hyperpigmented plaques in blacks (Figure 20.9). The most common sites to be affected are the face, neck and hands. A condition in which the skin of the nose, cheeks and ears becomes infiltrated, congested and purplish in color is now recognized as a manifestation of sarcoidosis (in older texts, it was referred to as lupus pernio).

The course of sarcoid is variable. The lesions may persist for a few months or many years. They may disappear leaving no residual signs, or there may be some scarring.

Treatment

The only drugs known to have a significant effect on sarcoidosis are corticosteroids. Topically, they have no effect because the lesions are in the dermis and not the epidermis. If the lesions are multiple, then systemic corticosteroids have to be given to produce any effect. However, since sarcoid usually runs a fairly protracted course, the dangers of long-term systemic corticosteroids must be considered. Generally speaking, if the skin is the only organ involved, the use of these drugs cannot be justified. If the lesions are few, intralesional injection of a corticosteroid may be helpful.

PURPURA AND VASCULITIS

Purpura is the extravasation of blood from the vessels into the skin or mucous membranes. It presents as a red patch in the skin and has to be distinguished from erythema, which is a red patch due to dilatation of the blood vessels in the skin. If the redness of the skin is due to extravasation of blood (purpura), the color of the skin will not change on pressure (a glass spatula is best as it permits the result to be seen while applying the pressure; Figure 20.10). If the redness of the skin is due simply to dilatation of the vessels, the skin will blanch.

The purpuric lesion may vary in size from a few millimeters to a few centimeters. The most common site due to whatever cause is the lower limbs (Figure 20.10) because this is the site of maximum venous or back pressure on the capillaries. The causes of purpura are numerous, but it must always be borne in mind that some of the causes are serious disorders and, thus, all patients must be carefully investigated. Essentially, the etiology of purpura is due to disorders of the blood or the vessel walls. The classification of purpura belongs to the realms of hematology, but Table 20.1 may serve as a useful guide, although it is by no means complete.

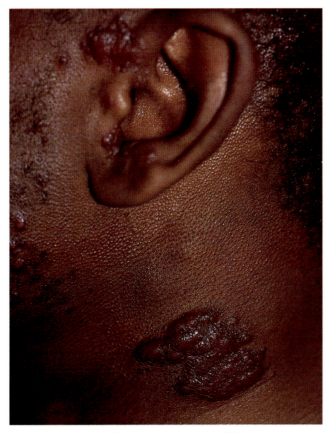

Figure 20.9 *Sarcoidosis. Hyperpigmented nodules and plaques on black skin*

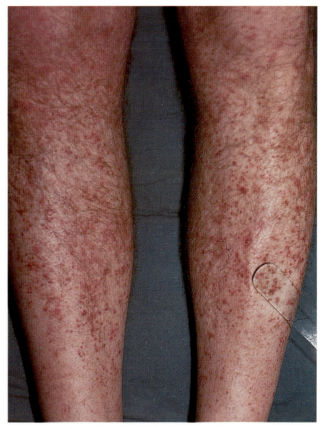

Figure 20.10 *Purpura. The eruption does not blanch on pressure, unlike erythema due to vasodilatation*

Table 20.1 Classification of purpura

Disorders of the blood	Disorders of the blood vessels
Deficiencies of platelets	Hereditary
Idiopathic	Aging (senile purpura)
Leukemia or carcinomatosis	'Allergic' (e.g. Henoch–
Vitamin B$_{12}$ deficiency	Schönlein)
Drugs (e.g. cytotoxics, gold,	Toxic
sulfonamides, chloramphenicol)	Vitamin C deficiency
Systemic lupus erythematosus	associated with emboli
Disorders of coagulation	(e.g. subacute bacterial
(other than platelet deficiency)	endocarditis)
Diseases producing cryoglobulins	Associated with eczema
and macroglobulins	Idiopathic capillaritis

Thus, it can be seen that the causes of purpura are numerous, and the treatment will depend on the cause. From a dermatological viewpoint, it is probably justifiable to stress those above-mentioned conditions which are most likely to present to the dermatologist.

Eczema

It is important to realize that any eczema may be associated with purpuric lesions. This is probably due to a combination of the inflammatory process and trauma (scratching).

Idiopathic capillaritis (Schamberg's disease)

This disease is characterized by discoid areas of purpuric lesions on the lower leg (Figure 20.11). Because of the continual leaking of blood into the skin, there is frequently residual pigmentation due to hemosiderin. The lesions may spread to involve the thighs and trunk, but are not associated with any internal disorder. The cause is unknown and there is no satisfactory treatment.

Henoch–Schönlein purpura

This disease frequently presents to the dermatologist with purpura on the legs and buttocks (Figure 20.12). There may be accompanying nephritis, arthritis and bleeding into the gut. The skin lesions in the severe forms may be papules, blisters and necrotic ulcers in addition to the purpura. Henoch–Schönlein purpura is probably what is termed an immune-complex disorder. A possible antigen is streptococcus.

Vasculitis

The term is used here to imply damage to arterioles and small arteries in the skin (cutaneous vasculitis). The disorder usually presents to the dermatologist as

multiple purpuric papules and/or blisters if the small superficial vessels are involved (Figures 20.13 and 20.14), or as deeper firm nodules if larger vessels are involved. As with other causes of purpura, the most common site for cutaneous vasculitis is the lower leg.

Occasionally, cutaneous vasculitis is associated with a chronic reticular cyanosis on the legs, so-called livedo reticularis (Figure 20.15). The causes of this type of lesion are often similar to those causing purpura. The most common etiological factors are 'allergic' (immune-complex, e.g. streptococci or drugs), toxic (e.g. drugs) and polyarteritis nodosa (cause unknown).

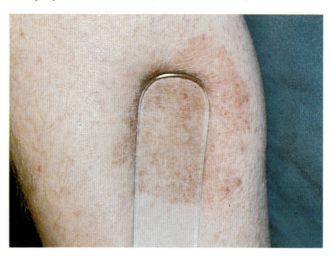

Figure 20.11 *Idiopathic capillaritis. Discoid purpuric eruption which may turn into a brown patch due to hemosiderin deposition*

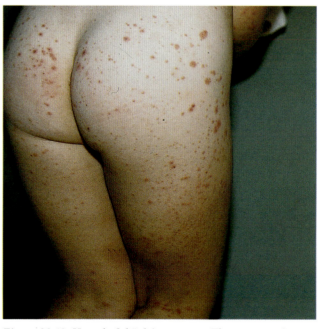

Figure 20.12 *Henoch–Schönlein purpura. The common sites are legs and buttocks. As well as purpura, the eruption is often papular and occasionally blisters are also present*

The treatment is first to define a cause if possible (e.g. drug or streptococcal infection). If this can be eradicated, the disorder is frequently self-limiting. However, if the disorder is continuous, systemic therapy will be required. Corticosteroids usually control the lesions and dapsone may also be effective. Other immunosuppressive drugs are sometimes necessary if there is no satisfactory response to either steroids or dapsone.

LESIONS IN THE SKIN DUE TO INTERNAL MALIGNANCY

Carcinomata

Acanthosis nigricans

In this condition, the skin becomes pigmented and thickened (usually due to epidermal hypertrophy) with a rough surface. The most common sites to be involved are the axillae (Figure 20.16), flexures of the limbs, and backs of the hands and neck. Although acanthosis nigri-

cans is certainly an indicator of internal malignancy, it is not always so, particularly in obese persons. However, in adults, the incidence is so high that all patients should be screened for carcinomas, especially of the stomach.

Secondary deposits

Secondary carcinomatous deposits in the skin are relatively rare. When they do occur, they present as firm nodules. The diagnosis is established by biopsy.

Lymphomas

Skin lesions in association with a lymphoma at other sites of the body are not infrequent. The lesions usually present as firm plaques or nodules. Leukemia, Hodgkin's disease and sarcomata may all give rise to nodular deposits in the skin (Figure 20.17). Occasionally, the skin lesion is the presenting sign. In chronic lymphatic leukemia, there is occasional infiltration of the nose (Figure 20.18) and ear lobes by the leukemic cells, which presents as a generalized firm swelling rather than a solitary nodule.

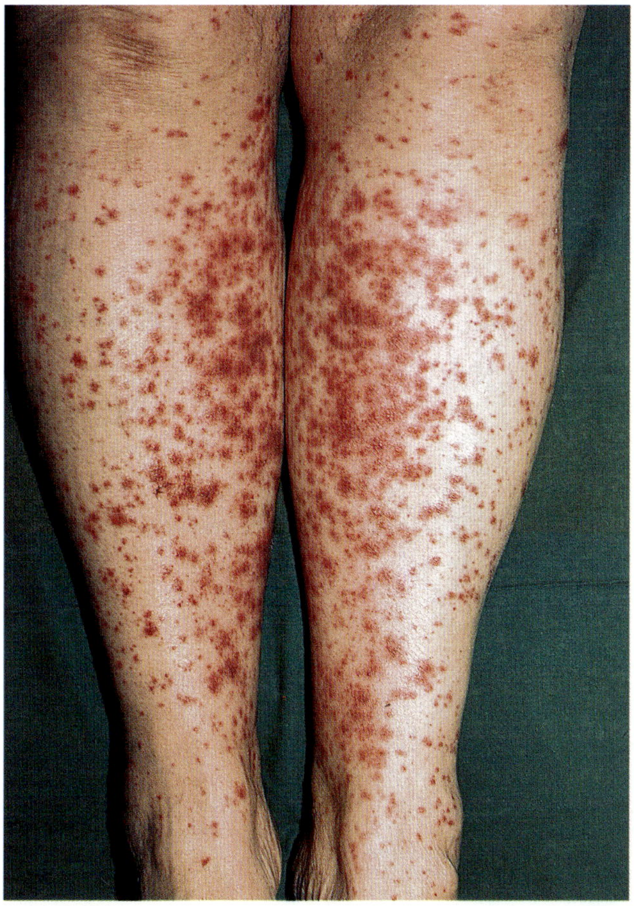

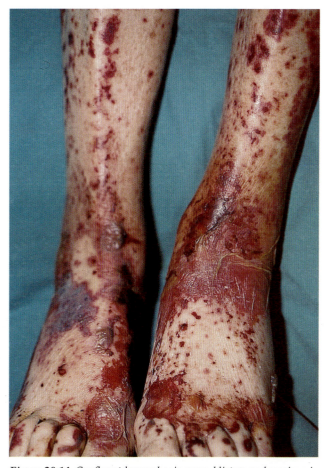

Figure 20.13 Purplish (purpuric) patches and papules on the legs in cutaneous vasculitis

Figure 20.14 Confluent hemorrhagic areas, blisters and erosions in a severe form of cutaneous vasculitis

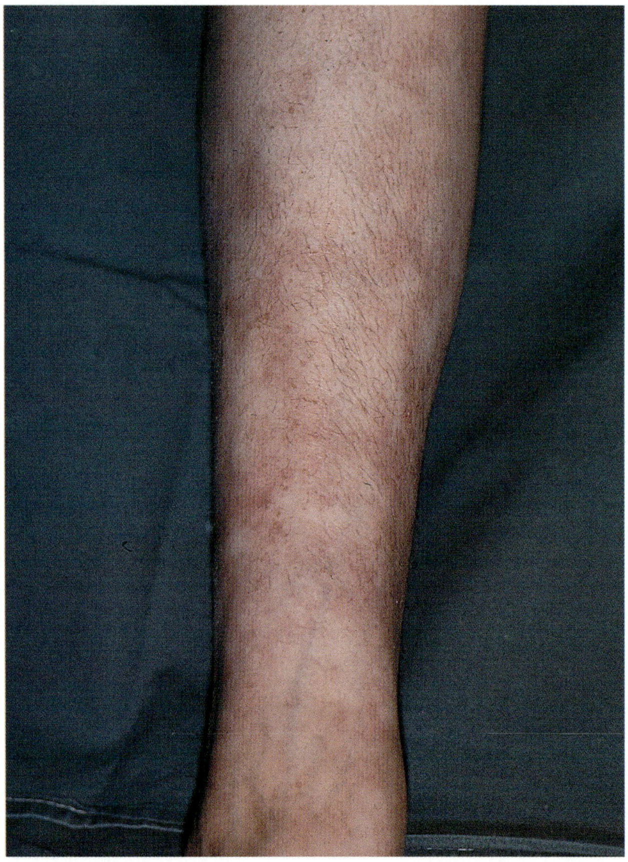

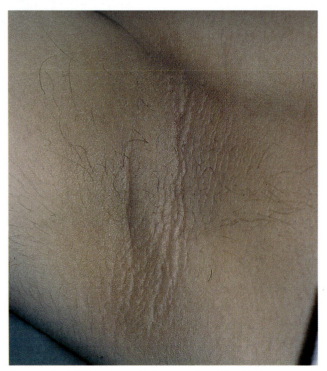

Figure 20.15 *Livedo reticularis*

PRURITUS

Patients who complain of generalized irritation with no obvious skin lesions (other than excoriations) have to be screened for internal disorders. The classical disorder to give rise to this symptom, possibly for years before there are any other signs, is Hodgkin's disease.

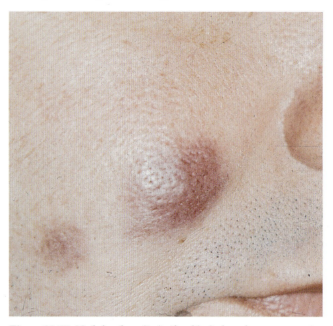

Figure 20.17 *Nodular deposits in the skin in lymphoma*

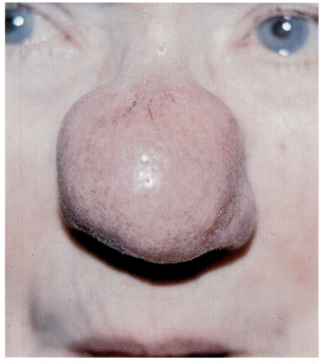

Figure 20.16 *Thickening and pigmentation of the skin in acanthosis nigricans*

Figure 20.18 *Infiltration of the nose with leukemic cells in chronic lymphatic leukemia*

Pruritus has also been recorded in association with other forms of lymphoma and carcinoma, renal failure and liver disease. In the latter, it has been attributed to the high level of bile salts in the skin but, more recently, a CNS cause for pruritus due to liver disease has been suggested.

Diabetes mellitus has also been mentioned as a cause of generalized pruritus, but this is questionable. The irritation here is usually due to *Candida* infection.

Pruritus due to psychiatric disorder is well recognized and has to be considered, but only after other causes have been excluded.

PYODERMA GANGRENOSUM

This is a distinct clinical entity which may be found in association with a number of underlying systemic disorders, the most common being ulcerative colitis and rheumatoid arthritis. However, it may also occur with Crohn's disease, Behçet's syndrome, leuke-mia and other disorders of the reticuloendothelial system. How these various diseases produce pyoderma gangrenosum is not known, but it seems likely that it is due to an immunological abnormality. Pyoderma gangrenosum may occur with no obvious underlying disease.

The typical lesion begins as a small, tender, red nodule or pustule which breaks down to form an ulcer (Figure 20.19). The ulcers rapidly increase in size and may eventually be 15–20 cm in diameter, although they usually stop enlarging once they have reached 4–5 cm in diameter. The outline of the edge of the ulcer is variable but, characteristically, there is an overhanging bluish edge (Figure 20.19). The ulcers may occur anywhere, but the trunk is the most common site. The ulcers may heal spontaneously, although scarring is common.

Treatment of pyoderma gangrenosum is with relatively high doses of systemic steroids, i.e. 60 mg prednisone daily. Cyclosporine has also been shown to be effective in pyoderma gangrenosum. An associated disorder should be sought if not apparent, and appropriate treatment given.

PRETIBIAL MYXEDEMA

As the name implies, the abnormality is most commonly seen on the front of the legs, although other sites may be involved. Pretibial myxedema presents as pinkish raised plaques (Figure 20.20). It may be associated with hyperthyroid, hypothyroid or euthyroid states. The long-acting thyroid stimulator (LATS)

hormone is often found to be elevated, but is not considered to be causally related. It is likely that another pituitary hormone is the causative factor. The skin lesions are due to infiltration of the dermis due to mucin. The condition often responds to topical (Group IV) steroids.

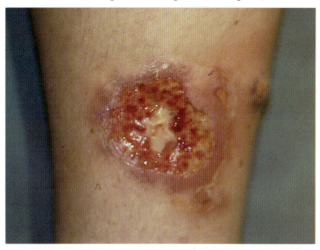

Figure 20.19 *Pyoderma gangrenosum. Ulcer with bluish edge. Small satellite lesions are present*

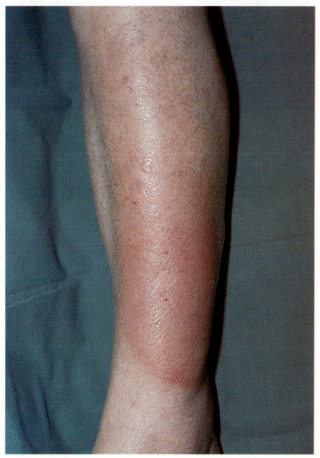

Figure 20.20 *Pretibial myxedema. Red infiltrated plaque on the anterior leg*

21

Parasitic infestations and insect bites

SCABIES

Scabies is one of the more commonly seen disorders in a skin clinic. Since it is a disorder with a potentially 100% cure rate with simple treatment, this implies that the referring doctor (usually the casualty officer or general practitioner) has missed the diagnosis or has not given the correct medication or instructions to go with it.

Etiology

The disorder is caused by a mite – *Sarcoptes scabei* var *hominis*. The female mite (acarus), which is only just visible with the naked eye, burrows into the keratin layer of the epidermis. In the burrow, the mite lays her eggs, which hatch after 3–4 days. Active larvae then emerge from the burrow and invade the adjacent epidermis. After 17 days, the male and female adult forms emerge. Copulation occurs and the gravid female then wanders over the skin surface before burrowing again and repeating the cycle. The female may live for 6–8 weeks in a burrow and lay up to 50 eggs.

The insect passes from one person to another when there is close bodily contact. The disease is highly contagious and the most usual way to acquire the infection is by sharing a bed with an infected person. Thus, invariably, there is a positive 'family' history of other members of the family, or a close friend, being similarly affected.

In the early stages of the disorder when the female mite makes her burrow in the skin, the patient will probably have no symptoms. However, after the eggs begin to hatch (usually 3–4 weeks after the infestation has been acquired), the patient develops a generalized irritating eruption. It is thought that this eruption is due to sensitization from a substance produced by the mite or possibly by the eggs themselves.

Clinical presentation

Symptoms
The first symptom of which the patient complains is a generalized irritation when going to bed at night. It appears to be fairly characteristic of scabies that the irritation is worse at night than during the day. Subsequently, the patient will be aware of a rash which may be fairly generalized and the irritation at this stage may also persist during the day.

Signs
The characteristic lesion of scabies infestation is the burrow. The classical appearance of a burrow is a grayish, linear or slightly curved, scaly lesion (Figures 21.1 and 21.2). It is usually 0.5 cm in length and rarely longer than 1.0 cm. Occasionally, at one end, a small vesicle may be seen. The most common sites for finding the classical burrow are the palms (Figures 21.1 and 21.2), between the fingers and on the wrists. Not infrequently, the classical burrow is not found, but superficially scaly lesions (the same size as burrows) are found between the fingers (Figure 21.3) or on the palms.

The lesions sometimes become secondarily infected and present as crusted lesions or pustules. Although the acarus may burrow at other sites, notably the breasts (in females), external genitalia (in males; Figures 21.4 and 21.5), buttocks (Figure 21.6) and umbilicus, the classical burrow may not be seen at these sites.

The lesions may present as firm, deep, red papules (Figures 21.5 and 21.6). There may be some superficial scaling or excoriation. The finding of this type of lesion on the male genitalia and buttocks is often as diagnostic as the typical burrow on the hands. In infants under 1 year of age, a common site of burrowing is on the soles of the feet. The lesions may present here as small blisters.

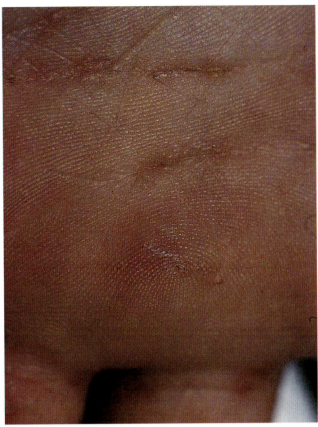

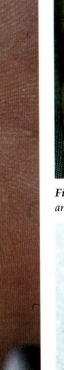

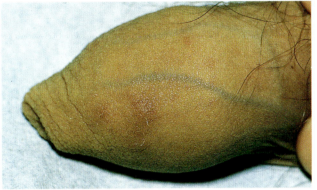

Figure 21.3 *Scaly, excoriated and inflamed area between the thumb and finger at the site of a burrow*

Figure 21.1 *Burrows in scabies presenting as linear scaly lesions on the palms*

Figure 21.4 *Burrows and erythematous papules on the penis in scabies*

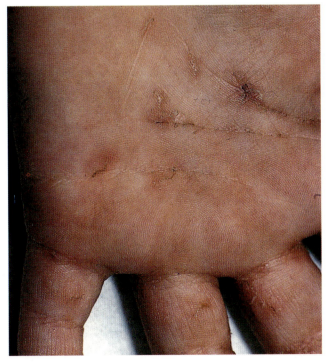

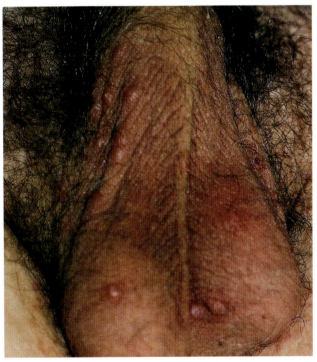

Figure 21.2 *Multiple burrows on the palm and fingers, the common sites in scabies*

Figure 21.5 *Multiple red indurated papules on the scrotum in scabies*

By the time the patient seeks medical advice, there is usually a generalized eruption on the trunk and limbs, but the head is never involved except in children under 2 years of age. The generalized eruption takes the form of excoriated papular urticarial lesions (Figure 21.7). On the trunk in children (Figure 21.8) and particularly around and in the axillae in adults, the lesion presents as firm red papules (Figure 21.9). These lesions are fairly characteristic of scabies. The generalized eruption in scabies is thought to be an allergic reaction to the contents of the burrow, either the mite itself, or its eggs or excreta.

It should be remembered that, because of the intense irritation and subsequent scratching, there is frequently secondary bacterial infection which presents as impetigo and boils, which destroys the typical structure and therefore the appearance of the burrows.

The most satisfactory way to confirm the diagnosis is to demonstrate the presence of the acarus (Figure 21.10) in a burrow on the hands or in a papule on the male genitalia or buttocks. This is best achieved by gently scraping the burrow with a blunt scalpel blade and examining the contents under low-power microscopy. Even if the acarus itself is not seen, eggs may be found. From the practical point of view, however, in general practice when a microscope is not available, the typical appearances and a positive family history are usually all that are required to make the diagnosis.

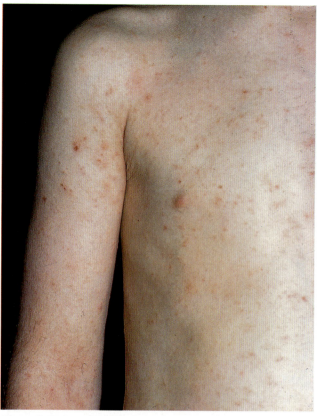

Figure 21.7 *Generalized excoriated papular eruption in scabies. This represents an 'allergic' reaction to the contents of the burrow*

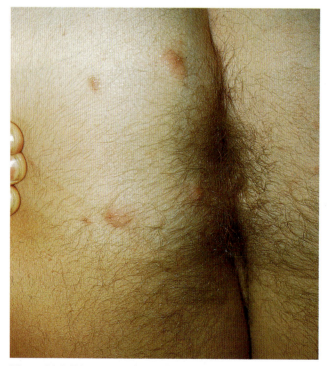

Figure 21.6 *Discrete papules on the buttock in scabies*

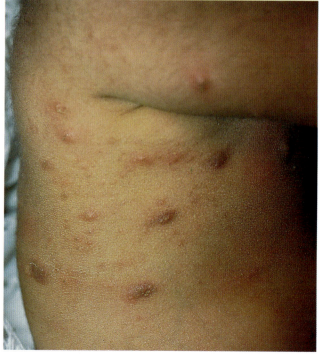

Figure 21.8 *Large red papules and nodules on the trunk in an infant with scabies*

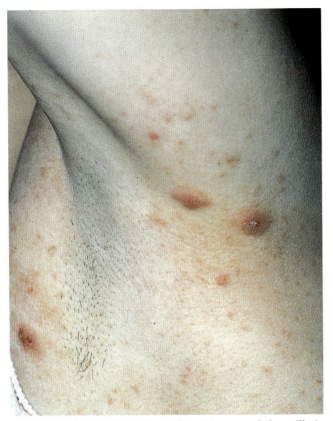

Figure 21.9 *Large red papules and nodules around the axilla in scabies. This is a similar cellular reaction to the lesions occurring on the buttocks and genitalia*

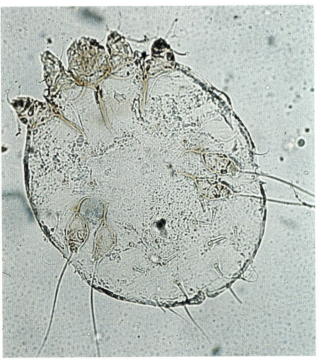

Figure 21.10 *The acarus isolated from a burrow, viewed by low-power microscopy*

NORWEGIAN SCABIES

This form of scabies is rare and has a completely different clinical picture from the disorder described above. It usually occurs in the elderly or in patients with mental deficiency living in institutions. The typical clinical appearance is a generalized scaly redness of the skin with thick hyperkeratotic crusting on the hands, feet and elbows.

It is important to be aware of this condition as it is frequently misdiagnosed as a generalized eczema and thus wrongly treated. Norwegian scabies is contagious and is often only diagnosed when a nurse or other care-worker of the patient develops scabies. The reason for the difference in the clinical appearance of Norwegian scabies from that of usual scabies is unknown, but must be due to host factors as the causal parasite is the same.

Treatment and management

Patients often arrive in a skin clinic from a general practitioner with the correct diagnosis of scabies, but with treatment having failed. There are two important points to remember in the treatment of scabies. First, the lotion must be applied to the *entire* skin surface, from the neck to the soles of the feet and, second, the whole household (including boyfriends and girlfriends) must all be treated simultaneously.

The preparations for scabies include benzyl benzoate (BP) application, gamma benzene hexachloride lotion 1%, malathion lotion 0.5% and permethrin cream 5%. Permethrin cream is the newest preparation and should only be used if the other preparations are not effective because of possible resistance of the mite to the other preparations.

Benzyl benzoate and gamma benzene hexachloride are not recommended for infants.

The treatment is carried out as follows:

(1) The patient is bathed and dried;

(2) The lotion or cream is then applied to the whole body apart from the head, except in children under age 2 years if lesions are present on the head. Lotions may be applied with either cottonwool or a paint brush;

(3) The preparation should be applied again after 24 h;

(4) 24 h after the second application, the patient is bathed again;

(5) The bedsheets and underclothes should be changed, but it is not necessary for outerwear or blankets to be laundered or dry-cleaned.

It is important to tell the patient that the irritation may persist for 1–2 weeks after treatment (due to an allergic reaction even though the mite has been killed). If patients are not told that the irritation may persist, they will usually continue to anoint themselves and produce an irritant eczema (particularly if using benzyl benzoate). Thus, although cured of scabies, they will continue to itch because of an iatrogenic eczema.

It is also important to realize that the papular lesions on the genitalia and around the axillae, particularly in children, may persist for many months after successful treatment. The papules represent an 'immunological' reaction in the skin with chronic inflammatory cells and do not disperse for a considerable length of time.

PEDICULOSIS (LICE)

Clinically, pediculosis may present as three distinct entities, depending on the species and variety of louse.

Pediculosis capitis (head lice)

This is a contagious disorder seen predominantly in children. The main symptom is pruritus of the scalp due to bites from the insect. Because of the irritation, there is continual scratching and this not infrequently becomes secondarily infected by bacteria. Thus, if a child is brought to the clinic complaining of scalp irritation or with impetigo of the scalp, and excoriations are present, it is most important to think of head lice as a cause of the symptoms and signs.

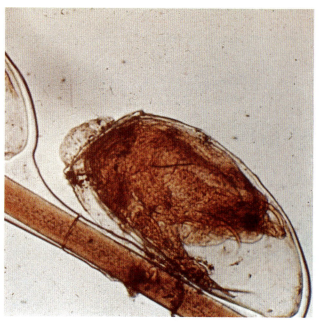

Figure 21.11 *Nit of a head louse attached to a hair, as seen on low-power microscopy*

The characteristic feature of head lice is nits on the hair shaft. The mature form of the insect has a relatively short life, but the female lays numerous eggs close to the scalp surface which develop into nits. Clinically, they are small white specks firmly attached to the hair shaft. The most common site is the hair behind the ears, but any part of the scalp hair may be involved.

The nits are approximately 0.5 mm in length and have to be distinguished from scales in the hair from seborrheic eczema (dandruff). Nits are firmly attached to the hair and cannot be brushed off whereas scales from dandruff can easily be removed. The nits can sometimes be slid along the hair shaft.

If a microscope is available, the diagnosis can be established by cutting off a hair with a nit attached and examining it under low power (Figure 21.11). The nit will be seen as an oval structure firmly attached to the hair by a sheath which completely encases the shaft. Very occasionally, the louse itself may be visible with the naked eye in the scalp.

Treatment
The preparations available for head lice include permethrin lotion 1%, malathion lotion 0.5% and gamma benzene hexachloride lotion 1%. The permethrin preparation should be applied after the hair has been washed and dried, left on the hair for 10 min and then washed off. Malathion is applied to the scalp and left for 12 h, after which the hair is then shampooed. Gamma benzene hexachloride application is left on the scalp for only 4 min before being shampooed.

After using any of these lotions, the hair should be combed with a fine comb while still wet. The treatment is repeated after a week. It is probably advisable to treat all members of the household, particularly children, at the same time even if they are asymptomatic.

Nits can be removed, even though they are not visible, with a nit comb – a fine metal comb. If this cannot be obtained from a chemist, some public health departments keep a supply.

Pediculosis corporis (body lice)

This has become a rare affliction and is usually only seen in persons whose personal hygiene is poor. It is now usually encountered in the homeless who attend a casualty department for one reason or another. The body louse is rarely found on the skin as it lives in the seams of clothing and leaves only for meals. The nits are firmly attached to the fibers of clothing. Thus, if pediculosis corporis is suspected, it is important to examine the clothes, particularly the underclothes, for the parasite, which is visible to the naked eye.

The characteristic skin lesion resulting from a bite is a small red macule. Occasionally, there is a papule with a central hemorrhagic punctum. The most frequent sites for bites are on the trunk. There is intense irritation and thus, on examination, the most obvious features are extensive and severe excoriations (Figure 21.12) and not the individual bites. There is frequently secondary bacterial infection. In severe and long-standing infestation, the skin becomes pigmented, dry, scaly and eczematized, and there are scars from previous excoriations. These features are sometimes referred to as 'vagabond's disease'.

Treatment

The clothing and not the patient require the treatment. High-temperature laundering and dry-cleaning are effective. Insecticides have also been used to treat the clothes and these have included permethrin and gamma benzene hexachloride.

Pediculosis pubis (pubic lice)

The principal site of involvement is the pubic hair, but the lice may involve other areas. Nits have been found attached to axillary and body hair (other than pubic), eyelashes and eyebrows. The main symptom is pruritus produced by the bites of the louse. Thus, on examination, there are excoriations and possibly secondary bacterial infection. The mature parasite is often visible to the naked eye.

Treatment

It is preferable to treat the whole body as the pubic lice frequently affect hair all over the body, including the axillae. Malathion, permethrin and gamma benzene hexachloride are all effective preparations.

INSECT BITES (PAPULAR URTICARIA)

The typical skin lesion produced by an insect bite, i.e. an urticarial lesion with a central punctum and surrounding flare (Figure 21.13), is easily recognized by lay persons. However, occasionally there is a different type of clinical response and this results in the person seeking medical advice. It is not possible to say which particular insect produces the lesions seen most frequently in a skin clinic but, undoubtedly, the different species are numerous, e.g. fleas, flies, mosquitoes, bedbugs, etc.

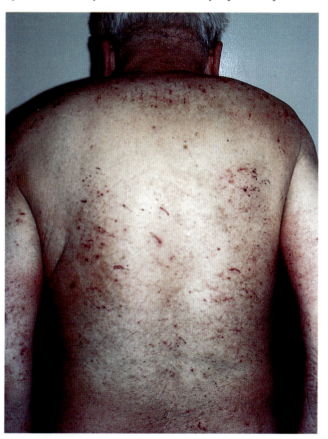

Figure 21.12 Extensive excoriations due to body lice

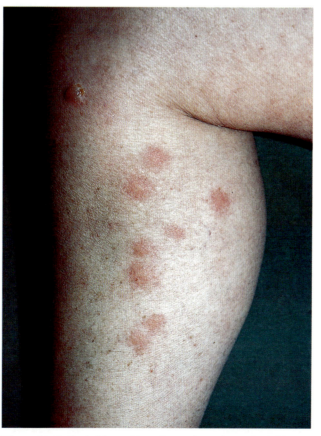

Figure 21.13 Typical insect bites. Grouped papular urticarial lesions

There are two main clinical patterns most commonly seen in a skin clinic. First, there may be an acute urticarial eruption with subsequent blister formation (Figure 21.14), the blisters being a few centimeters in diameter on occasions. Because of the size of the blisters, the patient will seek medical advice. The lesions are usually present on exposed areas, e.g. below the knees (Figure 21.14), on the forearms and hands and, occasionally, on the face.

The second type of clinical presentation is persistent papules, most commonly seen in children, on the arms and legs (Figures 21.15 and 21.16), but occasionally on the trunk. The papules are usually 2–3 mm in diameter and a clue to the diagnosis is often the presence of a central punctum. In the early stages, there is a central wheal, flaring and a central punctum characteristic of insect bites.

It is the persistence of the lesions beyond a few days which confuses both doctors and patients, and results in referral to a dermatologist. The cause of the persistence of the lesion is not certain, but is probably due to an altered immunological response on the part of the patient. The papules are due to a persistent cellular infiltrate and may take months to disappear.

The lesions are always discrete with normal skin in between and there is sometimes residual scarring. In blacks, this type of lesion invariably leads to post-inflammatory hyperpigmentation (Figure 21.16), which may persist for a few months, and is another cause for referral to a skin clinic. The hyperpigmentation eventually fades.

Treatment and management

Treatment of the acute blistering eruption is symptomatic with systemic antihistamines. The lesions usually settle within a few days. Dry non-adhesive dressings may be required when the blisters burst. Acute and widespread eruptions require a short course of systemic steroids.

In the second type of eruption with persistent small papules, it is often very difficult to convince parents that the lesions on the child are due to insect bites. There are probably two reasons for this. First, this type of lesion

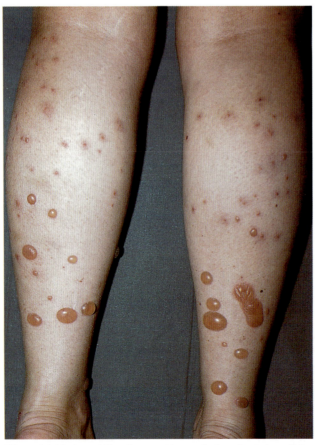

Figure 21.14 *Acute blistering eruption on the legs due to insect bites*

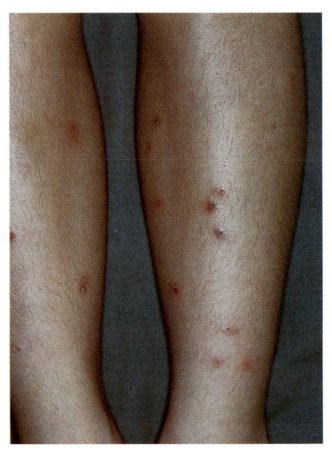

Figure 21.15 *Persistent papules on the legs due to insect bites. The lesions may last for months*

with its persistence is not what the parent associates with insect bites and, second, they cannot think of a source of the insects. If there is an animal pet at home, then this is frequently the source, but various types of insect may live in the furniture or in the gardens of the affected patients. The main problem is often not so much the source of the insects as the altered immunological response of the patient.

Treatment is often unsatisfactory. If the source can be identified, e.g. a domestic animal, this should be treated, if necessary with the help of a vet. Animals are often reinfested from other animals. If a pet is suspected of being a source, it is sometimes helpful to send brushings of its hair to a diagnostic entomological service. These institutes can detect the presence of insects on animals and determine whether these are pathogenic to humans. Insecticide powders containing pyrethrum are effective for treating furniture, etc. Insect repellents (in the form of dimethyl phthalate) are of limited help. Systemic antihistamines may relieve irritation, but do not appear to induce the lesions to resolve more quickly. Fortunately, the majority of children appear to lose this hypersensitive response to insect bites in due course.

CREEPING ERUPTION

This is sometimes referred to as larva migrans as it is due to the larva wandering in the skin. The condition is now seen more frequently in the UK as travel becomes more commonplace. It most commonly occurs in Central and South America, and in southeastern parts of the US. It is usually due to the larva of the hookworm *Ancylostoma braziliense* which penetrates the skin.

Sandy beaches are a common place to acquire the condition and, clinically, the lesions are most common on the feet. The lesions are produced by the larva's wanderings in the skin and consist of a red, slightly raised, irregular line (Figure 21.17). The condition is very irritating, and secondary infection may occur due to continual scratching.

The condition is self-limiting as the larvae have invaded a 'dead-end' host and will eventually die. The duration of creeping eruption is usually 4–6 weeks. No treatment is usually necessary, but 10% topical thiobendazole suspension under polythene occlusion is sometimes effective.

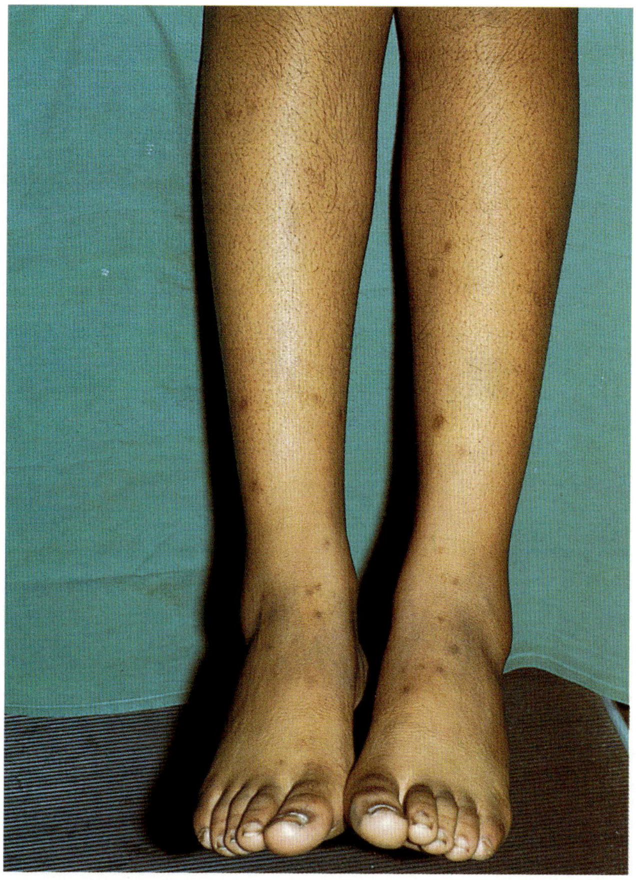

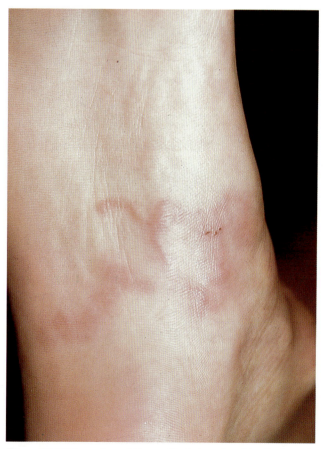

Figure 21.16 Persistent hyperpigmented papules in a black due to insect bites. The hyperpigmentation is postinflammatory and usually persists after the papule has resolved

Figure 21.17 Irregular red line on the foot produced by the larva in creeping eruption

22

Photosensitivity and tropical infections

With the increase in air travel and affluence, many more people are travelling abroad and patients now present with disorders attributable to different climates. Doctors must be aware of these problems.

The term 'photosensitivity' is used to imply an abnormal response to ultraviolet irradiation. It has to be distinguished from ordinary sunburn, which occurs in white people after prolonged exposure to sunlight (particularly strong sunlight) in those whose skin has not adapted to the sun by pigmentation, i.e. usually the first day of a holiday. As such, sunburn and the long-term effects of ultraviolet light on the skin are normal responses in whites, but are discussed here in some detail as they may present as a medical problem.

NORMAL REACTIONS TO SUNLIGHT

Sunburn

This is by far the most common adverse reaction produced by sunlight. The three important factors which determine sunburn are the degree of pigmentation prior to going into the sunlight (fair-skinned people are more at risk), the length of time exposed, and the strength of the sun (the more vertical the rays, the more damaging they are to the skin).

Sunburn is characterized by a biphasic erythema response. The initial erythema occurs during exposure and disappears shortly thereafter. The delayed erythema usually begins 2–4 h after exposure and reaches a peak after approximately 15 h and persists for up to 48 h. This stage is accompanied by pain and discomfort if the erythema has been severe. Very occasionally, there may be edema of the skin and blister formation. The erythema stage is followed by peeling of the skin.

Sunburn is a 'phototoxic reaction in the skin. The energy in solar rays causes the release of certain chemi-

cals in the skin and accounts for the inflammatory response. The sunburn reaction in normal subjects is caused by rays which constitute medium-wave ultraviolet light (290–320 nm; UVB).

Treatment and management

Once the patient has developed sunburn, treatment is symptomatic. Further exposure to sunlight must be avoided until the erythema subsides. Topical steroid creams may diminish the inflammatory response. For a short duration (2–3 days), one of the Group I or II steroid preparations should be used. A cream-based preparation should be prescribed as the cream itself may have a soothing effect, and should be applied three or four times a day. Mild analgesics and sedatives can be given if the patient is in severe discomfort.

Patients with fair skin should be warned not to stay exposed in the sunlight for long periods and given sunscreen preparations to use. There is now a large number of sunscreen preparations of varying protective strength (see Chapter 25). The skin protection factor (SPF) refers to protection against UVB, the sunburn fraction of ultraviolet light. The greater the protection required by the patient, the higher the SPF value.

CHRONIC EFFECTS OF SUNLIGHT

These effects are also within normal limits for whites who live in sunny climates. The changes vary with the degree of pigmentation (and thus protection) and duration of exposure. The changes include wrinkling due to damage to the elastic tissue, atrophy, hyperpigmented macules (lentigos; Figures 22.1 and 22.2), telangiectasia and actinic keratoses. In addition, ultraviolet irradiation is carcinogenic. Basal cell and squamous cell carcinomata are most commonly found on exposed skin and are more common in whites living in South Africa and Australia than in those living in England.

ABNORMAL REACTIONS TO SUNLIGHT: PHOTOSENSITIVITY

These may occur in the following three situations:

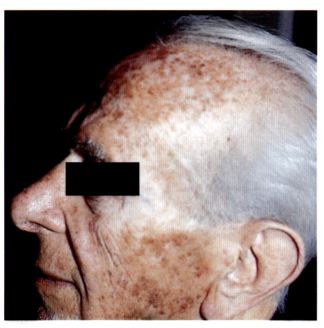

Figure 22.1 *Actinic lentigos. Hyperpigmented macules produced by years of exposure to strong sunlight*

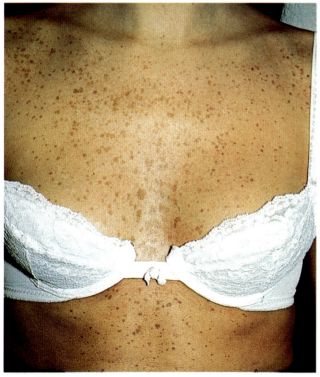

Figure 22.2 *Actinic lentigos on the chest in a young woman who lived in Northern Territory of Australia*

(1) When a known substance in the skin, either due to internal causes or applied externally, 'sensitizes' the skin;

(2) In disorders resulting in deficient protection; and

(3) With no known cause (at present) for the reaction.

Known photosensitizers

Porphyria

This is a disease in which abnormal porphyrin metabolism results in circulating porphyrins which become deposited in the skin. Some of the porphyrins cause photosensitivity.

The classification of porphyria is unsatisfactory. From a simple clinical point of view, porphyria may be classified into those cases in which the abnormal porphyrin metabolism is in:

(1) Bone marrow;

(2) Liver; or

(3) At both sites.

Alternatively, porphyria can be classified into that which involves photosensitivity and that which does not. The photosensitivity depends on the particular porphyrins produced which in turn depends on the basic biochemical abnormality present.

One type of porphyria associated with light sensitivity has recently been shown to involve abnormal iron metabolism. It is thought possible that an increase in the absorption of iron occurs and a raised serum iron concentration is frequently found. The cause for this abnormal iron metabolism is not known.

The skin lesions may present as an acute erythema or blisters in the light-exposed areas. The former is usually seen in young children and the latter in adults. There is increased skin fragility, and minor trauma produces blisters which break and form scabs (Figures 22.3 and 22.4). Scarring of the light-exposed skin is a common finding. In adults, there is occasionally an increase in pigmentation and excess hair growth (Figure 22.5).

Systemic drugs

A number of drugs taken orally cause photosensitivity. The most common drugs to elicit this response are the sulfonamides (Figure 22.6), sulfonylureas, tetracyclines (Figure 22.7), phenothiazines (particularly chlorpromazine), thiazide diuretics and nalidixic acid. The type of rash produced is usually an acute erythema (Figure 22.7), sometimes with accompanying blisters and subsequent peeling of the skin. It should be remembered that any drug can cause any rash and photosensitization may be the end result.

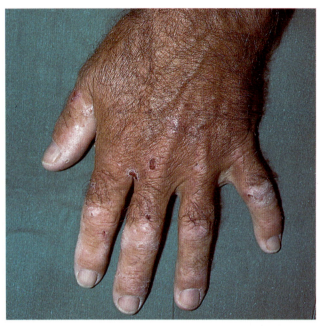

Figure 22.3 Small scabs on the back of the hand produced by minor trauma because of increased skin fragility in porphyria

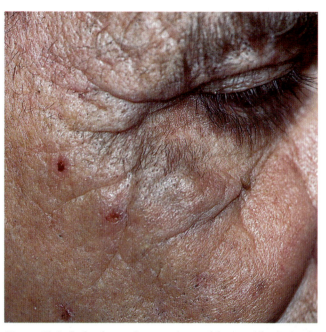

Figure 22.5 Scabs, hyperpigmentation and hypertrichosis on the cheeks in porphyria

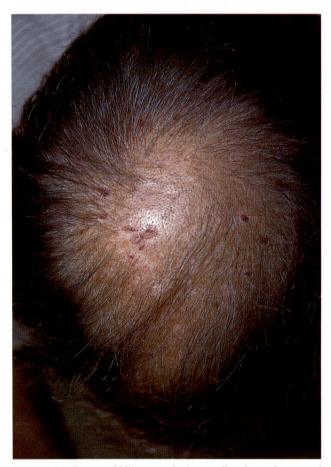

Figure 22.4 Ruptured blisters producing small scabs on the exposed part of the scalp in porphyria

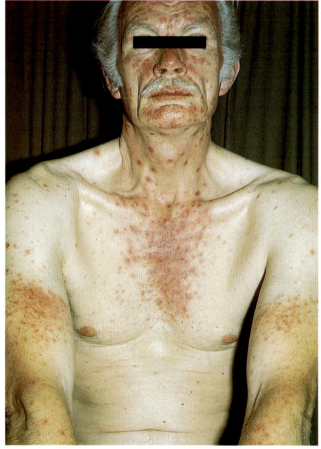

Figure 22.6 Photosensitive eruption due to a sulfonamide

Topical photosensitizers

Probably the most common topical photosensitizers are the essential oils in cosmetics. The one most frequently incriminated is oil of bergamot. This may cause acute erythema, blisters and subsequent pigmentation (Figure 22.8). Occasionally, only the excess pigmentation results.

The most common site for this pattern of reaction is the neck, as the result of perfume applied behind the ears and to the sides of the neck. Other topical photosensitizers are chemicals from plants, tar preparations, chemicals in shampoos, cosmetics (apart from perfumes) and industrial processes.

Adverse reactions from deficient protection

As has already been stated, melanin pigmentation offers protection from the damaging effects of the sun's rays. Thus, in disorders in which melanin formation is deficient or impaired, there will be abnormal reactions to sunlight. These conditions include albinism, oculocutaneous albinism, vitiligo and phenylketonuria, and affect persons with fair hair and light complexions.

In a rare condition called xeroderma pigmentosa, there is an abnormality in the repair of the skin cell DNA following damage due to exposure to sunlight. This failure to repair DNA results in malignant skin conditions at a very early age, usually in childhood.

Photosensitivity reactions with unknown causes

Systemic lupus erythematosus

Patients with this condition frequently develop an erythematous eruption in the exposed areas, particularly the face. The classical distribution is across the nose and cheeks – the so-called 'butterfly rash'. The eruption is usually an intense erythema (Figure 22.9), but urticarial and vesicular eruptions have also been reported.

Solar urticaria

As the name implies, the predominant skin lesion in some patients on exposure to sunlight is urticarial. This type of lesion usually develops on the exposed areas after a few minutes of exposure to sunlight. The urticarial lesions usually subside within 1 h after exposure.

Polymorphic light eruption

This is one of the most common photosensitive rashes and occurs predominantly in young adult women. The lesions appear on exposed areas, but not those normally exposed, i.e. face and backs of hands. The rash appears a few hours after being in the sun and lasts a variable

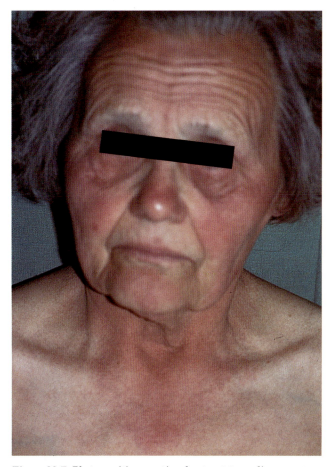

Figure 22.7 Photosensitive eruption due to a tetracycline

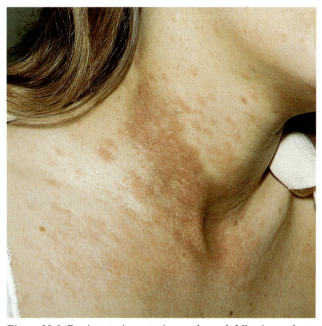

Figure 22.8 Persistent pigmentation on the neck following a photosensitive reaction due to perfume

length of time (a few hours to a few days) if no further exposure occurs. If the patient continues to be exposed to sunlight, the rash will persist, but may improve (although not necessarily) after a week of exposure. As the name implies, the rash varies in morphology. The most common lesions are small red papules (Figure 22.10), but erythematous plaques, patches and blisters may also occur. The rash is usually intensely irritating.

Hutchinson's summer prurigo

This is the term used to describe a condition which is usually seen in children and is characterized by grouped papules (Figure 22.11) on the nose and cheeks. The rash is photosensitive but, in severe cases, the rash also occurs on the body. The condition tends to disappear in adulthood.

Photosensitive eczema

This is most commonly seen in middle-aged and elderly men and presents on the face (Figure 22.12) and backs of the hands. If the condition is severe and remains untreated, the eczema will spread to the non-exposed areas of the skin.

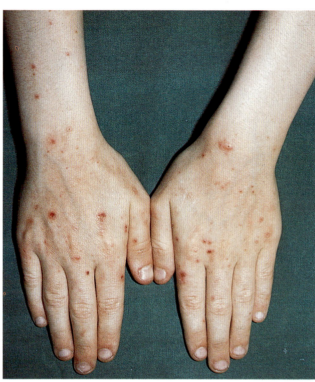

Figure 22.10 *Small scabbed red papules in polymorphic light eruption*

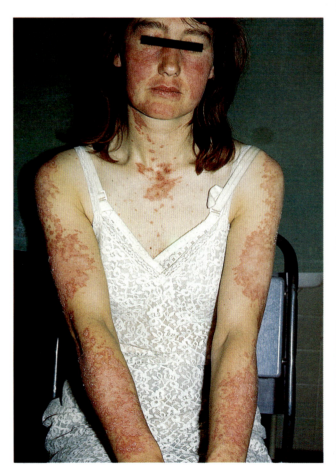

Figure 22.9 *Acute photosensitive eruption in exposed areas in systemic lupus erythematosus*

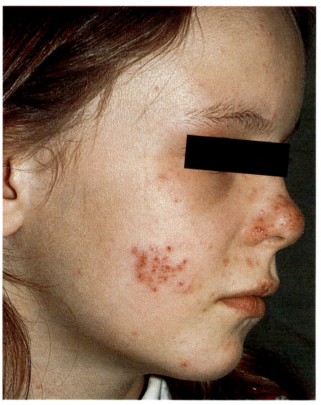

Figure 22.11 *Grouped erythematous papules on the nose and cheeks in Hutchinson's summer prurigo*

Treatment and management of photosensitivity

It is most important to enquire as to whether the patient has taken or is taking any drugs which are possible photosensitizers or whether any cosmetics, creams or lotions containing possible photosensitizers have been used. Enquiry should also be made regarding any contact with plants.

Unless an obvious cause for the photosensitivity is found, all patients should be screened for porphyria and systemic lupus erythematosus, the former by examination of blood, feces and urine for excess porphyrins, and the latter by examination of the blood for antinuclear antibodies. Simpler tests for porphyria screening have been developed, requiring only 5 ml of plasma and using spectrometry to screen for porphyrins.

If exogenous photosensitizers are considered likely, it is possible to carry out photo-patch tests with the suspected substances. The chemicals are applied to the subject's back and irradiated by ultraviolet light.

Treatment of photosensitivity will, to a certain extent, depend on the underlying cause. If it is due to systemic drugs or applied substances, these should be avoided if possible.

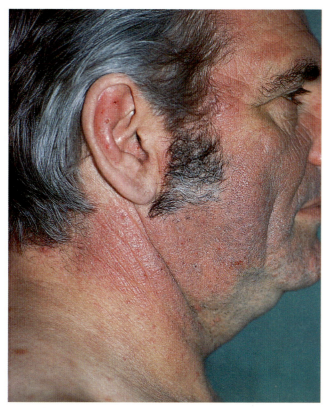

Figure 22.12 *Photosensitive eczema on the face and neck*

If the patient has porphyria, then further investigations will be required to determine if they have the type that is associated with abnormal iron metabolism. In light-sensitive porphyria associated with raised serum iron concentrations, the severity of the light eruption may be decreased and the lesions even prevented by lowering the serum iron levels by venepuncture.

If lupus erythematosus is found, then further investigations will be required before deciding on the appropriate treatment.

Unfortunately, topical sunscreens have not proved effective in preventing the endogenous photosensitivity skin disorders. It should be stressed that most sunscreens are only effective in screening out UVB (middle-wave ultraviolet light causing sunburn), but not UVA (long-wave ultraviolet light) or visible light. Sunscreens are also not 100% effective in screening out the ultraviolet light for which they were designed. Many of the endogenous photodermatoses are not confined to a narrow part of the light spectrum and, thus, it is difficult to screen out the offending rays with topical preparations. It is possible to test patients with a monochrometer to determine to which part of the spectrum the patient reacts, and this may be helpful in patients with disorders which prove difficult to manage. The eruption in porphyria, photosensitive eczema, drug eruptions and polymorphic light eruption is usually caused by long-wave ultraviolet light or visible light, so chemical sunscreens are of little or no use.

Polymorphic light eruption, one of the most common of the photosensitive disorders, can usually be prevented by a short course of PUVA treatment before exposure to the sun. The beneficial effects may last for up to 3–4 months, so patients should be treated in the spring or before they go to sunny climates for the winter. How PUVA prevents polymorphic light eruption is not known.

Systemic steroids in a dose of 20 mg daily will also prevent polymorphic light eruption, but a course of PUVA is preferable. The antimalarial drugs mepacrine and chloroquine have been used in the past to prevent or decrease the severity of photodermatoses. However, their use should be left to experts.

TROPICAL INFECTIONS

Leprosy

This is still an extremely rare condition to see in a skin clinic in the UK. However, because of the immigration into the UK of people from places where leprosy is endemic, a few patients with the disorder are encountered and, thus, the physician must be aware of the disease and its presenting symptoms and signs.

Leprosy occurs in tropical climates, but is most common in the subcontinent of India, West Africa, South China and Burma. The disease is caused by *Mycobacterium leprae,* although evidence is now accumulating that the disease process is influenced by immunological responses of the host. The skin, nerves, reticuloendothelial system, mucous membranes, eyes and testes may be affected by the disease.

The classification of leprosy is unsatisfactory at present but, for clinical purposes, it is usually divided into:

(1) Lepromatous leprosy: In this type, there is little immunity to the organism and thus the lesions contain many organisms. The course of the disease is often progressive;

(2) Tuberculoid leprosy: Organisms are rare and resistance to the organisms is high; the course is benign with a tendency to spontaneous cure;

(3) Intermediate or dimorphous leprosy: This group of patients do not have the classical features of either lepromatous or tuberculoid leprosy. It appears that, in this group, resistance is uncertain at first and the clinical course may follow that of either lepromatous or tuberculoid leprosy.

Lepromatous leprosy
The skin lesions have indistinct borders and there is a diffuse infiltration of the skin (Figure 22.13) and mucous membranes. Frequently, nodules develop in the skin particularly on the face and ears (Figure 22.14). The nasal mucosa is invariably affected and there is eventual destruction of the nasal septum and subsequent facial deformity. The skin may eventually ulcerate. The eye is also frequently affected. Erythema nodosum lesions frequently occur in lepromatous leprosy at the start of treatment with sulfones.

Tuberculoid leprosy
The lesions often present as infiltrated plaques (Figure 22.15), frequently on the face (Figure 22.16). The lesions are often hypopigmented and this may be the first sign causing the patient to consult a doctor (Figures 22.17 and 22.18). The lesions are often anesthetic and hypohidrotic due to nerve involvement.

Polyneuropathy is common in all types of leprosy and palpating the ulnar, lateral popliteal and posterior auricular nerves to ascertain whether they are thickened is often used as a clinical diagnostic aid. Because of the neuropathy, there may be atrophy and weakness of the muscles. In addition, because of sensory loss, ulceration

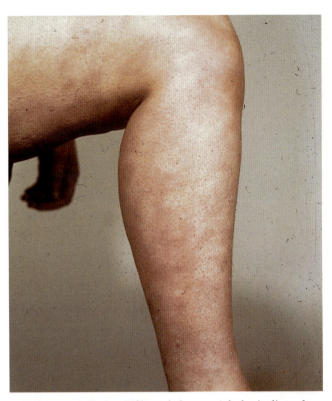

Figure 22.13 *Indistinct infiltrated plaques on the leg in dimorphous leprosy*

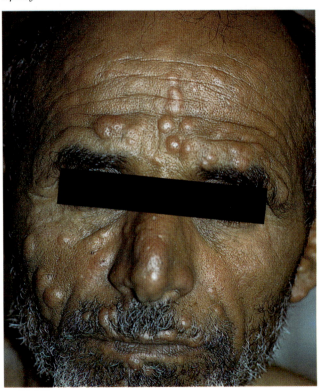

Figure 22.14 *Nodular lesions on the face in lepromatous leprosy*

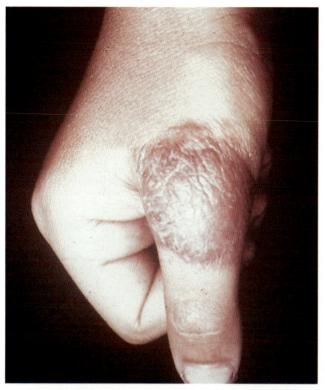

Figure 22.15 *Infiltrated plaque on the hand in tuberculoid leprosy*

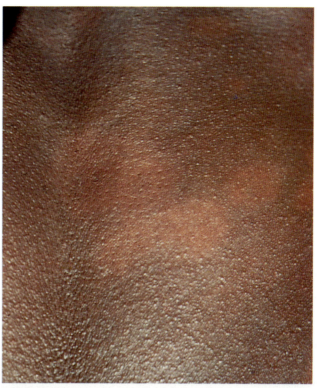

Figure 22.17 *Hypopigmented patches on the back due to dimorphous leprosy*

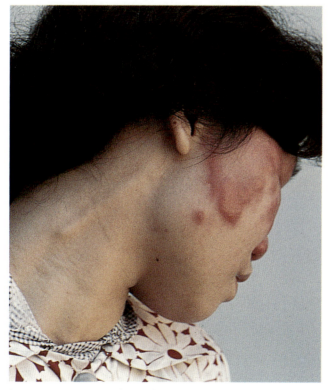

Figure 22.16 *Large infiltrated plaque on the face in dimorphous leprosy. The posterior auricular nerve is thickened and visible on the side of the neck*

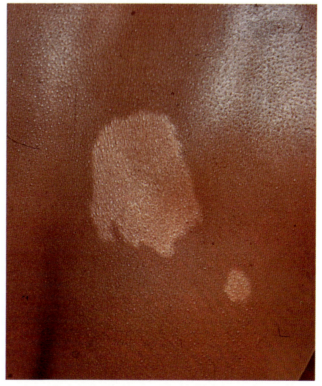

Figure 22.18 *Hypopigmented areas on the back in tuberculoid leprosy*

of the skin due to trauma is common. Gross destruction of the tissue also occurs due to the trophic changes which accompany severe neuropathies. The diagnosis of leprosy is made on the histological features of the skin lesion on biopsy and possibly on finding the organism in nasal smears.

Treatment

The drugs most commonly used in the treatment of leprosy are dapsone, rifampicin and clofazimine. Other drugs are available, but the treatment should be supervised by a leprologist.

Yaws

Although this is a disorder of tropical countries, because of immigration from the West Indies to the UK and air travel in general, some knowledge and awareness of the disorder is necessary.

The disease is caused by the spirochete *Treponema pertenue* and is indistinguishable on serological tests from *Treponema pallidum*, which causes syphilis. Like syphilis, yaws has three stages.

The primary lesion develops 3–4 weeks after the organism has entered the skin. The lesion begins as a small papule which then enlarges (Figure 22.19), or other papules develop around the original lesion and the whole area becomes a confluent crusted lesion.

Approximately 2–3 months later (in some cases longer), the secondary stage commences. This is usually a widespread papular eruption, but granulomatous lesions which ulcerate may also occur (Figure 22.20). The lesions fade and do not leave scars. The lesions in the secondary stage may persist for many weeks or months.

The tertiary stage of yaws begins after a few years. The skin and bones are the organs most commonly affected. The lesions include gummatous nodules, spreading ulcers (Figure 22.21), periostitis, tenosynovitis, and hyperkeratosis of the palms and soles.

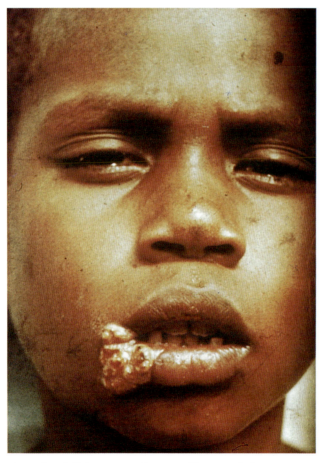

Figure 22.19 *Primary yaws. Large papillomatous lesion*

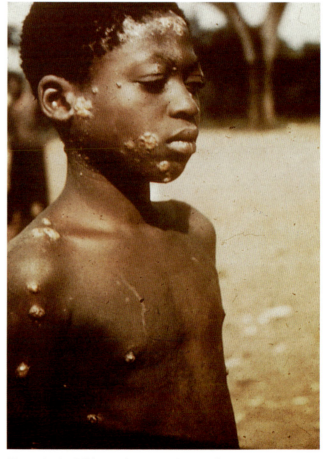

Figure 22.20 *Widespread eruption in secondary yaws. The lesions may be papular or granulomatous with ulceration*

Unlike syphilis, the heart and nervous system are not involved.

Treatment with penicillin is simple and effective.

Cutaneous leishmaniasis

Because holidays in the southern Mediterranean countries and Middle East are now relatively commonplace, it is important to be aware of this condition. The disease is also endemic in Africa, Asia, and Central and South America. Cutaneous leishmaniasis is caused by a protozoon. The organism affects animals and is carried by the sandfly.

Clinical features

The incubation period varies from weeks to months; thus, although the patient may not have been abroad during the last few months, the disease should still be considered if the lesion is suggestive. The lesion most commonly occurs on the exposed areas, e.g. face, neck and arms. It begins as a small papule which enlarges to form a nodule or plaque. It may become scaly and ulcerate (so-called 'oriental sore'; Figure 22.22).

After a few months, the lesion frequently heals spontaneously, leaving a depressed scar. As in patients with leprosy, it is thought that the course of the disease may be dependent upon the host immune responses at the time of the infection.

The diagnosis is made by biopsy and by finding the parasite on smears from the ulcer.

Treatment

In the majority of patients, the lesions are self-healing, and no treatment is required except for cosmetic reasons. Unfortunately, there is no simple effective treatment. Small lesions have been treated by cryotherapy, curettage and cautery, or by heating the lesion to 40–42 °C for a few hours a day. Local injections of steroids and antimony compounds have also been used. Systemic antimony compounds and steroids are used for widespread and persistent lesions.

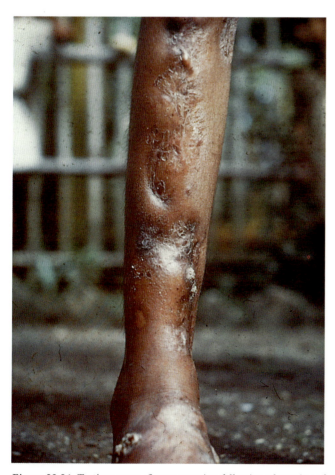

Figure 22.21 *Tertiary yaws. Severe scarring following ulceration of the legs*

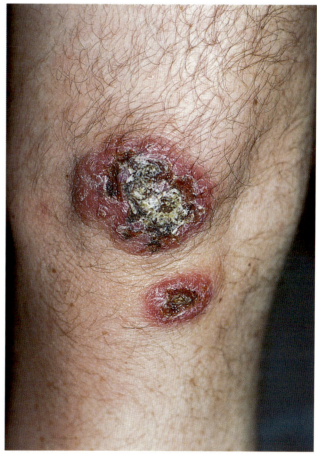

Figure 22.22 *Ulcerated plaques in leishmaniasis*

23

Hereditary disorders and dermatitis artefacta

HEREDITARY DISORDERS

The diseases discussed in this chapter are relatively rare but specific disease entities in which there are known genetic factors involved in their causation, whether the mode of inheritance be dominant or recessive. When discussing hereditary disorders, it must be borne in mind that many of the more common skin diseases, such as atopic eczema and psoriasis, also have strong genetic bases, and a number of the rarer disorders, such as familial hyperlipoproteinemia, epidermolysis bullosa and xerodermia pigmentosa, have already been described in other chapters. It is probable that many skin diseases are partly genetically determined and, thus, to consider only a few specific diseases as 'hereditary disorders' is somewhat misleading. It should also be stressed that the term 'genetic disease' should not be used synonymously with 'congenital disease' as many genetic diseases are not present at birth, but appear in childhood or even adult life.

Ichthyosis

Ichthyosis comes from the Greek word for 'fish', as the appearance of the skin in ichthyosis has been likened to the scaly skin of a fish. Ichthyosis is a condition of keratinization and is usually hereditary, although acquired ichthyosis may occur. There are a number of types based on clinical features and mode of inheritance.

Ichthyosis vulgaris

This is the most common form of ichthyosis. The disorder is not present at birth and rarely occurs before the age of 3 months. The skin is dry and scaly, and often gives the appearance of being cracked (Figure 23.1). Frequently, the skin appears darker than normal, and patients may be accused of not washing. It is usually found on the extensor surfaces whereas the flexures of the limbs are frequently spared (Figure 23.2), a distribution opposite to that seen in atopic eczema.

Ichthyosis vulgaris is inherited as an autosomal dominant and may be associated with atopy. The prognosis is usually good in that the condition often improves with age and may clear in adulthood.

Ichthyosis vulgaris is made worse by the cold and improves with a warm humid climate. Patients should

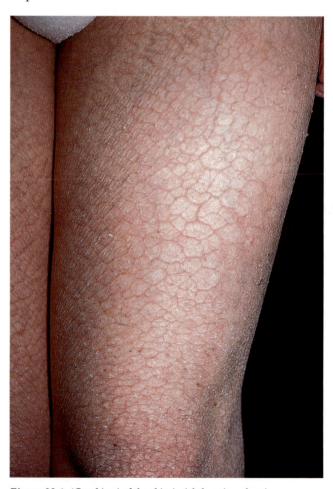

Figure 23.1 *'Cracking' of the skin in ichthyosis vulgaris*

be told to protect the skin, particularly of the hands and face, from the cold. Topical urea has been shown to improve the keratinization of this condition, although how this substance works is unknown; it may be related to keratin bonding. Urea 10% in a cream base should be applied once a day after bathing. Salicylic acid 2–5% in a cream base is helpful for any hyperkeratotic areas.

If secondary eczematization occurs, this should be treated with topical steroids. Claims have been made for the effectiveness of both lactic acid and mandelic acid at concentrations of 5% in a cream base. There has been improvement reported with the oral retinoid acitretin. However, it is better to attempt to control the condition with topical measures.

X-linked ichthyosis

This type of ichthyosis is only seen in men. It may be present at birth or occur within the first 3 months of life. The scales are large and brown and usually involve the whole body surface except for the palms and soles. It tends to be more severe on the trunk, face, and front of the neck and scalp. There is involvement of the flexures (Figure 23.3). In adults, the disease may become more severe, and it tends to persist with no evidence of remission. There is a high incidence of corneal opacities.

Urea 10% cream and lactic acid 5% cream have both been reported to be helpful. The oral retinoid acitretin has been found to be helpful in severely affected individuals. It must be borne in mind before starting retinoids that treatment may be lifelong.

Lamellar ichthyosis

This rare form of ichthyosis is transmitted by an autosomal recessive gene. The disease is usually present at birth or it presents in the first 3 months of life. It begins as a generalized erythema, and the skin then becomes thick and scaly (Figure 23.4). The scaling is more prominent in the flexures and persists throughout life. There is moderate hyperkeratosis on the palms and soles.

In severe forms, the baby may be stillborn or a collodion baby (*see below*). Cortical cataracts may occur.

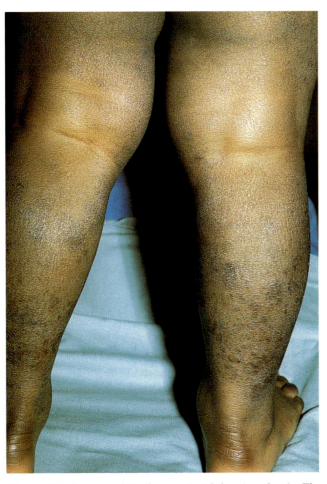

Figure 23.2 *Sparing of the flexures in ichthyosis vulgaris. The affected skin is darker*

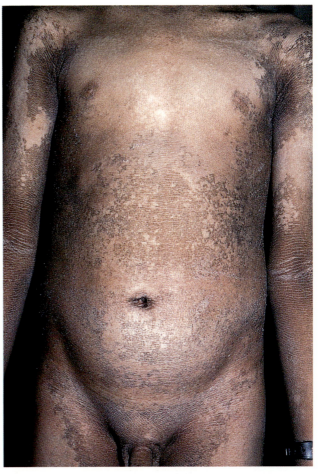

Figure 23.3 *X-linked ichthyosis. Extensive involvement including the flexures*

There have been reports of good responses with the retinoids acitretin and isotretinoin. However, treatment with retinoids has to be considered to last indefinitely. Otherwise, simple keratolytics such as 5% salicylic acid ointment should be used.

Bullous ichthyosiform erythroderma

This is a rare disorder transmitted by an autosomal recessive gene. Babies are usually normal at birth, but may be collodion babies (*see below*). The infant develops red scaly patches and subsequently blisters, ranging from a few millimeters to a few centimeters. The blisters are most common on the legs and become less frequent with age. The eruption may be generalized or localized to the flexures. The keratin is grossly thickened and becomes ridged (Figure 23.5). The palms may be involved.

The oral retinoid acitretin is helpful, but treatment is of indefinite duration, although some patients may show a spontaneous improvement around puberty. Keratolytics (e.g. 2–5% salicylic acid in a cream base) and emollients may provide symptomatic improvement.

Collodion baby

This is not a diagnosis of a particular type of ichthyosis, but may be due to underlying X-linked ichthyosis, lamellar ichthyosis or bullous ichthyosiform erythroderma. The babies are usually born prematurely with a red, translucent, shiny skin which feels hard and rigid. There is ectropion and a cellophane-like membrane covering the body, and distortion of the face. After

several days, the membrane is shed in large scales. The skin may then become normal or take the form of the underlying ichthyosis. Treatment consists of lubricating the skin with bland ointments such as white soft paraffin.

A point to remember in patients with ichthyosis is that there is often occlusion of the sweat ducts, and thus their tolerance to heat and exercise is reduced. Febrile episodes must be taken seriously particularly if the ichthyosis is extensive.

Neurofibromatosis (von Recklinghausen's disease)

This is a disorder affecting the skin and nervous system. The classical signs are light-brown macular lesions, so-called café-au-lait spots (Figure 23.6). There are usually several such lesions but, occasionally, there may be only a few.

Café-au-lait lesions may be present at birth and often precede the development of skin tumors by years. Occasionally, they are the only features of the disorder in the skin. If skin tumors develop, they usually do so

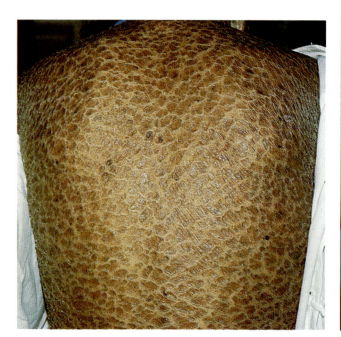

Figure 23.4 *Thick brown scales in lamellar ichthyosis*

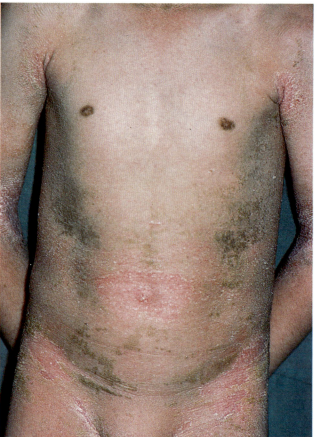

Figure 23.5 *Bullous ichthyosiform erythroderma. Thick brown hyperkeratotic areas peel to leave erythematous scaly areas*

around puberty. The tumors arise from the Schwann cells of the cutaneous nerves. These tumors may be few in number or numerous (Figure 23.7). The growths are usually skin-colored and vary in size from a few millimeters to a few centimeters. They may be small round elevations or pedunculated (Figure 23.7), or present as raised soft plaques. The tumors are usually painless, but may be painful if situated over a pressure area.

Neurofibromatosis affecting the skin is essentially a cosmetic disability, but of serious medical importance are the neurofibromata which may be found on the cranial nerves or in the spinal canal.

There is no treatment for this disorder but, if a tumor is particularly large or causes pain, it can be excised.

Epiloia (tuberous sclerosis)

This is a disease characterized by lesions in the central nervous system and skin. There are fibrous tumors in the brain whereas the presenting neurological features are mental deficiency and epilepsy. The skin lesions are characteristic and are not present at birth, but usually appear during the first decade of life. The lesions are small pink or skin-colored papules situated in the nasolabial folds (Figure 23.8) which may spread to involve the cheeks below the eyes, the nose and the chin (Figure 23.9). The lesions have been termed 'adenoma sebaceum'.

Other lesions in epiloia are flesh-colored or yellow plaques usually in the lumbar region which vary from

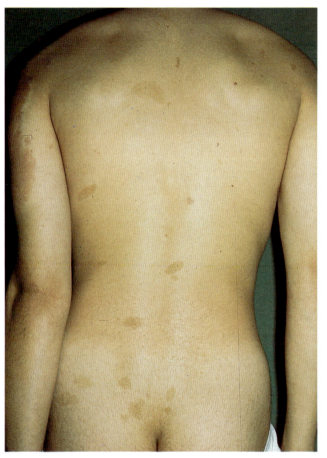

Figure 23.6 Pigmented macules (café-au-lait spots) in neurofibromatosis

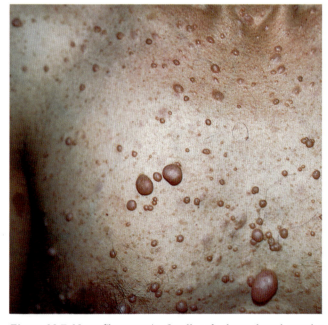

Figure 23.7 Neurofibromatosis. Small, soft, dome-shaped papules are seen with larger pedunculated lesions

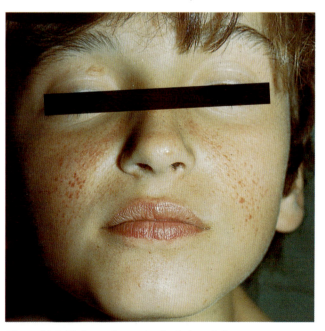

Figure 23.8 Pink papules on the cheeks in epiloia

1–10 cm in diameter. The lesions are due to alterations in dermal collagen. Occasionally, there are fibrous outgrowths beneath the nails on the fingers and toes.

Congenital ectodermal defect

This rare disorder is due to failure of development of the skin and its appendages. Numerous abnormalities may be present, or only one or two. The patients may present with bald patches in the scalp from birth due to absent hair follicles; the teeth may also be absent, reduced in number and abnormally shaped. The sebaceous and sweat glands may be unformed. The clinical importance of this latter feature is an intolerance to heat.

Darier's disease

This relatively rare disease leads to an abnormality of keratinization. It is inherited as an autosomal dominant gene. The disease usually begins in late childhood or adolescence. The typical initial lesions are small, brown, follicular papules (Figure 23.10). The lesions gradually coalesce to form scaly plaques. The common sites of involvement are the so-called seborrheic areas, namely, the face, neck, mid-chest (Figure 23.10), mid-back, groins and axillae. There may be small white papules on the mucous membranes which coalesce to form white patches. There may also be punctate keratoses on the palms and soles, and the nails are fragile and have longitudinal ridges.

Darier's disease responds well to the oral retinoid acitretin. This is the only effective treatment currently available. Treatment with retinoids must be considered indefinite, although some patients are happy to accept intermittent courses of treatment.

DERMATITIS ARTEFACTA AND NEUROTIC EXCORIATIONS

These are two disorders in which lesions are produced in the skin by the patient due to mental disease.

Dermatitis artefacta

In this disorder, the patient never admits to producing the lesions at the time the physician is taking the history. The diagnosis is often arrived at through negative reasoning as the skin lesions do not fall into any clinically recognized disease pattern, e.g. the symmetry of psoriasis or an endogenous eczema.

The lesions themselves have features which suggest that they have been produced by some physical or chemical agent, e.g. chemicals, burns (usually cigarettes) or trauma from a sharp instrument (Figure 23.11). There is usually ulceration or blister formation in the epidermis (Figures 23.11–23.14). The lesions are discrete (Figures 23.12 and 23.13) and usually asymmetrical.

The diagnosis of dermatitis artefacta is frequently missed at the first consultation. It is only when the

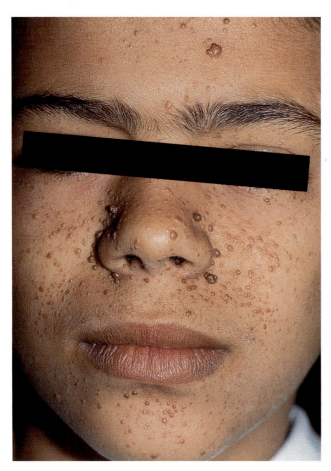

Figure 23.9 *Extensive papular eruption on the face in epiloia*

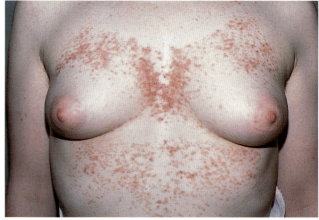

Figure 23.10 *Darier's disease. Reddish-brown hyperkeratotic papules over the sternum, chest and upper abdomen*

lesions fail to heal with conventional therapy and new lesions continue to appear that such a diagnosis is considered. To support the diagnosis, it is sometimes necessary to apply occlusive bandages (in extreme cases, plaster of Paris has been used) so that the patient can no longer inflict damage to the skin. The disease is more common in women than in men at all ages. The patient usually has an hysterical personality and requires psychiatric treatment.

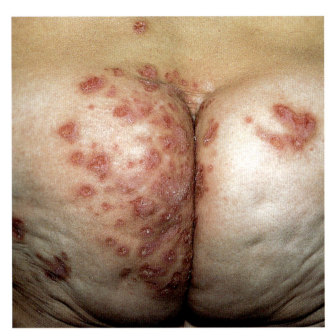

Figure 23.11 *Dermatitis artefacta. Deep ulcers on the buttocks produced by a nail*

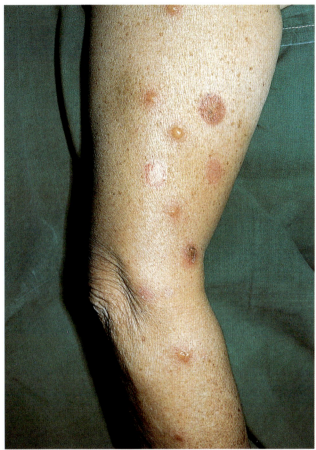

Figure 23.13 *Discrete blisters and erosions in dermatitis artefacta*

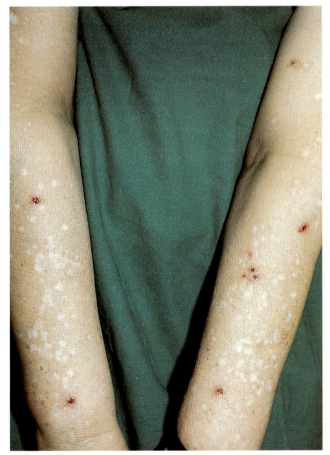

Figure 23.12 *Discrete ulcers and scabbed lesions on the forearms in dermatitis artefacta. Scarring from previous lesions is also seen*

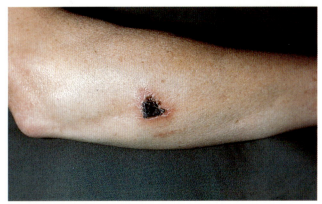

Figure 23.14 *Deep, solitary, scabbed lesion in dermatitis artefacta*

Neurotic excoriations

This is distinct from dermatitis artefacta because the patient admits to scratching and the lesions are usually produced by the fingernails, although some patients use mechanical aids.

The clinical presentation is that of superficial ulcers, although many will be in the healing stage and present as scabbed lesions. The lesions are usually found on the limbs and shoulders, and the center of the back is spared as the patient cannot reach this site (Figure 23.15). As in dermatitis artefacta, the lesions will heal completely with occlusive dressings. However, these dressings only serve to confirm the diagnosis. The patient may be helped by psychiatric treatment.

Prurigo nodularis

This is a distinct clinical entity which occurs most commonly in middle-aged women. The classical lesions are discrete discoid excoriations in which the skin becomes thickened and has a tendency to form nodules (Figure 23.16).

As in neurotic excoriations, the patient admits to excoriating the lesions, but the lesions produced are different. It is thought that these patients have an atopic tendency in which the skin becomes thickened due to trauma, as with other forms of atopic eczema.

The condition is persistent and resistant to most recognized forms of dermatological therapy, although some success has been claimed with PUVA. It is usually resistant to psychiatric treatment.

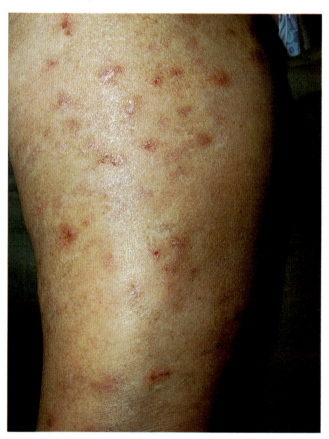

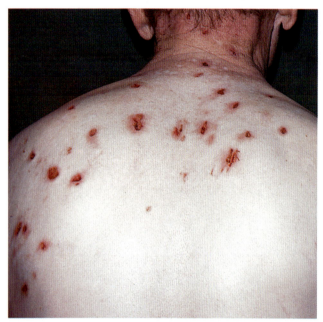

Figure 23.15 *Neurotic excoriations. The upper back is a common site whereas the center of the back is spared as patients find it difficult to reach*

Figure 23.16 *Prurigo nodularis. Excoriated nodular lesions on the arm*

24

Disorders of hair and pigmentation

DISORDERS OF HAIR

The disorders of hair seen in a skin clinic fall into two categories: loss of hair (alopecia); and excess hair (hirsuties). Hair loss can be classified into primary, where the fault lies in the hair or its production, or secondary, where the hair follicles are destroyed due to a disease affecting the dermis. Clinically, the latter type of alopecia is associated with scarring of the skin.

To understand the basis of a number of pathological conditions, it is necessary to have some knowledge of the growth cycle of hair. The growth cycle is divided into three stages – a growing phase (anagen), which is followed by a resting phase (telogen), during which the hair is shed and there is involution of the hair follicles and, finally, there is a stage of pronounced cellular activity of the hair follicle (catagen) prior to the actual production of the hair.

There are approximately 100 000 hairs on the scalp and the normal daily loss varies from 20–100 hairs. This means that up to 100 hair follicles enter the telogen phase every day.

Primary hair loss

From the clinical point of view, it is often useful to consider hair loss as either diffuse or patchy.

Diffuse hair loss

Male pattern baldness
Hair loss from the scalp in men is so common that it cannot be considered abnormal. However, a number of young adult men will present to their doctors or to skin clinics complaining of hair loss. There is a distinct pattern in this type of hair loss which should be distinguished from other causes of hair loss.

Normal male pattern baldness begins in the temporofrontal regions so that there is a receding frontal hairline. The next site to be affected is the vertex, particularly posteriorly and extending to the back of the scalp. If the hair loss is severe, the only remaining hair is at the sides and lower back of the scalp (Figures 24.1 and 24.2).

Male pattern baldness may begin in the late teens and, once it commences, is usually progressive. However, the time over which this progressive hair loss occurs is extremely variable. Some patients lose all the hair on the vertex and frontal regions of the scalp within 2–3 years; others may gradually lose some of the hair, but never become completely bald in the areas of the scalp involved.

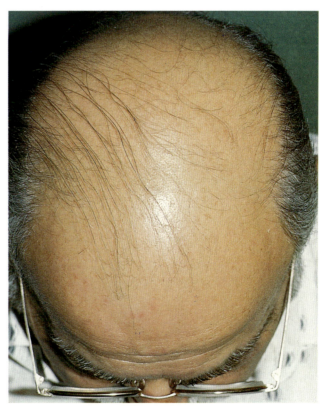

Figure 24.1 *Male pattern hair loss over the vertex*

179

Treatment is unsatisfactory. Topical minoxidil preparations used in men who are just beginning to lose their hair have been claimed to slow the process. However, it must be stressed that topical minoxidil has no permanent effect and, if discontinued, the patient's condition will be as if the treatment had never been used. Topical minoxidil is of no value in patients with established alopecia.

Hair transplants are clearly at the discretion of the patient.

Hair loss in women

So-called constitutional female alopecia is not an uncommon disorder to see in a skin clinic. It presents as a diffuse loss of hair from the scalp, but the loss is mainly from the vertex. Although the hair loss may be severe, it is not total as in men (Figure 24.3). The frontal hairline does not recede as in men.

This type of hair loss is seen most commonly in middle-aged and elderly women, but it can occur in young adults. The cause for this type of hair loss is as yet unknown, although it has been suggested that it may, like male pattern alopecia, be androgen-dependent. However, as in male pattern alopecia, it is likely to be an end-organ effect and does not indicate increased or abnormal androgen levels.

Occasionally, however, there is underlying systemic disease which may give rise to hair loss which is indistinguishable from the so-called constitutional form. The two disorders which are most likely to cause hair loss are hypothyroidism and iron-deficiency anemia, both of which are readily treatable so that women who complain of gradual diffuse hair loss should be investigated to exclude these disorders.

Another cause of diffuse hair loss in women is traction on the hair as a result of certain types of hairstyles. This is particularly common in blacks, and includes children whose hair is braided very tightly (Figure 24.4) and women who sleep in hair rollers. Thus, enquiry should always be made concerning these habits.

Unfortunately, there is no treatment for constitutional hair loss in women. If it is severe and the patient is distressed by her state, then a wig should be advised. If severe traction is the cause of the hair loss, then a change in hairstyle is all that is required.

Telogen effluvium

In this disorder, a large number of hair follicles suddenly enter the resting phase of the hair cycle (telogen) and thus the hair is shed. The most common causes of this type of hair loss are the postpregnancy state and diseases that are often associated with high fever. It has also been reported after stopping oral contraception.

Although this type of hair loss may be severe and alarming to the patient, the condition subsides spontaneously after a few months and the hair cycle returns to

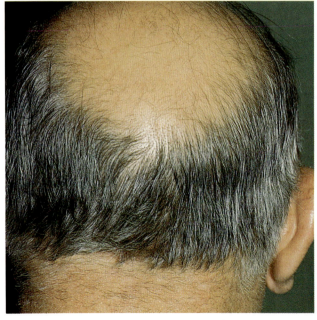

Figure 24.2 *Male pattern hair loss may extend from the vertex to the back of the scalp. However, even in the most severe cases, hair is always retained at the sides and lower back*

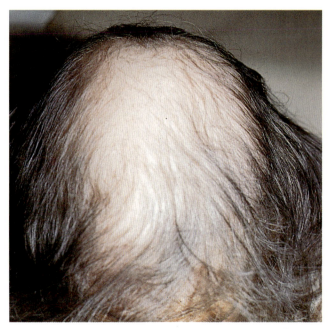

Figure 24.3 *Constitutional female hair loss usually affects the vertex, but the hair may also be thin elsewhere. The frontal hairline is retained in contrast to male pattern baldness*

normal. No treatment is available to stop the process, but the patient should be strongly reassured as to the eventual outcome of the process. Placebo therapy is sometimes helpful.

Drugs

A number of drugs may cause hair loss, but the most frequent offenders are the cytotoxic drugs. Hair loss has also been reported with oral retinoids, excess vitamin A intake and heparin.

Inflammatory dermatosis

Hair loss does occur in some patients with seborrheic eczema and psoriasis, but it is the exception rather than the rule. The cause of the hair loss is not known but, in some patients, an aggravating factor is the trauma from continual scratching. In these conditions, the hair loss is usually reversible.

Patchy hair loss

Alopecia areata

In this relatively common disorder, the patient suddenly notices a round or oval area of baldness (Figure 24.5).

The loss of hair may be complete, or so-called exclamation-mark hairs may be seen in the bald patch or at the edges. Exclamation-mark hairs are short, approximately 5 mm in length, and thicker distally with the shaft gradually tapering towards the proximal end (Figure 24.6). If these hairs are pulled with forceps, they come out easily with a small, white, round hair bulb attached to the proximal end.

Occasionally, the scalp is slightly erythematous in the part affected. The skin itself is non-scaly (Figure 24.5) compared with the bald areas seen in fungus infections of the scalp. In alopecia areata, there may be one or several bald patches. Occasionally, sites other than the scalp are involved, e.g. the eyebrows or beard area (Figure 24.7). In rare instances, all the hair on the head may be lost (Figure 24.8). This is termed alopecia totalis.

The most frequent course for alopecia areata is for the hair to regrow after an interval of time. The time to regrowth is variable, but is frequently 2–3 months. When regrowth does occur, the hair is often white but usually repigments over time. Occasionally, there is no regrowth of hair and, in other cases, the hair regrows,

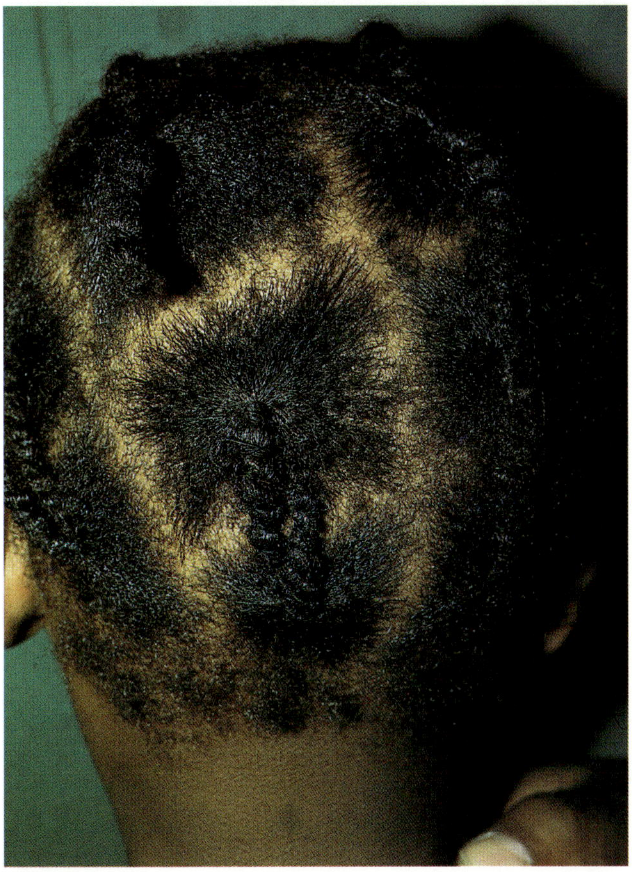

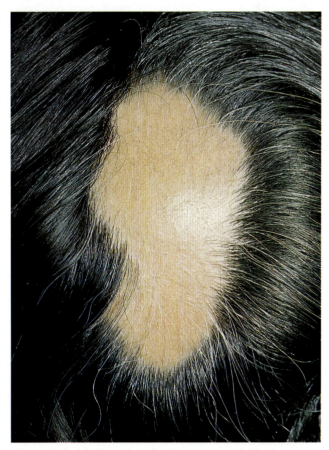

Figure 24.4 *Tight braiding of the hair may give rise to traction alopecia*

Figure 24.5 *A bald patch with otherwise normal skin in alopecia areata*

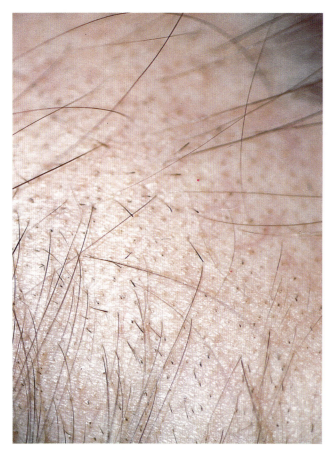

Figure 24.6 Exclamation-mark hairs in alopecia areata. The hairs are short, approximately 5 mm in length, and thicker distally, tapering towards the scalp

but new bald patches appear. Usually, the larger the area initially affected, the poorer the prognosis.

A feature sometimes seen in alopecia areata is dystrophy of the nails. This varies from a few pits to complete shedding. When such dystrophy occurs, it is usually in the more severe cases of hair loss and indicative of a poor prognosis.

Treatment
Topical steroids (particularly Groups III and IV) are widely used, but it is questionable as to whether they have any effect on the pathological process of alopecia or alter the final outcome.

Intralesional steroids injected into the affected areas often stimulate regrowth of hair, which should be apparent within 6 weeks. However, if the disease is very active, there may be no regrowth or, after initial regrowth, the hair is lost again.

PUVA to the bald areas is effective in a number of patients not helped by intralesional steroids. Sensitization and induction of eczema with dinitrochlorobenzene and diphencyprone have also been used with moderate results. However, as there is a high morbidity with these treatments, they should not be undertaken lightly. Systemic steroids are effective, but the hair tends to fall out again when the drugs are stopped.

Cyclosporine has been reported to be successful in reversing alopecia areata but, like systemic steroids, there is no permanent effect. When treating alopecia

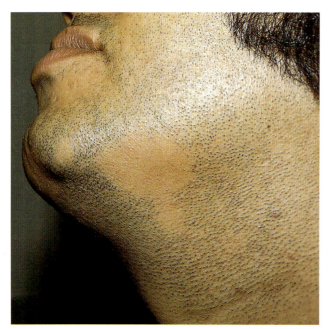

Figure 24.7 Alopecia areata involving the beard area

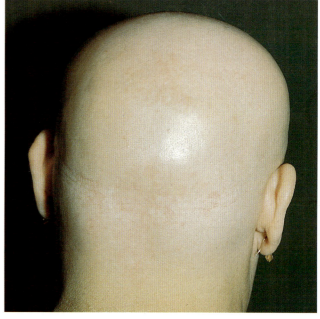

Figure 24.8 Total hair loss from the scalp in alopecia areata – so-called alopecia totalis

areata, it must be remembered that there is a good prognosis when the disease is mild, but a poor outcome when the condition is extensive whatever treatments are used. As there is no lasting effect after treatment is discontinued, it is doubtful whether systemic drugs are indicated.

Trichotillomania

This is a disorder in which the patient has the habit of rubbing a particular area of the scalp or pulling the hair from a particular area. The disorder is more common in children than adults. The presenting feature is a bald area but, on close inspection, it can be seen that the hairs have been broken close to the surface by trauma.

Most children grow out of the habit. If not, they should be referred to a psychiatrist.

Congenital

Bald areas occasionally are seen at birth. This is due to failure of the skin to develop normally in these areas and the hair follicles are absent.

Secondary hair loss

Scarring alopecia

In any disorder where there is severe inflammation of the dermis and subsequent scar-tissue formation, the hair follicles will be destroyed, resulting in baldness. This inflammation may be caused by burns, pyogenic infections or previous irradiation. These causes can usually be obtained from the patient's history.

A number of skin disorders, such as lichen planus, scleroderma and discoid lupus erythematosus, may affect the skin of the scalp and produce scarring alopecia (Figure 24.9). Scarring can usually be seen on examination of the scalp. The epidermis is frequently atrophic and the skin generally feels tight.

The only treatment that might be considered in some forms of scarring alopecia is plastic surgery, but this is only applicable if the area involved is small and due to a non-recurring cause, e.g. a burn.

Hirsuties

Excessive hairiness may be localized or diffuse. In the vast majority of people complaining of excessive hairiness, there is no disease. Female patients present to doctors with this complaint because society does not accept excessive hairiness in women as normal, but accepts it in men.

Localized hirsutism

This is most frequently found in association with benign pigmented nevi. Occasionally, localized overgrowth of hair is found on the back, and over the sacrum and lower lumbar spine.

Essential hirsutism

The amount of facial and body hair in women is partly genetically determined. Some facial hair and increased hair on the limbs is the norm among Asians and in southern Mediterranean countries.

Excess hair growth in women may be the presenting symptom of an endocrine tumor producing androgens. This is usually a tumor of the ovaries or adrenals. It must be stressed, however, that this cause of hirsuties is extremely rare.

As yet, the cause of essential hirsuties in women is unknown. No excess androgenic steroids or their precursors have been found in the serum, but this could be due to the fact that the appropriate techniques have not yet been developed. Apart from the excess production of androgens in the endocrine glands, there is now some evidence that the skin itself may be able to produce active androgens and, thus, hirsuties may be primarily a disorder of the skin itself.

When excess hair growth occurs in women, it is found at sites similar to where body hair growth occurs in men, namely, the upper lip, beard area, lower abdomen from the pubis to the umbilicus and around the areolae on the breasts.

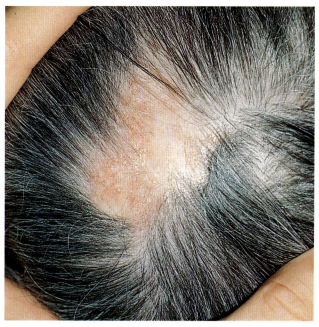

Figure 24.9 *Scarring alopecia secondary to discoid lupus erythematosus*

Treatment

It is important not to miss an endocrine abnormality as the cause of hirsuties in women. It is debatable whether all patients with hirsuties should be investigated. However, if patients present with this complaint, a physical examination for other signs of virilization or hyperadrenalism is necessary. A detailed history particularly of menstrual problems is obligatory. If there are any features to suggest an underlying endocrinological problem, then measurement of serum androgens and female sex hormones, and referral to a gynecologist for examination and ultrasound of the ovaries should be undertaken.

Removal of the excess hair in essential hirsuties is not satisfactory. Temporary removal can be effected by plucking, depilatory creams or, in severe cases, shaving. The only permanent method of hair removal is by electrolysis. This is a time-consuming procedure and must be carried out by an experienced person to be effective.

The most effective drug in the treatment of hirsuties is the anti-androgen cyproterone acetate. In premenopausal women, this is given combined with estrogens in a reversed sequential regimen. The dose of cyproterone acetate is 100 mg daily for 10 days, starting on the fifth day of the menstrual cycle. Ethinylestradiol 30 μg should be given for 21 days, starting at the same time as the cyproterone acetate.

COMMON DISORDERS OF PIGMENTATION

Lack of pigment

The most common type of depigmentation of the skin seen in a skin clinic is postinflammatory (Figure 24.10). The inflammation may have been due to any of the common skin disorders, e.g. eczema (Figure 24.11), psoriasis, pityriasis rosea. These depigmented areas usually become apparent once the dermatosis has cleared. One of the most common sites for this phenomenon is the face in young children (Figure 24.11). If a careful history is taken, there is usually a story of erythema and scaling preceding the eruption and frequently, on examination, scaling will be seen. Fortunately, the pigment returns after a few months and the only treatment required is to suppress the primary inflammatory dermatosis.

Vitiligo

This is a distinct clinical entity. At present, the cause is not known, but there is increasing evidence that vitiligo is an immunological disorder which results in the inhibition of the formation of melanin by the melanocyte.

There is a higher incidence of vitiligo in patients with autoimmune diseases, e.g. pernicious anemia, and some forms of thyroid and other endocrine diseases associated with autoantibodies, than in those without such diseases.

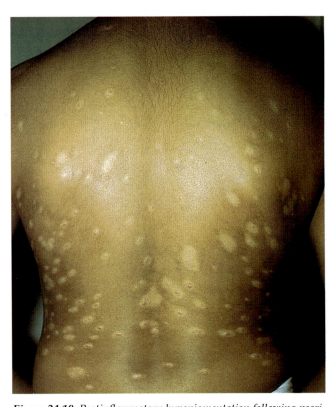

Figure 24.10 *Postinflammatory hypopigmentation following psoriasis*

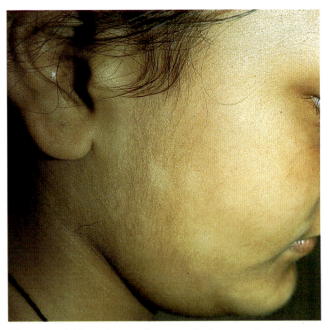

Figure 24.11 *Hypopigmented areas on the face secondary to eczema*

Vitiligo presents as oval or irregular white patches (Figures 24.12 and 24.13) that are frequently symmetrical (Figures 24.12–24.14). Occasionally, there may be a solitary patch of vitiligo or the disease may be very extensive, involving large areas of the skin (Figure 24.14). Very rarely, the whole of the skin is affected.

The white patches of vitiligo are usually distinguishable from other causes of depigmentation because the texture of the skin is normal. In some patients, the hair becomes white in affected areas.

Treatment

Vitiligo can be an embarrassing disorder for the patient if the depigmented areas are visible (Figure 24.13). Although treatment is difficult and may fail, it is certainly worth the attempt if the patient is particularly concerned about the appearance of the skin.

Two types of drugs are used in the treatment of vitiligo: corticosteroids and psoralens. Corticosteroids are used topically in a lotion or cream base. Only the potent topical corticosteroids appear to be effective in repigmenting the skin. Unfortunately, the cure rate with corticosteroids is low at no higher than 20%. The treatment usually has to be continued for many months and, thus, patients must be closely supervised because of the possible side effects of the steroids. If there is no evidence of repigmentation within 3 months, treatment should be discontinued. Vitiligo on the face is more likely to respond than that elsewhere.

The psoralens used in vitiligo are administered using the same regimens as are used in PUVA (see Chapter 25). If PUVA machines are not available, ordinary ultraviolet lamps as obtainable at pharmaceutical shops are also effective. The supervision of vitiligo treatment is best undertaken by a specialist.

Blacks and Asians respond to treatment of vitiligo better than do whites. If repigmentation does occur due

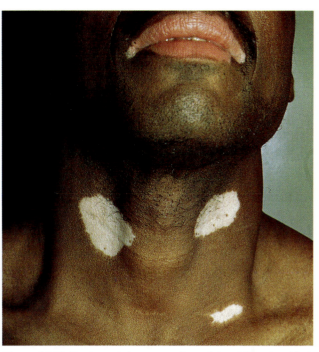

Figure 24.13 Depigmented areas on the neck in vitiligo in a black man, a severe cosmetic disability

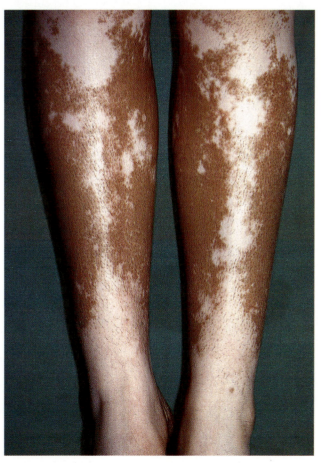

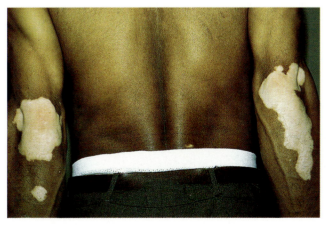

Figure 24.12 Symmetrical depigmentation in vitiligo

Figure 24.14 Extensive symmetrical depigmentation in vitiligo

to either psoralens or topical steroids, it will first appear as small spots of pigment within the depigmented areas. This is a useful sign as it is indicative of a good prognosis, and treatment should be continued. It is thought that repigmentation occurs when the melanocytes around the hair follicles migrate to the surrounding skin and then spread across the depigmented areas.

If treatment with psoralens or topical steroids is not effective, then the affected areas can be stained brown by the topical use of a number of substances, most usually, dihydroxyacetone.

If the vitiligo is extensive and the patient is embarrassed by the 'patchwork' coloration, it is worth trying to remove the pigment from the unaffected areas with a cream containing 20% monobenzyl ether of hydroquinone.

Increased pigmentation

This condition is most commonly postinflammatory, usually following one of the common dermatoses (Figures 24.15 and 24.16), particularly lichen planus.

This well-documented phenomenon of postinflammatory hyperpigmentation is particularly seen in blacks.

Patches of increased pigmentation may occur on the face and neck of women as a number of cosmetics are photosensitizers, which increase the pigmentation of the skin following exposure to sunlight.

Increased pigmentation may be found in association with a number of systemic disorders, e.g. Addison's disease (Figure 24.17), malabsorption states, carcinomatosis, renal failure, Peutz–Jeghers syndrome, Albright's disease, hemachromatosis and neurofibromatosis. These disorders belong to the realms of general or internal medicine, and their description is left to the appropriate texts, although the dermatologist must be aware that altered pigmentation of the skin may be the presenting feature in these diseases.

Chloasma

This is increased pigmentation, usually on the cheeks and forehead, which occurs during pregnancy and in some patients taking the contraceptive pill. This type of

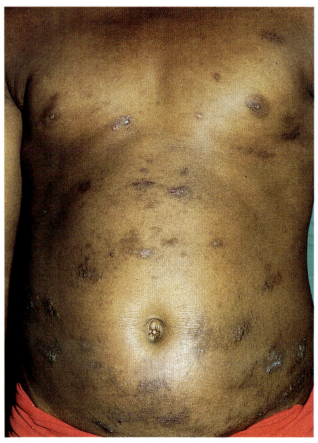

Figure 24.15 *Postinflammatory hyperpigmentation secondary to eczema*

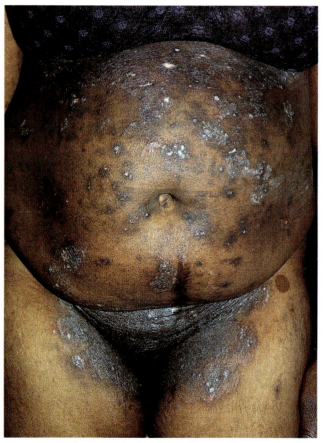

Figure 24.16 *Postinflammatory hyperpigmentation secondary to a fungus infection in a black woman. Such pigmentation may be the presenting symptom*

pigmentation may also occur in women who are not pregnant or taking the oral contraception and is sometimes referred to as melasma (Figure 24.18). It is more common in relatively dark-skinned people, particularly Asians, than in whites. Chloasma after pregnancy in fair-skinnned people usually fades spontaneously.

Treatment
In simple postinflammatory hyperpigmentation, the color of the skin usually returns to normal. If melanin hyperpigmentation of whatever cause persists, the skin can be depigmented by the use of hydroquinones applied topically. They should be used with caution under the direction of a dermatologist. Topical sunscreen agents should also be used in sunny climates.

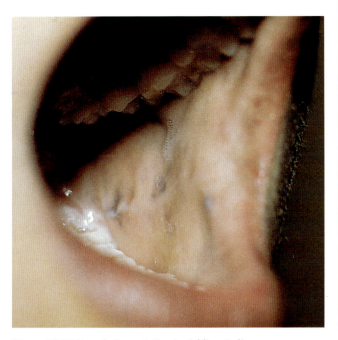

Figure 24.17 Buccal pigmentation in Addison's disease

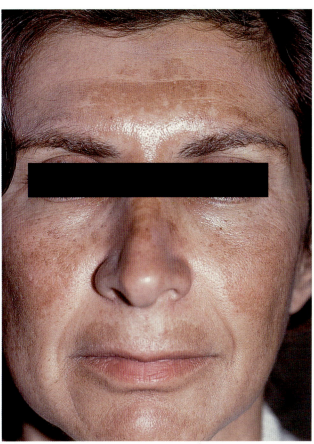

Figure 24.18 Pigmentation on the forehead, nose and cheeks in melasma

25

Guides to treatment

There are a number of therapeutic agents which are predominantly used in the treatment of skin diseases. It is important that students and physicians have some knowledge of these treatments as well as learn how to diagnose spots and rashes. In addition, as the skin is the most accessible organ of the body, many common drugs are used topically and the pharmacological principles of topical therapy are rarely taught to medical students.

In deciding whether topical or oral treatment should be used, the following points should be remembered. If the lesion is dermal rather than epidermal, then topical measures will be of little or no use.

Clinically, a lesion is dermal and not epidermal if there is no scaling, crusting or weeping of the skin surface. Topical measures are of little value in dermal disorders for two reasons: First, if the epidermis is intact, it is unlikely that a sufficiently high concentration of the drug will penetrate the skin barrier (normal keratin); second, if the drug does penetrate the epidermis and reaches the dermis, it is then absorbed into the tissue fluid and bloodstream, and is rapidly diluted at the site where it is expected to act.

If the lesion is mainly or partly epidermal, as suggested on clinical grounds by scaling, crusting or weeping of the skin surface, then topical preparations are indicated. Topical preparations are likely to be more effective in these cases because the epidermal barrier has been destroyed by the disease process and, as the epidermis has no blood vessels, systemically administered drugs can only reach the epidermal cells by diffusion through cells and intercellular fluid. Thus, a higher concentration of the drug is often obtained in the epidermis by topical rather than systemic administration.

The clear advantage of topically applied drugs compared with those systemically administered is that the diseased organ is specifically treated while the rest of the body is not exposed to the drug (or to only a very small concentration).

VEHICLES FOR TOPICAL PREPARATIONS

Students and practitioners are often confused because they need to know not only which drug to use for the disorder, but also with which vehicle to administer the drug. Basically, topical preparations can be divided into four groups: solutions; creams; ointments; and pastes.

Solutions

The drug (e.g. steroid) should be used in solution form when the skin is acutely inflamed, as manifested by weeping or exudation from the skin surface. Solutions are also indicated for dermatoses in the intertriginous areas (i.e. where two skin surfaces are in apposition, e.g. groins, axillae and between the toes).

It should be appreciated that solutions will evaporate quickly if applied to the skin surface and, thus, the duration of action of the drug on the diseased area is relatively short, perhaps only half an hour. Thus, if continuous treatment of the skin surface is required, lotions have to be applied frequently (e.g. hourly).

Creams

These are emulsions of either water dispersed in oil or oil dispersed in water. They have a relatively high content of water compared with oil. Clinically, this means they are pleasant and non-greasy to use, and the patients find that they are well absorbed into the skin. A cream should be chosen as the vehicle for a drug in sub-acute conditions, e.g. when there is slight exudation, and in disorders affecting the intertriginous areas.

The duration of action of the drug can be expected to be longer than that of a solution, but shorter than that of an ointment, probably around 4–5 h. Thus, if continuous treatment of diseased skin is required, the cream should be applied every 4–5 h.

Ointments

Clinically, these substances are 'greasy'. Chemically, there are three different types: those which are water-soluble; those which emulsify with water; and those which do not mix with water.

However, it is their clinical properties that are important. Because these substances are greasy, they should not be used in cases with acute weeping or subacute skin disease, or in the intertriginous areas, particularly the groins and under the breasts.

The main indication for their use is the presence of 'dry' chronic dermatoses. The duration of action of the drug in an ointment base is longer than that in a cream and needs to be applied 2–3 times a day for continuous action of the drug on the skin. As a general rule, a drug (particularly a steroid) in an ointment base is more effective than the same drug in a cream base.

Pastes

These are ointments to which zinc oxide has been added, giving them a stiffer consistency. They are used only in chronic dermatoses, e.g. psoriasis. They will remain on the skin surface for a considerable length of time and need only be applied once a day. They are not pleasant for the patient to use.

QUANTITY OF TOPICAL PREPARATION

When prescribing topical preparations, it is essential that patients be given the appropriate quantity to carry out the treatment correctly. In practice, it is useless to prescribe a standard 30-g tube of ointment for a patient with extensive skin disease.

It is important that the physician assess the area of body surface affected by the disease. As a guide, it takes approximately 30 g of cream or ointment to cover the entire body surface of an average adult. Thus, if it is estimated that 30% of the skin is involved with the disease, then 10 g will be required at each application and, if the preparation has to be applied twice daily, the patient will require 20 g per day or 140 g per week.

Patients often ask how much ointment or cream should they apply to their rashes, but it is difficult to give a clear and concise response. Drug companies are now making containers with instructions stating that a given 'length' of cream from the container will be sufficient for a given area, e.g. forearm or leg. This should prove helpful to patients.

TOPICALLY APPLIED DRUGS

Topical steroids

These are the most widely used drugs in dermatology. Steroids have many actions, and how they work in an individual disease is not always fully understood. They have potent anti-inflammatory activity; they break down collagen and inhibit fibroblast activity, and they suppress the body's reaction to infections. They may affect factors controlling cell division and influence a large number of processes in the immune system.

An important point to remember is that, if the dermatosis does not improve with topical steroids, then the possibility of an infective disorder, whether bacterial, viral or fungal, should always be considered.

Over the last few years, topical steroids have received a great deal of adverse publicity because of side effects, and patients are now reluctant to use them. These side effects are usually avoidable and arise because physicians fail to appreciate the wide range of activity of the various topical steroid preparations available.

The steroids used in topical preparations can be assayed and their strength compared with 1% hydrocortisone. From the practical point of view, it is convenient to assign the multitude of available topical steroid drugs into four groups. The practicing physician can then learn about one from each group, which is all that is necessary to know. To appreciate the wide range of steroid activity available, the comparative strengths of steroids are given in Table 25.1, where the strength of hydrocortisone is equivalent to 1 unit of steroid activity.

Table 25.1 Comparative strengths of steroids

	Strength (units)	Example
Group I	1	Hydrocortisone (1%)
Group II	25	Clobetasol butyrate (0.05%)
Group III	100	Betamethasone 17-valerate (0.1%)
Group IV	600	Clobetasol propionate (0.05%)

Apart from knowing the strength of the steroid and the base required for the drug, the site to which the drug is to be applied is also important because of the variation in skin thickness and moisture. Thus, the thinner the skin, the less connective tissue present and, therefore, the greater the risk of clinical damage to the skin. The face and genitalia are probably the areas with the thinnest skin and, as a rule, only Group I steroids should be used at these sites. There is increased moisture in the intertriginous areas, which hydrates the epidermis and increases the absorption of drug into the dermis. Thus, in the intertriginous areas, only Group I and II steroids should be used.

These are only general guidelines as there are instances when a skin disorder on the face or genitalia has not responded to weak (i.e. Group I or II) steroids. Stronger steroids will then be necessary and justified, although there should be close supervision of the patient. In general, Group III and IV topical steroids should not be given on repeat prescriptions without the physician first seeing the patient.

In clinical practice, it is often necessary to give large quantities of steroid preparations in the treatment of chronic dermatoses. In these cases, it is often cheaper to dilute a Group III or IV steroid with a suitable diluent. Which diluent depends on which proprietary preparation is to be prescribed. The appropriate diluent can be found in the *External Diluent Directory*. It is best to learn one diluent for one particular steroid ointment and another for one particular cream, and keep to them. Recently, the pharmaceutical industry has realized the need for large quantities of Group III topical steroids and are supplying already diluted preparations.

Side effects of topical steroids

The clinical side effects are proportional to the *strength of steroid used* and *duration of use*, and are also influenced by *skin thickness* and *skin moisture*.

As has already been mentioned, steroids suppress the formation of new collagen and cause atrophy of the existing collagen, which gives rise to a number of clinical appearances. The skin becomes thin and wrinkled, and the subcutaneous veins become prominent (Figure 25.1). Purpura develops (Figures 25.2 and 25.3) at sites of minor trauma, particularly on the backs of the hands and forearms (Figure 25.2), and on the legs. Striae may develop, particularly in the intertriginous areas (Figure 25.4) due to greater absorption of the steroid, although non-intertriginous skin may also be affected (Figures 25.5–25.7). Where the skin is particularly thin, e.g. on the face, telangiectasia may appear (Figures 25.1, 25.8 and 25.9). Acne may be induced by the use of Group III or IV topical steroids.

Circumoral dermatitis is a clinical entity which is now almost exclusively seen following the use of Group III or IV (and occasionally Group II) topical steroids on the face.

The history is fairly typical. The patient is usually an adult female with seborrheic eczema for which she has used potent topical steroids. Initially, the eczema clears

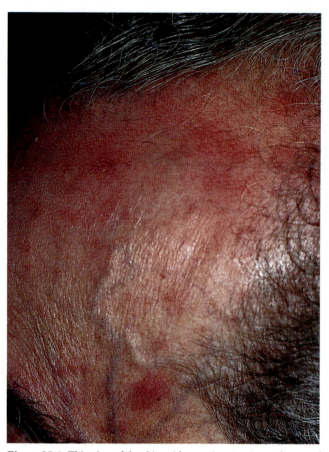

Figure 25.1 *Thinning of the skin with prominent veins and areas of telangiectasia due to prolonged use of potent topical steroids*

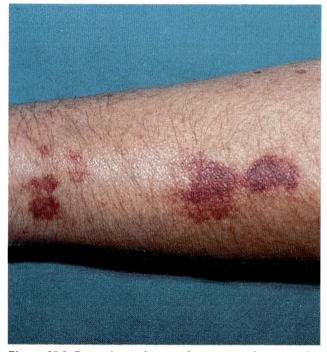

Figure 25.2 *Purpuric patches on the extensor forearms after prolonged use of topical steroids*

well but relapses fairly quickly when the treatment is discontinued and, on further use of the potent steroid, the drug loses its effect. Eventually, a papular eruption occurs around the mouth (Figure 25.10) which may spread upwards and outwards to the rest of the face (Figure 25.11). If the steroid is stopped at this stage, there will be a flare-up of the condition with pustules, and the clinical picture is not unlike rosacea.

The treatment of circumoral dermatitis is to continue with topical steroids, but gradually to decrease the strength of the steroid over a period of 3 months while at the same time giving oral tetracycline at a dose of 250 mg twice daily.

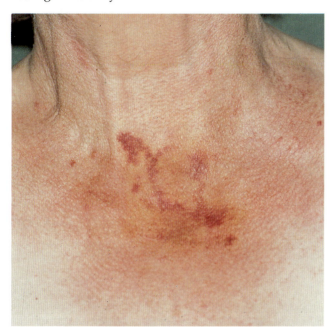

Figure 25.3 Purpura and telangiectasia on the neck after prolonged use of potent (Group III) topical steroids

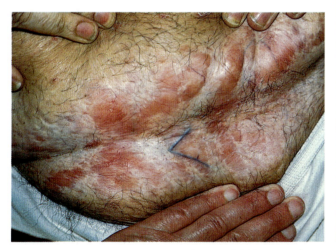

Figure 25.4 Striae developing in an abdominal fold, an intertriginous area

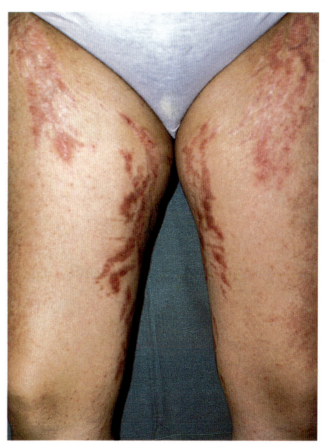

Figure 25.5 Striae on the thighs after Group IV topical steroids. The medial parts of the thighs are a common site for this problem

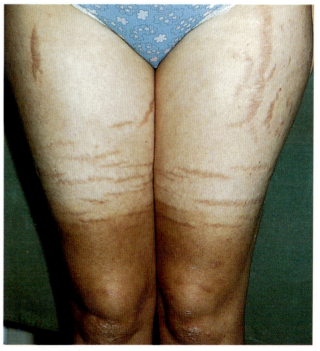

Figure 25.6 Striae on the thighs after unsupervised use of Group IV topical steroids

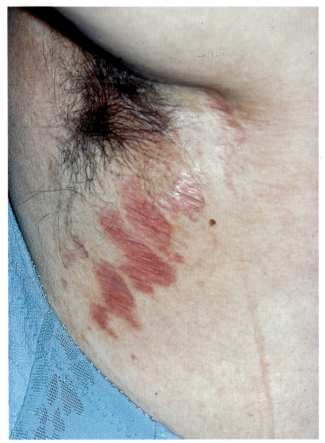

Figure 25.7 *Striae just below the axilla, another common site, after prolonged use of potent topical steroids*

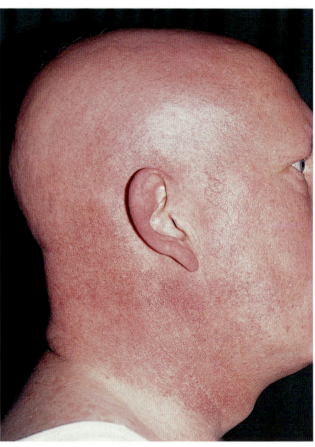

Figure 25.9 *Telangiectasia of the scalp, face and neck after 4 years of using a Group IV steroid lotion on the scalp for alopecia totalis. The lotion ran down the face and neck*

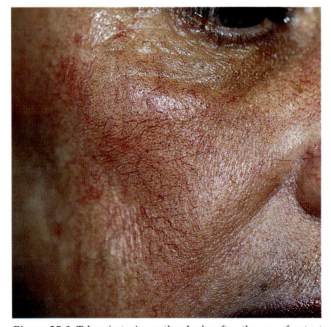

Figure 25.8 *Telangiectasia on the cheeks after the use of potent topical steroids which should not have been prescribed for eczema*

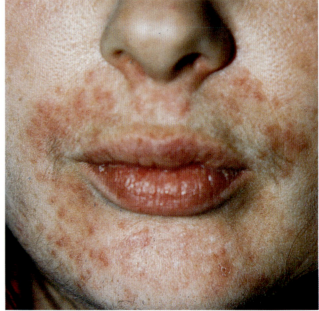

Figure 25.10 *Circumoral dermatitis. A red papular eruption around the mouth after the use of Group III topical steroids for seborrheic eczema*

If topical steroids are used for fungal or bacterial infections, they may mask the usual clinical presentation and lead to diagnostic difficulties. This is particularly so with fungal infections of the skin in which the scaling and annular configuration is lost (Figures 25.12 and 25.13). Viral infections, particularly herpes simplex infection, may spread if topical steroids are used in the management of the condition.

Care is needed when topical steroids are used for treatment of dermatoses on the eyelids. Increased ocular pressure has been reported as a result of topical steroid being absorbed through the conjunctiva into the eye.

Systemic side effects following the use of topical steroids are extremely rare. The side effects are proportional to the potency of the topical steroid times the quantity of steroid used. Thus, the risk is greater when potent steroids are used over large areas of skin. The most common side effect is suppression of the adrenal–pituitary axis. There are a few reports of Cushing's disease and even diabetes mellitus being precipitated by topical steroids.

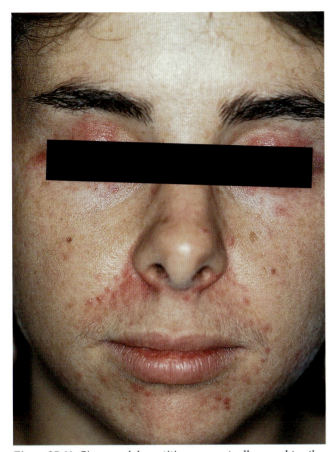

Figure 25.11 *Circumoral dermatitis may eventually spread to other parts of the face, particularly around the eyes*

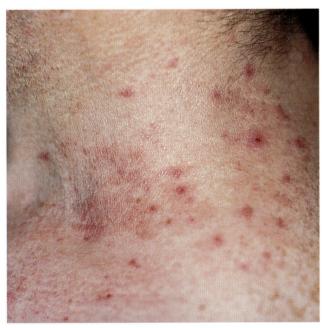

Figure 25.12 *Tinea incognito. Fungal infection on the side of the neck treated with topical steroids. The characteristic scaly annular edge is absent. The eruption has non-specific features*

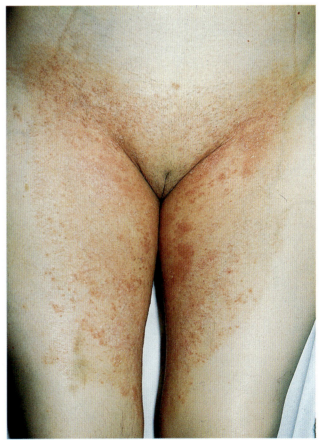

Figure 25.13 *Fungal infection of the groins which has spread down the thighs and up to the lower abdomen. The inflammatory component of the rash and scaling are absent*

Topical antibiotics

These are used less frequently than they used to be. Many topical antibiotics (particularly neomycin and soframycin) are potential sensitizers, and the risk of strains of bacteria developing resistance to these antibiotics has also contributed to the decline in their use.

Fusidic acid and mupirocin have a low incidence of sensitization and are effective against superficial staphylococcal infections. Topical antibiotics should be avoided on chronic leg ulcers and eczema as there is an increased risk of sensitization.

Topical antihistamines and topical local anesthetic preparations

These have no part to play in the treatment of skin disease. They are potential sensitizers, and topical steroids are more effective in controlling inflammation and irritation associated with epidermal disorders.

Tar preparations

These still have a definite part to play in the management of some patients with psoriasis. They may occasionally be helpful in persistent eczematous lesions.

In psoriasis, crude coal tar is usually used at a concentration of 5% in an ointment base (soft paraffin) or paste (Lassar's paste).

Fifteen per cent coal tar solution in emulsifying ointment BP is helpful in the treatment of chronic eczematous lesions. It should be applied in liberal quantities to the trunk and limbs prior to bathing, and the use of soap should be avoided. When this preparation is used, the patient should stay in the bath for 15 min and use the ointment as a soap substitute as it has some cleansing properties.

Potassium permanganate soaks

At a dilution of 1:8000, potassium permanganate solution is effective in helping to control acute inflammatory dermatoses, e.g. weeping or blistering eczematous lesions, or fungal infections.

Magenta paint

This is a relatively old-fashioned remedy, but it is often helpful in controlling a dermatosis affecting an intertriginous area. It has mild antifungal, antibacterial, anticandidal and astringent properties.

Patients should be warned that it will stain the skin temporarily, and clothes more permanently, red.

Topical antifungal preparations

There has been a significant increase in the number of topical antifungal preparations over the last few years. Physicians should become familiar with a limited number and learn the spectrum of their activity (and their cost).

Nystatin is only effective against yeasts and has no activity against dermatophytes (ringworm fungi).

Imidazoles are broad-spectrum agents active against yeasts (*Candida*), dermatophytes and *Pityrosporum orbiculare* (the fungus causing pityriasis versicolor), and *Corynebacterium minutissimum* (erythrasma).

Terbinafine is effective against dematophytes and *P. orbiculare*.

Aluminum chloride

An alcoholic solution of 25% aluminum chloride hexahydrate is an effective agent in inhibiting sweating, and is very useful for essential hyperhidrosis involving the axillae and, to some extent, the palms and soles. In the axillae, the solution need only be used once or twice a week at night whereas, on the palms, daily treatment may be necessary.

Keratolytics

These are chemicals which break up keratin. They are most commonly used in acne to break down excess keratin around the pilosebaceous orifice. The most commonly used keratolytics are salicyclic acid and benzoyl peroxide. The strength may vary according to the type of problem treated. They are usually used in a lotion or cream base.

PUVA (psoralen–ultraviolet A) treatment

Psoralens are naturally occurring substances found in plants but, recently, they have also been synthesized. Psoralens are potent photosensitizers and, in the presence of ultraviolet light, they also have a number of actions on cellular function. The combination of psoralens and ultraviolet light has been shown to stimulate melanocytes, impair cell division of epidermal cells, and affect the function of Langerhans cells and lymphocytes, thereby altering immune reactions.

Lamps emitting only long-wave (320–400 nm) ultraviolet light (UVA) are used for treatment with psoralens as medium-wave (90–320 nm) ultraviolet light (UVB) is responsible for the sunburn effect of ultraviolet light. Thus, by omitting UVB, the risk of sunburn is removed. However, a phototoxic reaction may occur with high doses of UVA and psoralens that is similar to a sunburn reaction. Thus, PUVA treatment is always begun with a small dose of UVA which is gradually increased only if there is no burning.

The psoralen usually used in PUVA treatment is 8-methoxypsoralen, and the dose depends on body weight. The drug has to be taken 2 h before the patient is irradiated with UVA. Treatment is usually carried out 3 times a week.

PUVA was originally used for the treatment of psoriasis, but is now also used for vitiligo, refractory eczema, lichen planus, alopecia areata and cutaneous T-cell lymphoma (mycosis fungoides). In vitiligo, the action is on the melanocytes but, in the other conditions, the clinical effects are obtained by an action on cells of the immune system.

Side effects
A number of side effects of PUVA have been noted. The most common is gastric irritation from the drug, which may be eased by taking the psoralen with food, particularly milk. Metoclopromide is also helpful and should be taken with the psoralens. If the nausea persists, a change from the commonly used 8-methoxypsoralen to 5-methoxypsoralen may stop or decrease the nausea.

If the dose of UVA light is too high, there may be redness and soreness of the skin and, in severe cases, blistering of the skin.

A rare side effect seen mainly in middle-aged men is itching and hyperesthesia over the upper trunk. If PUVA is given for any length of time, the effects as seen with overexposure to sunlight may occur, e.g. lentigos and degeneration of elastic tissue.

As ultraviolet light is potentially carcinogenic, there is a risk of skin cancers with PUVA. However, so far, the only increase of skin cancers reported is that of squamous cell carcinomata on the male genitalia. Thus, male patients are now advised to cover their genitalia with appropriate clothing during treatment.

SYSTEMIC DRUGS

Retinoids

These drugs have been introduced into dermatology over the last few years. They are derivatives of vitamin A (retinol). It has long been known that vitamin A is necessary for the growth, differentiation and maintenance of epithelial tissues. Vitamin A has been used in a number of dermatological conditions over the years, but was not particularly effective and, in high doses, is toxic,

causing the hypervitaminosis A syndrome, which includes raised cerebrospinal fluid pressure, hepatomegaly, splenomegaly, dry scaly skin, dryness of the mucous membranes, bone pain and anorexia.

Retinoids have long been synthesized and have been shown to have biological effects on many epithelia, including that of the skin. There are two retinoids in current use – isotretinoin and acitretin. The latter drug is mainly used in psoriasis, Darier's disease and some of the ichthyoses. Isotretinoin is used mainly for acne. Retinoids have been of considerable benefit to dermatological practice, and newer retinoids with other actions are likely to be developed. Unfortunately, as with all drugs, retinoids are not without side effects.

Side effects
The most common side effects are cheilitis (dry cracked lips), dry skin, dry mucosal surfaces, hair loss and mild eczematous patches. The most serious side effect of retinoids is teratogenicity. Thus, women of childbearing age must be warned, and adequate contraception is essential. Patients should also be told that, although it takes *1 month* for isotretinoin to be excreted from the body after cessation of treatment, it takes *2 years* for excretion of acitretin.

If retinoids are given for psoriasis or genodermatoses, they may be taken for long periods or even indefinitely, and there are a number of possible long-term side effects. Retinoids tend to raise serum lipids and, thus, fasting lipids should be checked before commencing long-term treatment and then at 6-month intervals. There is also a slight risk of hepatotoxicity and, thus, liver function must be monitored. Retinoids may also affect the musculoskeletal system. Transient arthralgia and muscle pain may occur particularly after strenuous exercise. Premature closing of the epiphysis has been reported in children. Finally, although rare, the diffuse idiopathic interstitial hyperostosis (DISH) syndrome may occur, with ossification of ligaments and accretion of bone onto vertebral bodies, raising the question of periodic radiographic examinations, the place of which is still to be determined.

How retinoids work and why they should be effective in diseases with different pathologies is not known but, with more research and a better understanding of the disease processes, retinoids are likely to be important drugs in the future.

Cyclosporine

In dermatology, cyclosporine was first used for psoriasis and, more recently, for atopic eczema. It has a specific action on activated CD4 T lymphocytes. Thus, skin diseases which are mediated by these cells should respond to cyclosporine. Cyclosporine tends to be reserved for widespread and persistent disease which does not repond to other treatments.

Cyclosporine is a highly effective drug for both psoriasis and atopic eczema. However, like most of the currently available effective treatments, there are side effects. The two most serious are nephrotoxicity and hypertension. Thus, prior to commencing treatment, it is essential to establish that patients have normal renal function. During treatment, both renal function and blood pressure must be monitored.

Methotrexate

This drug has been used for many years for severe psoriasis, for which it is highly effective. Immediate side effects are nausea, lethargy, gastrointestinal ulceration and bone marrow depression. The most important long-term side effect is hepatotoxicity and, thus, liver function must be monitored. Periodic liver biopsy may be necessary in long-term treatment.

Antifungal drugs

Griseofulvin is only effective against dermatophyte infections. It has to be taken for 1 month for skin infections, 6 weeks for scalp infections and 6 months for fingernail infections. It is not effective for toenail infections.

Terbinafine is effective against dermatophyte infections. Its main indication is toenail infections, for which it is especially effective.

Itraconazole and *fluconazole* are broad-spectrum antibiotics effective against yeast as well as dermatophyte infections. They are also effective for nail infections when taken *weekly* for 9 months. Itraconazole has an 80% chance of clearing pityriasis versicolor after 1 week of treatment.

Antibiotics

Apart from their use to treat skin infections, antibiotics are used extensively in the treatment of acne. The tetracyclines are still the most common drugs used for this purpose as well as for the management of rosacea and perioral dermatitis.

Antihistamines

These drugs have an antipruritic action. Many of them make patients drowsy, which is useful at night but not during the day. Their main indications are in the control of pruritus and in the treatment of urticaria.

Steroids

The main point concerning systemic steroids in the treatment of skin disease is that the indications for their use are few.

Cyproterone acetate

This is an antiandrogen that is used to treat women with acne or hirsuties. In those of childbearing age, it should be taken in conjunction with estrogens to maintain contraception and regular menstrual periods.

Dapsone

This sulfone has been used in the treatment of leprosy for many years. It is effective in clearing the lesions of dermatitis herpetiformis as well as in a number of other conditions with an immunological basis, particularly cutaneous vasculitis.

The main side effects are hemolysis and methemoglobinemia.

Sunscreens

Ultraviolet light is that part of the solar spectrum which tends to cause most skin problems. Ultraviolet light is divided into UVC (short waves that are screened by the ozone layer), UVB (medium waves) and UVA (long waves).

UVB is responsible for the sunburn effect, but UVA may cause a number of photodermatoses. UVB is definitely carcinogenic and UVA is probably likewise. UVA is thought to play an important part in photo-aging as it damages the elastic tissue of the dermis and causes wrinkles.

Most sunscreens currently in use are absorbent, i.e. they work by absorbing the energy of ultraviolet light. They are effective against UVB, but have little or no action against UVA. The main compounds used in absorbent sunscreens are esters of para-aminobenzoic acid, esters of cinnamic acid and benzophenones.

Substances which reflect ultraviolet light are protective against UVB and UVA. Examples are titanium dioxide and zinc oxide.

The skin protection factor (SPF) of sunscreens refers to UVB. The SPF number is the ratio of the time needed to produce minimal erythema with the sunscreen (Tp) compared with no protection (T); thus, SPF = Tp/T. None of the sunscreens are totally effective in screening out either UVB or UVA.

Appendix

TOPICAL CORTICOSTEROIDS

Generic name	Trade name (UK)	Trade name (USA)
Group I (weak)		
Alclometasone dipropionate (0.05%)	Modrasone	Aclovate
Hydrocortisone (0.5%, 1% and 2.5%)	Efcortelan	Carmol HC
	Hydrocortistab	Cortisporin
	Hydrocortisyl	Eldecort
		Hytone
		Nutracort
		Penecort
		Synacort
		Vioform
		Vytone
Group II (intermediate strength)		
Clobetasone butyrate (0.05%)	Eumovate	NA
Fluocortolone pivalate (0.1%) + fluocortolone hexanoate (0.1%)	Ultradil	NA
Flurandrenolone (0.0125%)	Haelan	NA
Flurandrenolone acetonide (0.025%)	NA	Cordran
Fluticasone propionate (0.05%)	Cutivate	Cutivate
Hydrocortisone butyrate (0.1%)	Locoid	Locoid
Mometasone furoate (0.1%)	Elocon	Elocon
Group III (strong)		
Beclomethasone dipropionate (0.025%)	Propaderm	NA
Betamethasone dipropionate (0.05%)	Diprosone	Diprosone
	Diprosalic	Lotrisone
	Lotriderm	Maxivate
Betamethasone valerate (0.1%)	Betnovate	Betatrex
		Beta-Val
		Valisone
Diflucortolone valerate (0.1%)	Nerisone	NA
Diflucortolone valerate (0.3%)	Nerisone Forte	NA
Fluclorolone acetonide (0.025%)	Topilar	NA
Fluocinolone acetonide (0.025%)	Synalar	Fluonid
		Synalar
		Synemol
Fluocinonide (0.05%)	Metosyn	Lidex

Fluocortolone pivalate (0.25%) + fluocortolone hexanoate (0.25%)	Ultralanum	NA
Halcinonide (0.1%)	Halciderm	Halog
Triamcinolone acetonide (0.1%)	Adcortyl	Aristocort
		Kenalog

Group IV (very strong)

Clobetasol propionate (0.05%)	Dermovate	Temovate
Fluocinolone acetonide (0.2%)	NA	Synalar HP

Index

Note: Page numbers in italics denote illustrations and
tables